HEALTHY
BODY

A practical guide to body care

HEALTHY
BODY

A practical guide to body care

GEORGE D. PAMPLONA-ROGER

Doctor of Medicine and Surgery (University of Granada, Spain)
Board-certified General and Digestive Surgeon (Accredited by the European Union)
Specialist in Health Education (UNED University, Spain)
Master of Public Health (Loma Linda University, California, USA)
Member of the International Union for Health Promotion and Education (IUHPE)

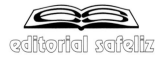

editorial safeliz

Disclaimer

The information contained in this book is intended for educational purposes and cannot replace the functions of a qualified health professional in any way. The advice and treatments provided in this book are general in nature, and therefore cannot take into account each person's particular circumstances. Only a qualified health professional may diagnose disease, therefore self-treatment of symptoms of illness is not advisable. The author, publishers, and distributors of this work are not liable for any adverse effect or outcome that may result from a reader's individual application of treatments and advice presented in this book.

Collection: **Life and Health**
Title: **Healthy Body**
Original title in Spanish edition: *Cuerpo saludable*

Autor: George D. Pamplona-Roger
Translation: Jennifer de la Cruz
Design and layout: CIF B-83217315
Photographs and illustrations from MedicalRF/Jupiterimages

All rights reserved © **Editorial Safeliz, S. L.**
Pradillo, 6 · Pol. Ind. La Mina
E-28770 · Colmenar Viejo, Madrid, Spain
Tel.: [+34] 91 845 98 77 · Fax: [+34] 91 845 98 65
admin@safeliz.com · www.safeliz.com

May 2010: 1st edition in English language

ISBN: 978-84-7208-174-1

PRINTED IN THAILAND

*Dedicated to my parents who,
at the age of nearly 90 and still full
of life, continue to teach me how
to care for the precious gift that is
the body.*

To the Reader

For a surgeon, the human body is his natural workplace. In everyday practice and in the operating room I have seen, inside and out, sick bodies, broken bodies, bodies that are worn out by age or bad habits, bodies that have been mistreated, as well as bodies that are well cared for; bodies of every shape and size.

But in all of the bodies, no matter what their condition, even in those damaged by disease or misuse, one can appreciate a certain order, an intelligent design, and even a beauty that inspires awe and admiration. In seeing the wonder of the human body up close, it is not difficult to perceive within it a reflection of the divine, which serves as motivation to care for and protect it even more.

For this reason, upon seeing how every day the media displays atrocities committed against the body; seeing how commonly it is subjected to mistreatment and violence, in both the fiction of movies and the truth of cruel reality; and after having witnessed time and again the negative consequences of a lack of care and respect for the body ignoring the principles of good health, I have been moved, dear reader, to present this "Practical Guide to Body Care".

Editorial Safeliz has put forth its best, using the most advanced technology to achieve an educational and practical publication on an international level.

The most sincere wish of this author is to inspire respect for the human body, and to motivate people to care for each part of it according to the latest scientific research.

Dr. George D. Pamplona-Roger

LAYOUT OF THIS WORK

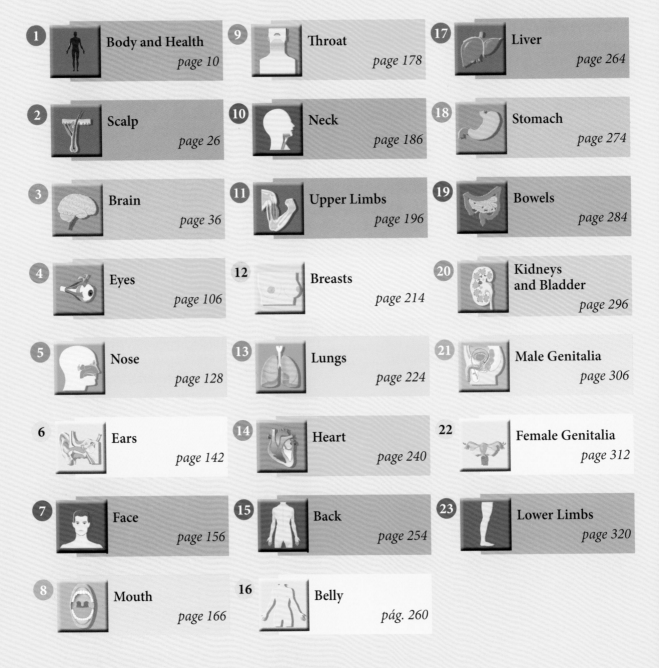

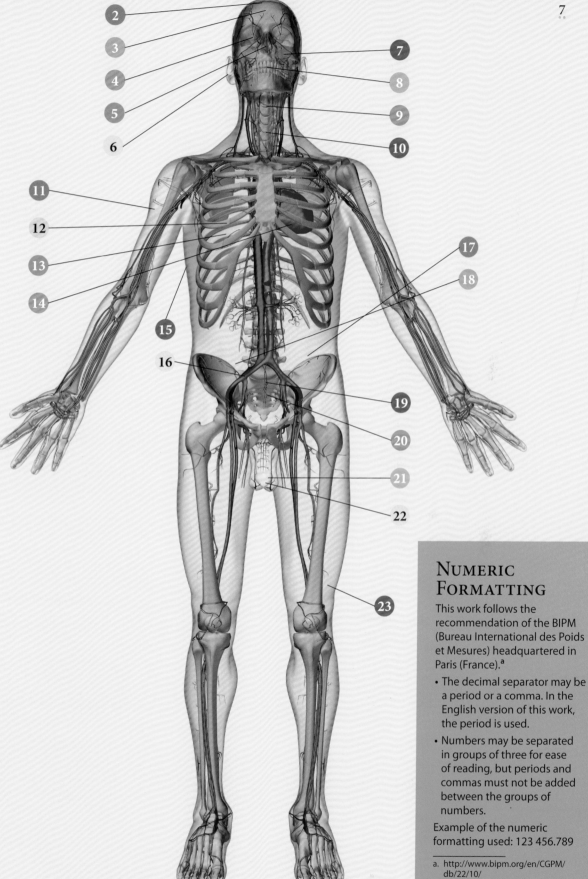

NUMERIC FORMATTING

This work follows the recommendation of the BIPM (Bureau International des Poids et Mesures) headquartered in Paris (France).[a]

• The decimal separator may be a period or a comma. In the English version of this work, the period is used.

• Numbers may be separated in groups of three for ease of reading, but periods and commas must not be added between the groups of numbers.

Example of the numeric formatting used: 123 456.789

a. http://www.bipm.org/en/CGPM/db/22/10/

FOREWORD

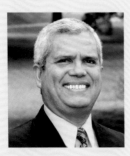

ABRAHAM A. ACOSTA MD., MPH.

*Dean School of Health Sciences
Universidad Adventista del Plata.
Libertador San Martín,
Entre Ríos, Argentina*

"This morning I was called upon for the most unusual consultation I've had since entering the medical profession," my ophthalmologist friend told me, peering over his glasses. "A 17 year-old young man came to me for what he considered a serious health problem. He said 'Every time I smoke marihuana, my eyes get red. I'm really worried. What can you prescribe for my condition?'" Intrigued, I asked my colleague, "So, what did you tell him?" "Well… to stop smoking marihuana! And he answered, 'Anything but that', then turned and walked out of my office."

This young man's behavior is representative of the conscious or unconscious attitude that thousands of people have about their health: They want clear lungs, free of any risk of cancer, yet refuse to stop using tobacco; they want a functionally healthy liver, free of any risk of cirrhosis, yet they keep drinking alcohol; they long to enjoy a heart that serves them by beating warmly in the chest for many years, yet insist on eating habits that stop it before its time as a result of blockages from cholesterol within the fragile arteries nourishing it; they want a clear mind that allows them to make sound decisions in our complex world, yet insist on denying it the nocturnal rest that it desperately needs for better functioning; they want to have an attractive figure and strong muscles, bones and joints that allow them to move freely from place to place, yet never dedicate time to a program of regular physical exercise; basically, they want to enjoy good health, but are not willing to pay the price for a lifestyle that brings them closer to such a worthy goal.

Health is not a matter of sheer coincidence, and does not come by chance. In most cases, it is the result of respect or obedience to the laws of human health and happiness; it is the result of decisions that we incorporate into daily living, about certain widely recognized factors that are essential to a longer, healthier life. The truth is, the way we live today determines, in many cases, the health we will enjoy tomorrow.

The importance of lifestyle and personal skills that support good health has been a topic examined in several reports and international forums. The Lalonde Report, for example, which came out of Canada in 1974, already held that lifestyle and environmental conditions are more significant to the health of Canadians than medical care, yet the resources available to the healthcare industry were oriented mainly toward medical care instead of actions designed to change those conditions. Four years later, in the Alma-Ata Declaration, a document that defined Primary Care Medicine as a strategy to achieve the goal of Health for All by the Year 2000, the WHO pointed out, in the same context, the importance of being responsible for oneself and community participation. The concepts of this declaration were taken up again by the WHO just a few years later, on the 25th Anniversary of the launching of this strategy. On the other hand, in the 80s, in the Ottawa Letter, a document that gives rise to Health Promotion, which is considered by some to be a new Public Health model, the "development of personal skills that promote health" is defined as one of its five operational areas. The other areas have to do with the development of healthy public policy, the creation of health-friendly environments (physical, social, economic, political and cultural environments), the strengthening of community action and the redirection of health services. The proposals of these declarations continue to make up the strategic backbone of health policy in many countries around the world.

It is in this context where the book HEALTHY BODY, by Dr. George D. Pamplona-Roger, holds a timely and rightful place as an important tool that allows the reader to reinforce his skills in promoting good health. In order to achieve this goal, the author offers a clear and practical description of the structure and function of the main organs and systems of the human body, as well as practical tips in providing the care required to keep them healthy. In his efforts, the author also demonstrates, through a masterful offering of interesting facts, the complexity of the human body as a living machine, leading us to face, almost without realizing it, the reality of a wonderful Creator to whom we must answer for how well we care for it in consideration of the tremendous worth that it has been given.

For reasons that are surely didactic, the author approaches the care of the body as it refers to each organ and system –which does not mean that this living machine, the greatest work of all creation, is simply the sum of its parts. When considering the whole of the work, it goes to assume that the author considers the human being to be a bio-psychosocial-spiritual entity, whose nature is whole and that, as with any other system, when something affects one aspect of its composition, it affects the whole. From this perspective, positive results of a functionally healthier body, derived from the practical advice offered in this book, will also reach the other dimensions of the whole being.

The publication of the book HEALTHY BODY by Editorial Safeliz, is backed up by the broad and renowned career of Dr. George D. Pamplona-Roger as a writer and as a physician. His prior publications, some of which have been translated into multiple languages, have been widely distributed and accepted in several places around the globe. It is my sincere wish that this new publication be as successful as the others have been in improving readers' health.

Abraham A. Acosta MD., MPH.

Body and Health

Human beings do not just "have" bodies, rather they "are" bodies. Health and wellbeing depend primarily on knowledge about those bodies, and how to care for them.

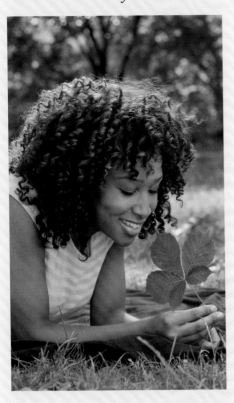

*I*n the entire universe, no known structure is as complex, as perfect and at the same time as beautiful as a healthy human body. Familiarity with its unique characteristics is essential to caring for it and enjoying it for a lifetime.

- **Organization**: The human body is a highly organized structure on different levels. The word "organism", used to refer to a living being, specifically implies organization, resulting from intelligent planning.
- **Continuous Renewal**: Human beings are in a continuous state of transformation, continually replacing cells and chemical components. In spite of this, their shape and some characteristics remain constant throughout life.
- **Self-Healing**: The human body has been given the ability to repair itself. With the right care, the body can become healthy again after an injury, poisoning, infection or other condition.
- **Individuality**: No two human bodies are identical –not even identical twins. In addition to fingerprints and the veins of the retina at the back of the eye, the sound of the voice, the face, and facial expressions make each human being unique, and therefore infinitely valuable.
- **Integration**: The mind and the body make up a complete and inseparable functional unit.

Because the human body is so complex, unique and fascinating, it is well deserving of our greatest respect and utmost care.

Facts and Figures About the Human Body

120 days	Time it takes for erythrocytes (red cells) in the blood to completely replenish themselves.
206	Number of bones in the body.
30 000	Number of dead cells that slough off the skin each minute.
96 500 km	Combined length of all of the blood vessels in the body.
75 000 000 000 000 (= 75 trillion)	Number of cells in the human body.

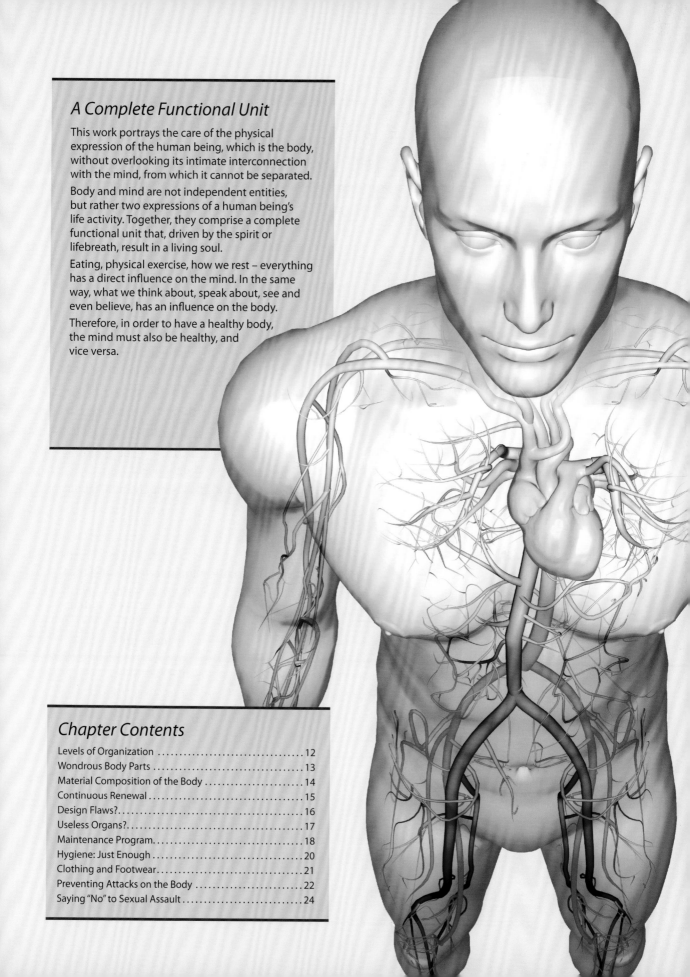

A Complete Functional Unit

This work portrays the care of the physical expression of the human being, which is the body, without overlooking its intimate interconnection with the mind, from which it cannot be separated.

Body and mind are not independent entities, but rather two expressions of a human being's life activity. Together, they comprise a complete functional unit that, driven by the spirit or lifebreath, result in a living soul.

Eating, physical exercise, how we rest – everything has a direct influence on the mind. In the same way, what we think about, speak about, see and even believe, has an influence on the body.

Therefore, in order to have a healthy body, the mind must also be healthy, and vice versa.

Chapter Contents

LEVELS OF ORGANIZATION

In this world, there is nothing that is better organized than the healthy human body. From its systems and organs, to the atoms that comprise its matter, everything is equipped for optimal functioning.

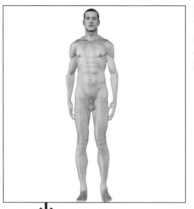

The Human Body as a Whole
The body is comprised of several systems that function in conjunction with each other in order to maintain a fulfilling and healthy life.

Systems
A system is a group of organs capable of carrying out complex and wide-ranging functions. For example, the digestive system is able to transform foods to the point that they can be absorbed and enter into the bloodstream.

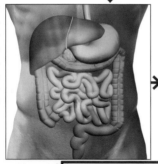

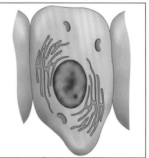

Organs
An organ is an anatomic unit comprised of various tissues that is designed to perform specific functions within a system.

Tissues
A tissue is comprised of many similar cells that are interconnected to perform a specific function.

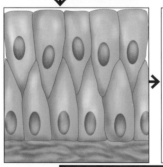

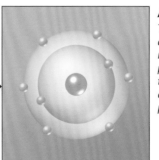

Cells
Cells are the smallest living units. Each cell is a complex world in itself, containing millions of chemical molecules that constantly interact with one another.

Molecules
A molecule is the smallest quantity of a substance that continues to preserve all of its chemical properties. Molecules are comprised of a variable number of atoms, ranging anywhere between two and several thousand.

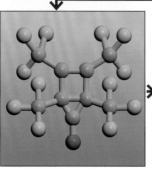

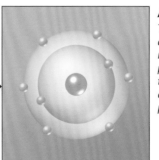

Atoms
The atom is the smallest unit of a chemical element. The atom is not divisible by way of chemical processes. By its very nature, the atom is undividable and is comprised of mostly electrons, protons and neutrons

WONDROUS BODY PARTS

Only a body that is a product of intelligent design would be able to survive in such a hostile world as ours. Thousands of adaptation mechanisms work in a simultaneous and coordinated fashion for the preservation of life.

Skin Cells: Protection on Demand
They secrete the necessary amount of melanin to protect itself from excess solar radiation.

Heart: Dynamic Adaptation
It adapts its rhythm to the needs of the body. Its various arteries dilate or contract according to the needs of each organ or body part.

Brain: Selective Memory
Among its many surprising abilities is its ability to forget, automatically erasing any trace of irrelevant memories.

Kidneys: Chemical Regulation
The concentration and composition of urine fluctuate in order to keep the blood composition constant.

Hypothalamus: Precision Thermostat
This part of the brain is in charge of keeping the body temperature constant, whether in an icy igloo or in the torrid desert. It does this by increasing or decreasing the sense of thirst, the breathing rate, perspiration and blood flow to the skin.

Blood: Liquid to Solid, As Needed
It remains fluid continually, becoming solid only if there is a hemorrhage that it needs to stop.

Bronchi: Self-Cleaning
The cells that line the inside of the bronchi send out a layer of mucous that dust or smoke particles, germs and other contaminants adhere to when they are brought in with air. This layer of mucous is carted out by tiny vibrating hairs as if it were a tapestry on wheels.

Liver: Selective Filter
It detects and eliminates dangerous or foreign substances circulating in the bloodstream, such as alcohol, and stores useful substances, such as certain vitamins.

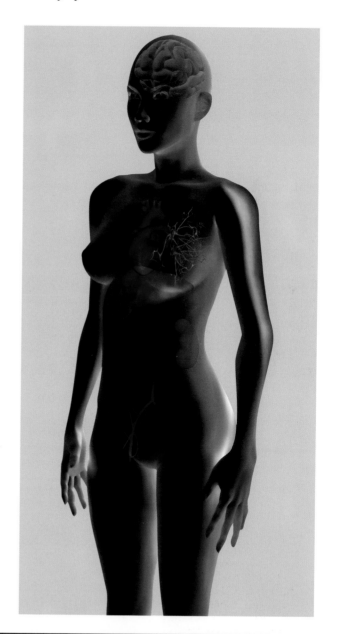

For You formed my inward parts; You covered me in my mother's womb. I will praise You, for I am fearfully and wonderfully made; Marvelous are Your works, And that my soul knows very well.

David, the Psalmist (NKJV, Psalms 139: 13, 14)

MATERIAL COMPOSITION OF THE BODY

*All of the chemical elements that comprise
the human body are found in the dust of the earth.*

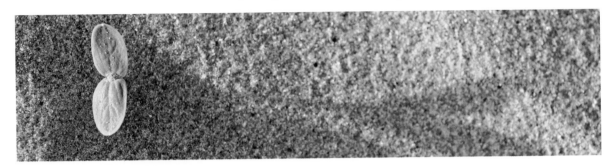

The human body is comprised of the atoms of 35 different chemical elements. They are all part of the 92 elements of the Periodic Table occurring spontaneously in nature.

The three most abundant elements, oxygen, carbon and hydrogen, comprise 94% of body weight. A combination of 15 elements makes up 99.83% of body weight, as shown in the adjacent table.

The small percentage that remains (0.17%) is made up of 20 mineral elements, called trace elements. Some of them, such as iodine, perform extremely important functions in the body, despite being found in very small quantitie. Without the 14 mg of this mineral in the body, the thyroid gland could not produce hormones and a child's brain would never develop. Other minerals, such as nickel, magnesium or gold, are known to exist in very small quantities as well, but their exact function is not known.

Chemical Composition of the Human Body

Element (Atomic Number)	Weight in a 70 kg Man	% of Total Weight	Primary Location
Oxygen (8)	42 700 g	61%	Whole Body
Carbon (6)	16 100 g	23%	Whole Body
Hydrogen (1)	7 000 g	10%	Whole Body
Nitrogen (7)	1 820 g	2.6%	Muscles and Bones
Calcium (20)	980 g	1.4%	Bones, Teeth
Phosphorus (15)	770 g	1.1%	Bones, Brain
Potassium (19)	140 g	0.2%	Cells
Sulfur (16)	140 g	0.2%	Cartilage
Sodium (11)	98 g	0.14%	Extracellular Fluids
Chlorine (17)	84 g	0.12%	Blood, Stomach
Magnesium (12)	18.9 g	0.027%	Bones
Silicon (14)	18.2 g	0.026%	Connective Tissue, Skin
Iron (26)	4.2 g	0.006%	Blood
Fluorine (9)	2.59 g	0.0037%	Bones and Teeth
Zinc (30)	2.31 g	0.0033%	Prostate, Pancreas
TOTAL	**69 878 g**	**99.83%**	

How Much Is the Human Body Worth?

If all of the elements that comprise the human body were purchased in a chemical products warehouse, the price would not be over a few hundred dollars. But… is that really all we are worth?

Of course not. The extraordinary organization of all those atoms of chemical elements that form molecules, cells, tissues, organs and systems, gives tremendous value to the matter that forms us. Moreover, add to that the fact that such organization of matter allows us to think, feel and love, and its worth becomes colossal.

Organization is never the result of chance, or the sum of small spontaneous changes, but rather of intelligent planning. Having a healthy body begins with appreciating its true worth. This is what makes the human body worthy of the utmost respect and care.

CONTINUOUS RENEWAL

The body is undergoing a continuous process of renewal of its material composition and of the cells that comprise it. Despite this, it preserves a constant organization and identity.

CONTINUOUS RENEWAL OF MATTER

Each day, between one and three liters of matter in the form of food, water and air enter the body. About the same amount of matter leaves the body each day, mainly through feces and urine.

Every year, it is believed that a majority of atoms that make up the matter of a human body has been renewed. During this time, despite this change in matter, the mystery of life causes us to continue to be the same person.

CONTINUOUS RENEWAL OF CELLS

Despite its relatively constant appearance, the human body is not at all static. The body's cells, its basic units of life, are also continually being renewed. Millions of them die every minute, whether due to apoptosis (natural cell death) or necrosis due to an infection, lack of circulation or some other pathology.

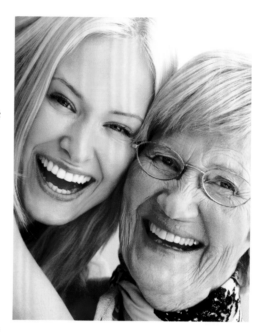

The dead cells, whatever their cause, are replaced automatically through a continual process of regeneration, whether in the skin, the bones, the stomach mucosa or the blood.

Of all of the body's cells, only the neurons in the brain remain constant all throughout life. For this reason, in order to have a healthy body, the brain must be cared for more than anything else, as shown in Chapter 3, the longest in this work.

Life Expectancy of the Body's Cells

Cells	Average Life Expectancy	Destination After Cell Death
Enterocytes (cells of the intestinal mucosa)	4 days	Eliminated through the digestive tract as part of stool.
Cells of the stomach mucosa	5 days	Eliminated through the digestive tract as part of stool.
Skin Cells	30 days	Eliminated through skin cleansing.
Hepatocytes (liver cells)	42 days	Digested by microphages, a special type of white blood cells responsible for eliminating dead cells. Microphages literally eat the cells of the body as they are dying, thereby keeping it clear of waste.
Hematities (red blood cells)	120 days	
Osteocytes (bone cells)	90 days	
Leukocytes (white blood cells)	1 year	
Neurons in the Brain	Up to 90 years or more (the entire life of the body)	In a healthy brain, neurons live as long as the body lives.

DESIGN FLAWS?

Some scientists have called certain apparently badly made or defective body parts "design flaws" or "bungles". At least two arguments can be made to interpret those apparent defects in the design of the body.

ARGUMENT 1: INABILITY TO EXPLAIN

The fact that modern science cannot explain the reason for a certain body structure design does not mean that the body part is poorly made. After all, can modern science really explain everything? How many times have scientists already had to modify their positions when faced with new findings?

It is very realistic to think that some of the apparent faulty designs in the human body are simply structures that modern science is unable to understand or figure out. The most common example is the human eye that, incomprehensibly, has optic nerve fibers in front of the retina. Nevertheless, despite this apparent design defect, it achieves extraordinary visual acuity, and is a marvel of functional design.

ARGUMENT 2: REGRESSIVE EVOLUTION

Although in recent decades human life expectancy has been extended, mainly in Western countries, there are many indicators that physical strength has been diminishing over time.

This "regressive evolution" of the human body is, in reality, a negative microevolution within the same species. According to this theory, the human body, just like all of nature, lost its original vitality and has been deteriorating over time. Were it not for the intervention of modern medicine, human life would actually be shorter and of poorer quality than that of our ancestors.

These are some examples of the defects of the human body, not due to an error in its original design, but rather to misuse and unhealthy habits:

- **Osteoarthritis**: Due to postural changes, obesity and an acid-producing diet rich in animal proteins.
- **Inguinal and femoral hernias**: Due to tissue atrophy –not to erect posture, as some have said (quadruped animals also suffer from this condition).
- **Herniation of intervertebral disk**: Due to postural changes, constipation and tissue degeneration due to a poor diet.
- **Impacted teeth** that do not erupt, such as the third molars: Due to underdevelopment of the mandible from a lack of chewing exercises in children who eat only soft foods.

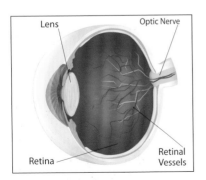

The design of the human eye has incomprehensible aspects, but that does not make it a flaw or a bungle.

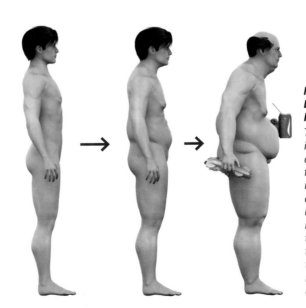

Regressive Evolution of the Human Body
The current trend in condition is not due to a design flaw, but rather to misuse. In order to develop a healthy body, it is now more important than ever to care for it well, thus preventing this tendency toward reversal that is affecting humanity.

USELESS ORGANS?

More than 100 organs or body parts had been considered useless leftovers until scientific research began revealing their important functions.

COCCYX

The last stretch of the spine has been considered by some as the remains of the tail or tailbone of vertebrate animals.

However, the coccyx is not the leftover of some atrophied tailbone, but instead, a part of the spine designed to carry out important functions:

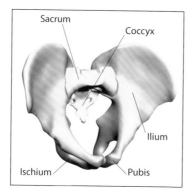

- Stabilization of the pelvis.
- Insertion point for the ligaments and muscles that make up the pelvic floor, upon which fecal and urinary continence depend.
- In women, it moves backward to widen the birth canal.

APPENDIX

In decades past, the cecal appendage was considered a useless organ that had no function except providing work for surgeons.

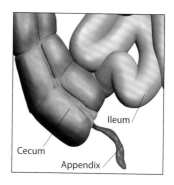

We now know that the appendix is a lymphatic organ producing defenses against intestinal infections, and that it should only be removed when it is truly infected.

TONSILS

These are accumulations of lymphatic tissue in the throat that defend against infections. Up until a few decades ago, the tonsils were considered useless organs that should be removed if they became infected.

It is now known that the tonsils perform important defensive functions:

- Protection against entry of bacteria or viruses through the airways or digestive tract.
- Removal increases the tendency to suffer colds and sore throat.
- Necessary for proper functioning of the immune system. A tonsillectomy (removal of the tonsils) triples the risk of Hodgkin's disease, a form of cancer that attacks lymphatic tissue.

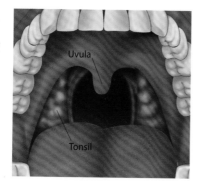

THYMUS

It used to be considered a vestigial organ –an evolutionary leftover. However, it is now known that it performs very important functions for the immune system, especially in children and adolescents.

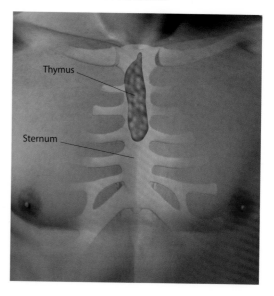

Maintenance Program

*To preserve the body's machinery in a healthy state,
a daily maintenance program must be followed,
based on the eight remedies provided by nature.*

1. Take Some Deep Breaths

Just getting up is an ideal time to take some deep breaths. During the night, breathing movements are shallow, and secretions tend to build up in the airways.

With deep breathing, the brain becomes oxygenated and alert, the bronchial tubes are cleansed, and the entire respiratory system becomes prepared to provide the body with its most pressing need: oxygen.

Ten deep breaths upon just waking up also remind us, throughout the day, of the need to correctly breathe in fresh air.

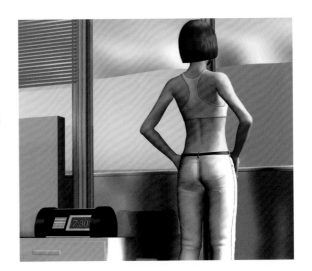

2. Drink Water and Take a Shower

After doing the breathing exercises, it is good to start the day by drinking a glass or two of water. This hydrates the body, cleanses the stomach and promotes good circulation after a night of rest.

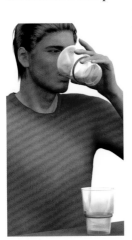

These are just the first of the 6-8 glasses of water that are needed throughout the day, primarily before meals.

Water should be on the outside of the body as well as on the inside. Therefore, it is good to take a shower that cleanses and hydrates the skin and promotes good circulation.

Scottish showers, which are done by alternating hot and cold water, are especially good for building up the immune system and protecting against colds, flu and other infections.

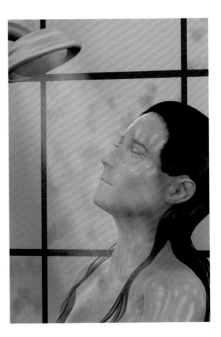

3. Get Some Sun

Each day it is necessary to be under the sun for a little while. If only the hands and face are uncovered, half an hour can be enough for light-skinned people to synthesize enough Vitamin D. Dark-skinned people may need 50-60 minutes of exposure.

In addition to promoting Vitamin D synthesis in the skin, which is needed for calcium absorption and strong bones, sun exposure stimulates blood production and fights depression.

4. EAT WELL

Each day, our bodies need certain chemical substances, called nutrients, which can only be obtained properly through food. Meat is a food that is not needed, nor even recommendable, for children as well as adults.

- **A Healthy Breakfast**: Fresh fruit; whole grain cereals in the form of bread, muesli, or flakes; nuts, almonds, or other nuts; vegetable "milks", such as soy or oat milk.
- **A Healthy Lunch**: Fresh vegetable salad; legumes, potatoes, rice, pasta or other energetic dish; cooked vegetables or vegetable meat; optionally, a piece of fruit.
- **A Healthy Dinner**: Optional for adults, but should always be light: Salad, soup or fruit.

5. PHYSICAL ACTIVITY

Each day, a period of at least half an hour must be set aside for physical activity. Ideally, it should be enough to break a sweat, which helps eliminate toxins and prevent obesity. Tending to a vegetable or flower garden, or walking at a vigorous pace, are two of the most recommendable activities for the body and the mind.

6. SELF-CONTROL

Each day, there are opportunities to exercise self-control over our appetite. The goal is to educate our appetite so that we will like those foods that are good and healthy, such as those shown in Chapter 3.

For some, it will be necessary to resist the allure of tobacco, alcoholic beverages, and other drugs; others will have to confront the temptation to eat between meals or overeat; some will need to avoid certain foods or products that are harmful to them; and others will have to fight the tendency toward being sedentary. All of this requires exercising of self-control through willpower.

Health depends mainly on the habits of daily life. No medication or surgery can make up for the consequences of unhealthy habits.

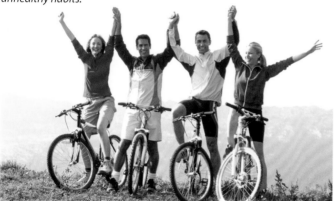

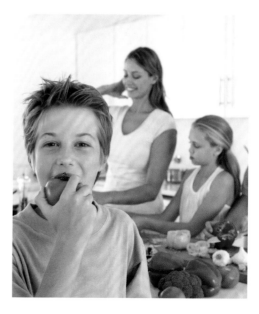

7. HOPE

All human beings need to have hope in order to achieve complete health. Believers have the privilege of placing their hope each day in a loving Father. Dedicating time each day to meditation and prayer also contributes to a healthy body.

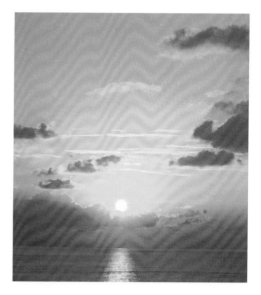

8. REST

Six to eight hours of rest are needed each day, and a day is needed each week. Sleeping well requires a comfortable bed, a well-ventilated room, and a light dinner. As the old adage goes, "Sleeping well is good nutrition."

HYGIENE: JUST ENOUGH

Hygiene is necessary, but being too clean can have negative health consequences, especially during childhood.

Humanity has bathed for millenniums, but only in last few decades has there been running water in every household. The ability to bathe daily and year-round has been a decisive factor in the eradication of many infectious diseases. While a lack of hygiene and body cleansing promotes infections, doing it in excess can also have undesired effects.

TIPS FOR HEALTHY HYGIENE

- Shower at least once per day. However, water alone is not enough to completely cleanse the skin, since it does not eliminate oily secretions and the residues of environmental pollution. This is why soap or gel need to be used, but in moderation.
- Do not use soap or gel more than once per day. Excessive soap or gel eliminates the protective oily covering of the skin, causing dryness.
- Wash certain parts of the body more often (it is not necessary to use soap or gel each time):
  – Face
  – Armpits
  – Groin and genitals
  – Anus (after every bowel movement)
  – Hands
  – Feet
- Do not use ordinary soap or gel to wash the female genitalia, as they alter the necessary vaginal acidity, promoting infections (see Chapter 22).

THE BODY'S SCENT

All bodies, even those recently cleansed or showered, give off a certain scent. This is normal and trying to completely suppress the body's scent through overuse of deodorants or antiperspirants can cause infections and other skin changes.

However, sometimes the body's scent can become excessive and unpleasant, and must be controlled.

Common Causes of Body Odor

- Poor skin hygiene, allowing the proliferation of certain bacteria in moist areas, such as the groin or armpits.
- Drinking alcohol or smoking.
- Taking certain medications.
- Kidney or liver disease.

Tips to Control Body Odor

- Shower often.
- Use an antibacterial soap.
- Apply apple vinegar in the armpits to stop the growth of odor-producing bacteria.
- Shave or wax the armpits.
- Use talcum powder in the armpits, the groin, under the breasts, or other moist areas. Moisture promotes bacterial development.
- Wear cotton undergarments, and change them daily.
- Diet: This greatly influences body odor. Avoid meat and strong or spicy condiments, as well as sugared candy and cakes and refined flour.

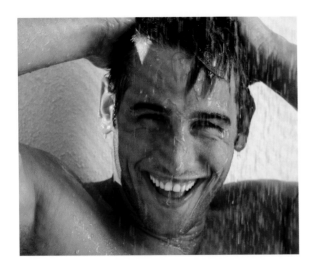

EXCESSIVE HYGIENE

Excessive hygiene or cleansing also eliminates the necessary beneficial bacteria from our skin and intestines, and weakens the immune system.

Several research projects done in recent years show that excessive hygiene promotes allergies, including asthma and atopic dermatitis, and autoimmune diseases.

Excessive hygiene would be, for example, sterilizing children's dishes and silverware, or trying to overprotect them by repeatedly cleaning the items around them with chemicals.

Clothing and Footwear

The body needs clothing and footwear for physical protection and warmth. In addition, clothing contains the body secretions, preventing them from reaching others and promoting public health. Clothing and footwear also highlight the body's natural beauty.

However, some clothing or footwear can be harmful to health, and should be avoided, even if they are fashionable.

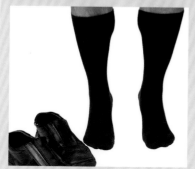

Girdles
They became fashionable in the 19th Century in Europe and North America. They cause breathing difficulty and affect the organs in the abdomen.

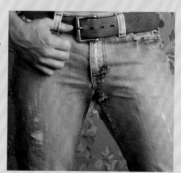

Tight Bras
Statistics show a relationship between continually wearing a bra and the risk of breast cancer. The bra should be removed at least for sleeping.

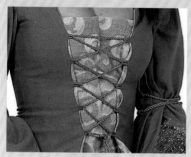

Tight Hosiery and Socks
They impede blood circulation to the legs and can be a cause of venous thrombosis (blood clots in the veins).

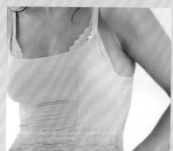

Tight Jeans
In men, they can be a cause of male infertility. When the testicles are pressed up against the body, their temperature increases and sperm production stops.

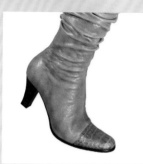

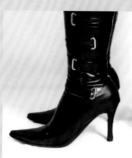

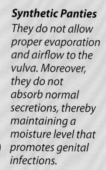

Synthetic Panties
They do not allow proper evaporation and airflow to the vulva. Moreover, they do not absorb normal secretions, thereby maintaining a moisture level that promotes genital infections.

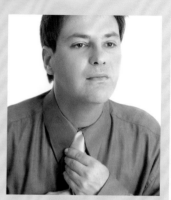

High Heels
They can cause injury to the front part of the foot due to excess pressure, as well as back pain.

Tight Shoes
They change the normal support of the foot, and promote hallux valgus (bunions) and hyperkeratosis (calluses).

Tight-Collared Shirts
They can compress the nerves in the neck and cause fainting.

PREVENTING ATTACKS ON THE BODY

*A structure as perfect and unique as the human body is deserving
of the utmost care and respect. For a healthy body,
any attack on its integrity must be prevented.*

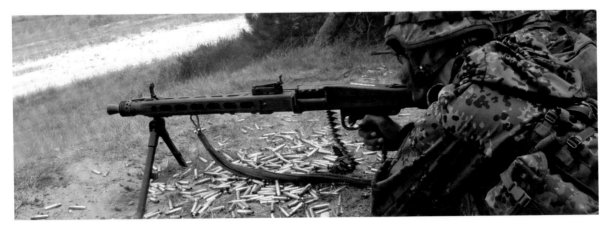

WAR AND TORTURE

Because it seeks to destroy the bodies of the enemy, war itself is an attack on the human body. War is followed or accompanied by torture, an especially malicious and brutal attack on the body that crushes human dignity.

The Preamble to the United Nations Charter, signed in the North American city of San Francisco on June 26, 1945, opens with, "We the people of the United Nations determined to save succeeding generations from the scourge of war…". [a] But despite this laudable declaration of intentions, war continues to be the primary threat to the integrity of the human body around the world.

Many more initiatives that aim to preserve peace and prevent war are needed, as they constitute a practical way to respect and dignify the human body.

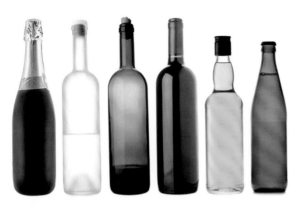

*A night spent partying with drinking
is an attack on the body, especially on the brain.*

USE OF ALCOHOL AND OTHER DRUGS

The use of any type of drugs, whether legal or illegal, constitutes an attack on the body –a sort of slow suicide (although sometimes it is quick).

Studies by the University of North Carolina (United States) show that acute alcohol poisoning or drunkenness, such as occurs after a night of carousing or "binge drinking", causes the death a certain number of neurons.[b] The consequence of neuron degeneration and loss is a major or a minor degree of cognitive deterioration, with a loss of intellectual performance.

a. http://www.un.org/en/documents/charter/preamble.shtml
b. Mechanisms of neurodegeneration and regeneration in alcoholism. Crews FT, Nixon K. Alcohol Alcohol. 2009 Mar-Apr;44(2):115-27. Epub 2008 Oct 21. Review. PMID: 18940959

BODY PIERCING

The fact that many cultures throughout history have practiced piercing does not legitimize its use. Torture and slavery have also been common, yet that does not justify them.

Body piercing done to insert of a piece of metal is a way of attacking and degrading the body, whether it's done for looks, superstition or fad. The truth is, historically, body piercing has much more often been used as a sign of slavery and submission than as an accessory.

The Risks of Body Piercing

- **Bacterial infection**: Occurs in 20% of piercings. Infections from tongue or mouth piercings are much more serious, as they are easily spread to vital areas.
- **Viral infection**: Piercing can spread the viruses of hepatitis B, hepatitis C and AIDS (HIV). Even the use of sterilized materials and proper procedures (which does not always occur), there is a risk of acquiring a viral infection through the open door caused by the perforation in the skin and subcutaneous tissue. The risk is even greater with the use of piercing guns, which are not easily sterilized.
- **Allergic reactions** to hygiene products when they are used close to the piercing or to the chlorine in pools, when swimming with a piercing.
- **Tears and injuries** if the piercing accidentally becomes entangled with other objects.
- **Unsightly scars** and keloids.
- **Risks in specific areas**: In addition to all of the above, piercings in certain areas have additional complications:
  - **Nipple** piercing can cause fibrosis of the milk ducts and the inability to breastfeed.
  - **Mouth** piercing often causes gum inflammation and the loss of pieces of tooth.

ABUSE

Abuse occurs when a person fails to respect the physical, emotional or sexual integrity of another person. Abuse generally includes an attack on the body in some way or another. Victims of abuse are generally women, children and the elderly, as well as many animals.

Points to Keep in Mind
- All forms of abuse, including, of course, domestic violence between spouses, is a crime.
- There is no reason or excuse that can justify abuse.
- Although the abuser generally believes he owns the person being abused, he has to be reminded that human beings –body included, of course– is not an object that can be possessed by another person. Every human being is a creature endowed with intrinsic value and deserving of the utmost respect– physical, emotional and sexual.

Abuse Prevention

Abuse happens in all cultures and social classes. Preventing it is everyone's responsibility, through these and other potential strategies.

- Education, primarily of children and adolescents, that emphasizes the unique worth of the human body and the respect that, as such, it deserves.
- Avoid corporal punishment upon children. An abused child has a greater risk of becoming an abuser. An abused girl is at higher risk of becoming an abused woman.
- Speak out about abuse– do not let this issue be kept silent. Reporting of known cases should be encouraged, always for the protection of victims.

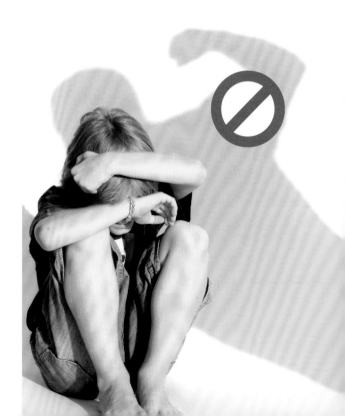

SAYING "NO" TO SEXUAL ASSAULT

*Sexual assault is also an attack on the body and a person's dignity.
All types of sexual assault must be prevented and fought.*

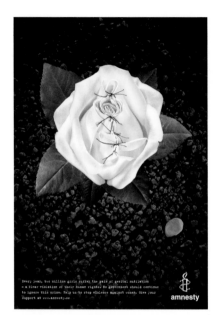

*Image used in Sweden against female
genital mutilation.*
Designer/idea: Yasin Lekorchi
och Malin Åkersten Triumf
Photograph: Niklas Alm/Vostro
Retouching: Sofia Cederström/Vostro
Volontaire, www.volontaire.se

FEMALE GENITAL MUTILATION

According to WHO (World Health Organization), female genital mutilation includes all procedures performed intentionally and for non-medical reasons in order to change or cause injury to the female genitalia.[a]

Female genital mutilation is considered a crime in most countries around the world, constituting an assault on a woman's body under the guise that it is a cultural practice.

Types of Mutilation

1. **Clitoridectomy or "sunna"**: Partial or total removal of the clitoris.

2. **Excision**: Removal of the clitoris and the labia minora.

3. **Infibulation**: Total removal of the external genitalia, leaving only a small opening for the passage of urine and menstrual blood. This type of mutilation prevents penetration, and requires a painful additional procedure to allow for sexual intercourse and childbirth. Infibulation makes up 15% of all mutilations performed around the world.

4. **Other harmful procedures** with non-medical ends, such as perforation, incision, scraping, or cauterization of the genital region.

a. http://www.who.int/mediacentre/factsheets/fs241/en/index.html

Misconceptions About Female Genital Mutilation

Misconception	Reality
"It is a ritual that is necessary in order to be considered an adult woman."	Traditions that include physical violence against the body such as this should be stopped. Genital mutilation does not make a woman valuable, but rather subjects her to an increased risk of infection and other disorders.
"It increases a man's sexual pleasure."	Quite the opposite: genital mutilation makes penetration uncomfortable for men, and even bothersome. For a woman, the penetration is quite painful.
"Eliminating a woman's sexual pleasure promotes her chastity and faithfulness."	The elimination of sexual pleasure does not protect against infidelity, as this tends to occur due to reasons that are not strictly sexual.
"It improves the appearance of the female genitalia by eliminating body parts that are considered masculine or dirty."	No part of a woman's body should be considered masculine or dirty. Every part of the female body has its specific and necessary function.
"It makes conception and childbirth easier."	Quite the opposite: it promotes sterility and increases the risks associated with childbirth and death in newborns.
"It's a religious principle."	No religion in the world, not even Islam or others, includes female mutilation as a principle.

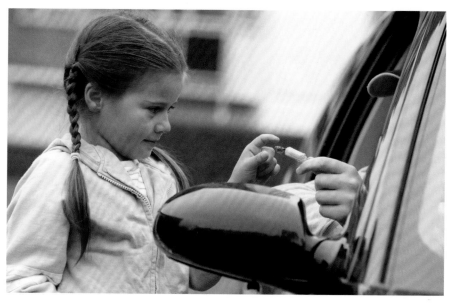

Child sexual abuse is one of the most repulsive forms of aggression to a child.

Rape is the crime of forcing someone to have sexual relations with another person without their consent.

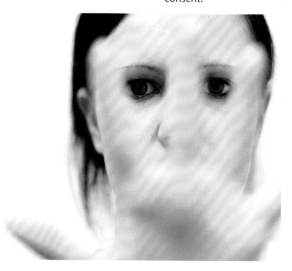

SEXUAL ABUSE OF CHILDREN

Child abuse for sexual purposes is one of the most repulsive forms of attack on the body and the person of the child. In 1989, the General Assembly of the United Nations approved the Convention on the Rights of the Child, which is currently in force.[a] Under Article 34, it states that all of the states parties undertake to protect children from all forms of sexual exploitation and sexual abuse. The so-called "sexual tourism" is one of the primary causes of child sexual abuse in the world.

Preventing Sexual Abuse of Children

• A watchful attitude by a child's parents or guardians: They must be aware of any adult that comes near the child, no matter who it is. The majority of abuse or rape cases in children are committed by adults that the parents and the victim know: family members, neighbors and trusted people from the family environment.

• Warn children starting at a young age that they should not allow any adult to touch their genitals.

• Warn children to avoid solitary and dark places, and never to get into a car with any adult they do not know.

• Warn children not to accept gifts from any adult without the knowledge of the parents.

a. http://www2.ohchr.org/spanish/law/crc.htm

RAPE

Rape is the crime of forcing another person to have sexual intercourse without their consent, using violence in the action, or threat of violence. It is also considered rape to have sexual intercourse with a minor who, although he/she may have agreed to it, is not of consenting age.

Rape is a physical attack on the body, generally on a woman, that can have the following consequences:

• Tears and injury to the genitalia, as well as trauma to other parts of the body.
• Genital infections.
• Unwanted pregnancy.

Scalp

*The skin on the head where hair begins to grow,
functioning as its physical and nutritional support.*

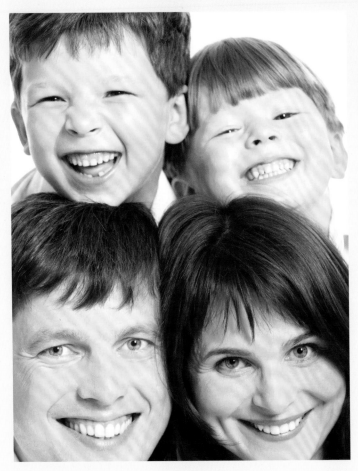

*T*he scalp and the hairs that originate within it are a reflection of the body's physical condition, and even of its mental state. Consequently, they are a reliable gauge of a person's overall health.

Hair is not an accessory on the outside of the body; rather, it is a living part of it –just like an eye or a hand. Hair carries out several functions, in addition to having aesthetic value: Physical protection for the head, a temperature regulator for the head, a solar shield and a sensory receptor to perceive the distance of objects or wind intensity.

Each one of the hairs is important, and carries out a function of its own. That is why in the Sermon on the Mount, Jesus said that "the very hairs of your head are all numbered."[a].

a. Matthew 10:30 (NKJV)

Facts and Figures About the Scalp

0.25 to 0.5 mm per day (9 to 18 cm or 3.54 to 7.09 in per year)	Growth rate of a single hair.
2 to 6	Average lifespan of a hair, in years.
40 to 80	Number of hairs lost each day, and that are usually replaced.
1 000	Number of hairs that, when braided, can support a person's body weight.
90 000 to 140 000	Number of hairs on the head.
540 000	Number of sebaceous glands on the scalp (500-600 per cm^2)

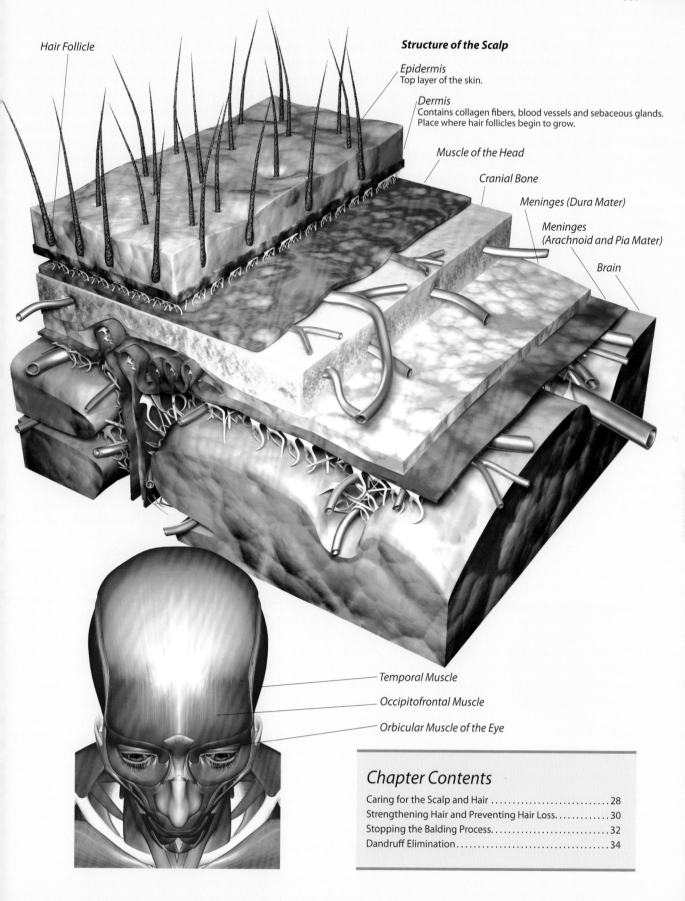

Hair Follicle

Structure of the Scalp

Epidermis
Top layer of the skin.

Dermis
Contains collagen fibers, blood vessels and sebaceous glands.
Place where hair follicles begin to grow.

Muscle of the Head

Cranial Bone

Meninges (Dura Mater)

*Meninges
(Arachnoid and Pia Mater)*

Brain

Temporal Muscle

Occipitofrontal Muscle

Orbicular Muscle of the Eye

Chapter Contents

CARING FOR THE SCALP AND HAIR

*The scalp is the support for the hair. In most cases, a good diet
and some basic care, such as that indicated in this unit,
are enough to achieve gorgeous hair.*

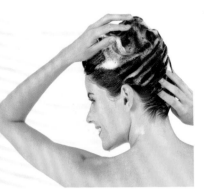

WASH HAIR REGULARLY

The scalp covering the head is exposed to the environment, so it becomes saturated with smoke, dust and other contaminants. In addition, the scalp secretes oil, which forms a thin layer of protection for the hair roots. All of this makes it necessary to wash hair with shampoo or a mild soap at least twice per week.

USE SOFT BRUSHES

Brushes or combs with hard tips that scratch the scalp stimulate the production of sebum and can promote hair loss.

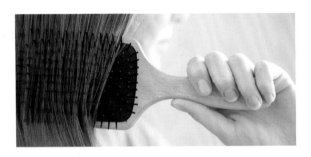

AVOID SHAMPOOS THAT CONTAIN A DETERGENT

Detergents added to shampoos achieve a better cleansing effect, but at the cost of stripping all of the natural oils that coat the scalp. When this happens, hair follicles lose their vitality and hair becomes brittle.

MASSAGE THE SCALP

Massaging the scalp stimulates circulation and improves the supply of oxygen and nutrients to the hair follicle cells where hair begins to grow.

How to Perform
- This can be done with or without help.
- Use the fingertips to make gentle movements, moving from the top to the bottom of the head, and from front to back.
- After finishing the massage, wash hair with a natural shampoo without detergent.

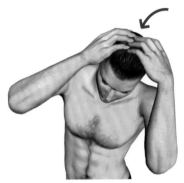

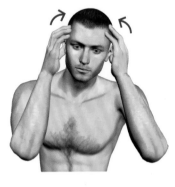

KEEP THE HAIR TYPE IN MIND

Oily hair requires care that is different from what is needed for dry hair. Before using a lotion on the hair, determine if it is oily or dry. In the unit "Dandruff Elimination", some lotions are given for each hair type.

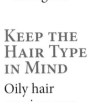

Clay Mask for the Hair

This mask cleanses the scalp, purifies it, and tones the hair follicles. It is good for all hair types, whether oily or dry.

1. Dilute very fine green clay with water in a wooden or porcelain container.

2. Add a few drops of essence of lavender or mint.

3. Add a tablespoon or two of olive or almond oil.

4. Mix well until a homogeneous paste is formed.

5. Apply a thin layer of the paste onto the scalp. Leave it in place for 15-30 minutes.

6. To finish the treatment, rinse with diluted lemon juice (one or two lemons per liter of water).

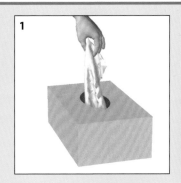

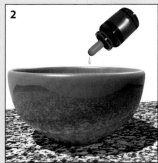

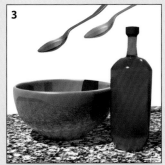

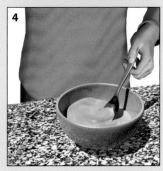

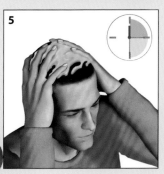

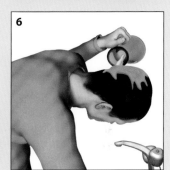

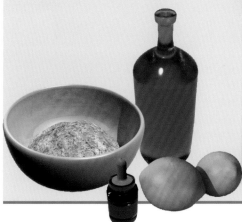

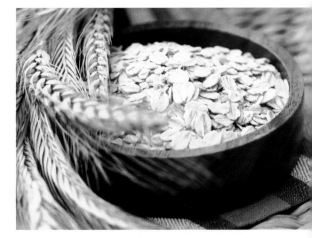

Lemon Is Better than Vinegar

Lemon juice diluted in water is ideal for rinsing the hair after applying a lotion, poultice or compress. This is because lemon preserves the acid levels needed by the scalp. The recommended dosage is one to two lemons per liter of water.

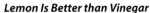

Taking wheat germ and brewer's yeast helps strengthen the hair, due to the vitamins and minerals provided by both supplements.

STRENGTHENING HAIR AND PREVENTING HAIR LOSS

It is normal to lose 40-80 hairs each day, but this should not be worrisome, since other hairs replace the hairs that have been lost. When this replacement does not occur, baldness ensues.

Hair loss in men, and to a lesser degree in women, is a normal process after a certain age. However, baldness may also be the first symptom of a skin disease, a vitamin deficiency, a thyroid malfunction or a constant state of stress.

The herbs and supplements in this unit can help stop hair loss, not only for male-pattern baldness, but also for the other causes of alopecia.

WAYS TO USE HERBAL TREATMENTS TO STRENGTHEN HAIR

Poultices

- Poultices are made by crushing the herb in a mortar, or by grinding it in an electric grinder.
- Spread the resulting paste onto a gauze pad.
- It is good to heat the poultice to body temperature before applying it. Using an iron is easiest.

- Leave it on the scalp for 5-10 minutes.
- After removing the poultice, rinse hair with lemon juice diluted in water (one or two lemons per liter of water).
- The poultices to strengthen hair can be made with watercress, stinging nettle, garden nasturtium, great burdock, or maidenhair fern.

Lotions

- Lotion is a liquid applied with a gentle massage on the skin; in this case, on the scalp.

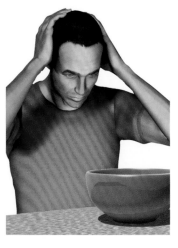

- Lotions are applied once or twice per day. After allowing it to dry for 10-20 minutes, rinse the scalp with diluted lemon juice (one or two lemons per liter of water).
- Lotions to strengthen the hair can be made with fresh juice or with an infusion of watercress, stinging nettle, common thyme, garden nasturtium, or maidenhair fern.

Compresses

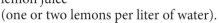

- Soak a cloth in the infusion or preparation of the herb cooled to body temperature, and apply it onto the scalp for 10-15 minutes, one to three times per day.
- Remove the compress, then rinse the scalp with diluted lemon juice (one or two lemons per liter of water).
- Compresses can be made with the infusion of any of the herbs recommended for strengthening the hair. Compresses with a preparation of quinine bark or burdock root are especially effective.

Medicinal Herbs for Strengthening Hair
(for external use)

WATERCRESS ("NASTURTIUM OFFICINALIS")

Due its sulfurated essence, watercress regenerates the hair follicles and stops hair loss. It can be applied as a lotion with the infusion or fresh juice from the herb, or as a poultice with crushed herb.

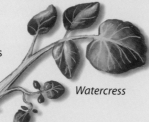

Watercress

STINGING NETTLE ("URTICA DIOICA")

Prevents seborrhea (excess oil) and strengthens hair, thanks to its histamine content, which stimulates circulation in the dermis. It may be applied as a lotion with the infusion or fresh juice from the herb, or as a poultice with crushed herb.

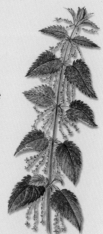

Stinging Nettle

COMMON THYME ("THYMUS VULGARIS")

Its essence tones the scalp and is antiseptic. The essence can be applied directly as lotion, or a preparation can be made with a handful of common thyme in a liter of water. Moisten the head with this infusion and leave it on for an hour or more, until it dries. Afterward, rinse with lemon juice diluted in water.

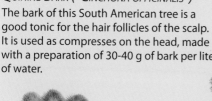

Common Thyme

GARDEN NASTURTIUM ("TROPAEOLUM MAJUS")

Hair revitalizer and antibiotic. It is applied as a lotion in the form of its fresh juice, infusion, or marinade (2 handfuls of flowers and leaves soaked in half a liter of alcohol for 2 weeks).

QUININE BARK ("CINCHONA OFFICINALIS")

The bark of this South American tree is a good tonic for the hair follicles of the scalp. It is used as compresses on the head, made with a preparation of 30-40 g of bark per liter of water.

Quinine Bark

Garden Nasturtium

GREAT BURDOCK ("ARCTIUM LAPPA")

Its root stimulates hair growth. It is used as a poultice or a compress.

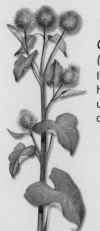

Great Burdock

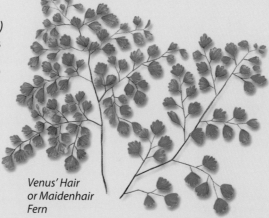

Venus' Hair or Maidenhair Fern

VENUS' HAIR OR MAIDENHAIR FERN ("ADIANTUM CAPILLUS-VENERIS")

Traditionally, this herb has been used as a poultice on the head to strengthen hair.

STOPPING THE BALDING PROCESS

Medicinal herbs and supplements help reduce hair loss without the side effects of many medicines for male alopecia, such as a reduction in libido and a tendency toward feminization.

MEDICINAL HERBS FOR MALE BALDNESS (FOR INTERNAL USE)

Saw Palmetto ("Serenoa repens")

The fruits of this small palm tree stop the production of dihydrotestosterone, the male hormone responsible for androgenic baldness and hypertrophy of the prostate. There are studies that confirm the ability of saw palmetto to stop the progression of male-pattern baldness, and even reverse it.[a] It is taken orally as extracts, 160 mg twice per day.

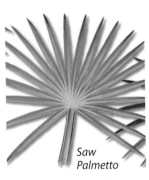

Saw Palmetto

African Plum ("Pygeum africanum")

The bark of this tree also stops the production of the hormone responsible for male baldness. It is taken as an extract (100-200 mg per day). Its effect is increased by taking it along with stinging nettle (*Urtica dioica*), as an infusion or as extracts (50-100 mg per day).

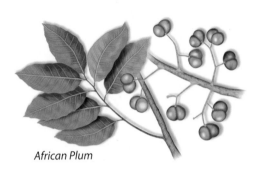

African Plum

Common Horsetail ("Equisetum arvense")

Due to its high silicon content, it strengthens the hair and stops hair loss. It is taken as an infusion or an extract.

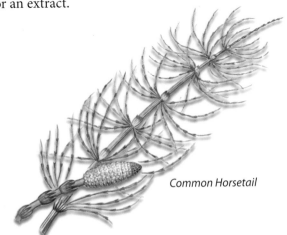

Common Horsetail

SUPPLEMENTS FOR STRONGER HAIR

B-Group Vitamins

All B-group vitamins strengthen hair, but especially biotin or vitamin B_3 (100-150 mg per day). Brewer's yeast, legumes, nuts and sunflower and pumpkin seeds are good dietary sources of these vitamins.

Zinc

Zinc stimulates hair growth within the hair follicle. The recommended dosage is 30-50 mg per day. Wheat germ, brewer's yeast, nuts and sunflower and pumpkin seeds are good dietary sources of zinc.

Omega-3 Essential Fatty Acids

Flaxseed, evening primrose oil, nuts and soy are rich in this type of fat that is needed for healthy hair.

---

a. A randomized, double-blind, placebo-controlled trial to determine the effectiveness of botanically derived inhibitors of 5-alpha-reductase in the treatment of androgenetic alopecia. Prager N, Bickett K, French N, Marcovici G. J Altern Complement Med. 2002 Apr;8(2):143-52. Erratum in: J Altern Complement Med. 2006 Mar;12(2):199. PMID: 12006122

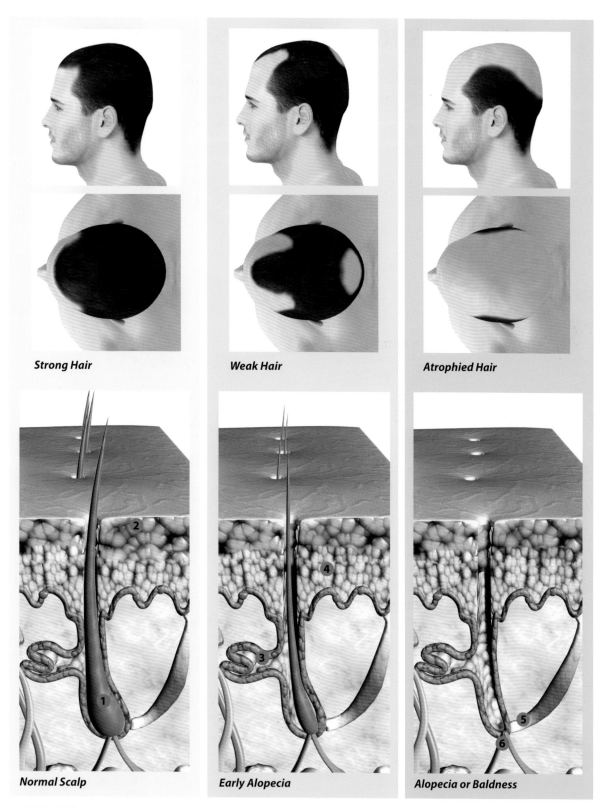

Strong Hair

Weak Hair

Atrophied Hair

Normal Scalp

Early Alopecia

Alopecia or Baldness

(1) Hair follicle
Place where hair is produced.

(2) Epidermis

(3) Sebaceous gland of the hair
Produces a fatty substance to protect the hair and keep it smooth and lustrous.

(4) Dermis

(5) Hair erector muscle
Each hair has a small involuntary muscles that can tense the hair or make it stand on end.

(6) Artery that nourishes the hair

DANDRUFF ELIMINATION

Dandruff accelerates baldness, making it very important to eliminate it in order to achieve healthy hair.

The flakes made by dandruff are the manifestation of inflammation in the sebaceous glands of the scalp that produce the protective oils. Dandruff elimination requires much more than simply using a certain shampoo.

AVOID THE CAUSE

The most frequent cause of dandruff is seborrhea or an excess of oil on the scalp, associated with inflammation of sebaceous glands. There are certain triggers that should be avoided:
- Hormonal or metabolic imbalance.
- Diet high in sugars and other carbohydrates.
- Nutrition deficiencies, especially of B-group vitamins, essential fatty acids (polyunsaturated) and selenium.
- Trauma or local irritation of the scalp.
- Stress and anxiety.

DIET

- Primarily raw diet, in which 50-75% of foods are fruits, grains, nuts and raw vegetables in their natural state or that are minimally processed.
- Avoid milk and milk products overall, as they increase oil production in the scalp, even if they are non-fat.
- Avoid fried foods, foods with added sugar, honey, white flour, chocolate and seafood, which increase sebaceous secretions.

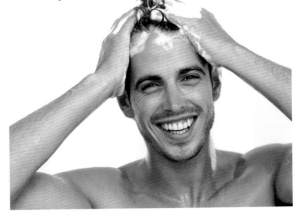

HAIR CARE

- Do not scratch the scalp, as this increases oil secretions.
- Wash hair no more than 2 or 3 times per week, with natural shampoos that do not contain detergents or alkaline chemical products that destroy the protective acid covering of the scalp.
- Avoid greasy ointments and creams on the scalp.
- Do not abuse selenium shampoos, because although they eliminate dandruff at the time of use, they irritate the scalp and can cause a rebound effect.
- Rinse hair after washing with vinegar diluted in water (about one 200 ml cup of vinegar per liter of water).

AVOID STRESS

Through nerve endings, emotions influence the skin overall, and especially the scalp. This is the reason that stress and anxiety increase fatty secretions, promoting dandruff.

A lifestyle change which increases contact with nature and its curative agents such as water, sunshine, exercise, etc., along with taking sedating medicinal herbal teas (valerian, passion flower, white thorn and others), are simple remedies to alleviate stress and anxiety.

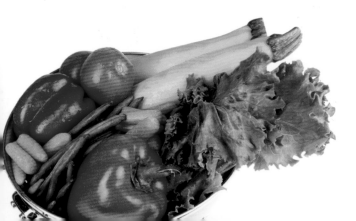

Lotions for Oily Hair

The scalp's sebaceous glands produce a special type of oil, needed to protect the hair follicles where hair is implanted. However, an excess of oil due to hormonal imbalance, deficient nutrition or stress, suffocates the hair follicles instead of protecting them.

To reduce oil production, one of these lotions can be applied:

- Pure or slightly diluted lemon juice.
- Poppy (*Papaver rhoeas*) infusion.
- Hamamelis (*Hamamelis virginiana*) infusion or water.
- Fresh stinging nettle (*Urtica dioica*) juice.

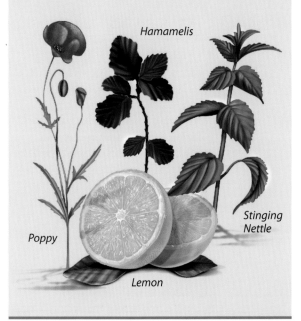

Hamamelis

Poppy

Stinging Nettle

Lemon

Lotions for Dry Hair

When the scalp does not produce enough oil, hair becomes dry and brittle. The application of a lotion made of egg or avocado nourishes the hair follicles and increases oil production.

EGG LOTION

Beat a whole egg in a glass of water with two tablespoons of apple vinegar, until foamy. Apply to the scalp and keep it there a few minutes. Rinse with diluted lemon juice (one or two lemons per liter of water).

AVOCADO LOTION

Finely mash an avocado and apply it directly to the scalp as a shampoo. Avocado oil can also be applied. After a few minutes, rinse with diluted lemon juice.

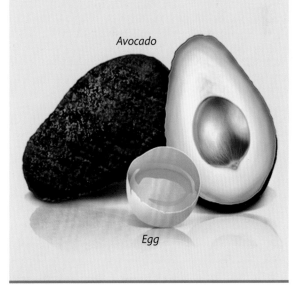

Avocado

Egg

How to Apply Hair Lotions

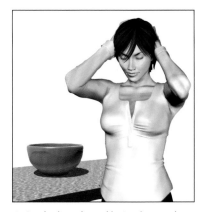

1. Apply the selected lotion by gently massaging it into the scalp.

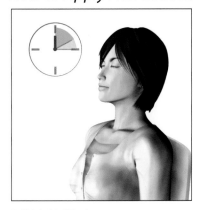

2. Wait 10-15 minutes.

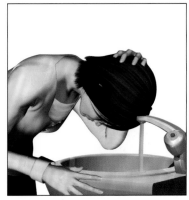

3. Wash and rinse hair.

Brain

*T*o Aristotle (4ᵗʰ Century B.C.), the brain was nothing more than a sponge designed to cool the blood. Anatomists of the Renaissance period considered the brain nothing more than a motor for moving the body. But today, we know that the brain is the control center for all bodily functions, not just movement; more importantly, it is the center of the mind and higher functions that are specific to humans.

The human brain is the most complex object in the known universe, and, at the same time, the least understood.

The human brain is so complex, so efficient in energy use, and so powerful, that evolutionist theories cannot explain its origin.

If a "simple" neuron, the body of which measures less than a tenth of a millimeter, surprises us by its organization and intelligent design, how much more surprising is the brain, being made up of millions of interconnected neurons which are capable of making decisions, thinking, loving and believing?

Facts and Figures About the Brain

0.1 volts	Average voltage of the electrical current between neurons.
2%	Percentage of the brain in relation to the rest of the body.
2 a 4 mm (0.08 to 0.16 in)	Weight of the gray matter of the cerebral cortex, where neurons are located.
4 minutes	Time that the body can continue living after becoming separated from the brain.
4.8 grams (0.17 oz)	Glucose consumed by the brain in one hour.
15%	Percentage of blood flow from the entire body going to the brain.
20%	Percentage of oxygen breathed going to the brain at rest.
45 liters (95.1 US pt)	Blood volume traveling through the brain in one hour.
120 meters per second (= 430 km/h or 267 mph)	Speed of transmission of nerve impulses.
1 300 grams (2.87 lb)	Average weight of the brain (1 450 g in men and 1 250 g in women)
2 300 cm² (356.5 sq in)	Surface of the cerebral cortex, equivalent to a square with sides measuring 48 cm.
10 000	Number of connections of each neuron has with the rest of the neurons.
1 600 000 km (994 194 mi)	Length of all of the nerve fibers in the brain.
100 000 000 000 (one hundred billion)	Number of nerve cells in the nervous system (brain, cerebellum, spinal cord). Of these, about 20 billion are neurons and the rest are glial or support cells.

Frontal Lobe
Center of the mind's higher functions, unique to humans, such as reasoning, judgment, self-control and language.

Parietal Lobe
Receives and processes the tactile sensations of the entire body, and controls body movements.

Temporal Lobe
Receives and processes auditory information. It is the center of recall and memory.

Occipital Lobe
Receives and processes visual information.

Cerebellum

Spinal Cord

Chapter Contents

Caring for the Brain

General Overview

The brain directs all bodily functions.
By taking care of the brain and meeting its needs,
the health of the rest of the organs and body parts is promoted

Well-Protected, But Very Needy

No organ in the body is better protected physically than the brain; and no other performs such complex functions and requires so much care.

The brain is also the most threatened organ in these special times in which we live. Trauma, infections, unbalanced diets, toxins and environmental contaminants, addictive drugs, and stress all pose an increasing threat to the brain's ability to perform its higher and complex functions.

As a result, the brain is currently the organ that requires the most protection and care.

In the units that follow, much of its needed care is described, from physical protection to psychological care and diet..

Taking Care of Basic Needs (pg. 40)
Oxygen and glucose are the brain's two basic needs. Without these substances, the brain simply does not work.

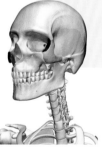

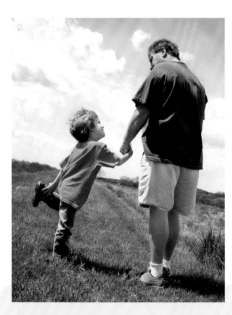

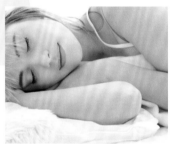

Physical Protection (pg. 46)
Despite the fact that it is better protected than any other organ in the body, all physical aggression against the brain should be avoided.
Electromagnetic radiation is also a physical agent that can affect the brain.

Chemical Protection (pg. 48)
Alcohol, drugs, and certain neurotoxic plants easily deteriorate brain function.
In addition, aggressive molecules called free radicals deteriorate the neurons and cause degenerative diseases such as Alzheimer's. Fortunately, with the use of antioxidants it is possible to neutralize free radicals.

Healthy Habits (pg. 44)
Good hydration, regular rest, physical activity and breathing fresh air, among other habits, promote good brain function.

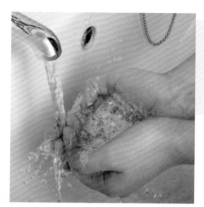

Microbiological Protection (pg. 56)
The brain is sensitive to a number of viruses, bacteria and other germs that can damage the structure and function of the brain, even permanently. Certain basic hygiene standards, and protection against mosquitoes and ticks, are very effective for protecting the brain against bacteria and viruses.

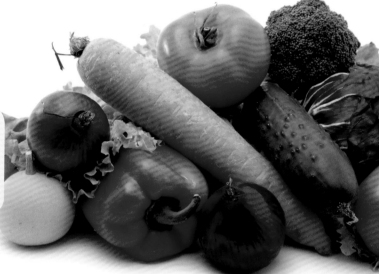

Food for the Brain (pg. 62)
Foods definitely influence brain function. Some foods and certain plants have a confirmed neuroprotective effect, and their regular use keeps neurons in good condition.

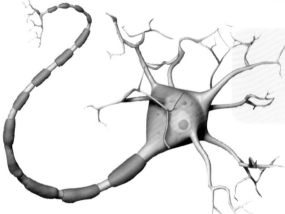

Psychological and Spiritual Care (pg. 74)
For good functioning, the brain also needs psychological and spiritual care. All humans need to love and be loved, and in this way, brain performance improves.

Reasons You Must See a Doctor

- Headache with nausea or vomiting, loss of balance or visual disturbances.
- Any headache that does not resolve within a week.
- Loss of strength in the arms or legs.
- Difficulty in coordinating walking movements.
- Progressive memory loss.
- Hand tremors.

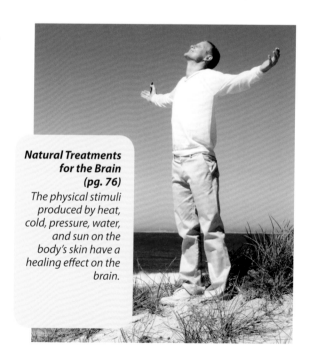

Natural Treatments for the Brain (pg. 76)
The physical stimuli produced by heat, cold, pressure, water, and sun on the body's skin have a healing effect on the brain.

BASIC NEEDS OF THE BRAIN - 1

OXYGEN

A steady supply of oxygen is the brain's first and most important need. Without this vital gas, which comes from clean air, the brain cannot perform any of its functions.

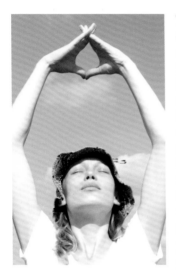

The brain is a big oxygen consumer, surpassed only by the liver. Although its weight is only 2% of the body's weight, it consumes 20% of all of the oxygen carried by the blood. This means that it consumes 10 times more oxygen than the average for the rest of the body.

In addition to needing lots of oxygen, the brain requires a steady, uninterrupted supply of it. Without oxygen, neurons die within a few minutes. A complete lack of oxygen occurs in cases of asphyxia or sudden blockage of a cerebral artery, and can lead to death.

The more common disorder, however, is when the blood supply to the brain is poorly oxygenated or some partial arterial blockage causes slowed blood flow (usually due to atherosclerosis). If this happens, mental abilities are affected in a way that is similar to a low dose of alcohol:

- Decreased willpower.
- Slowed thinking.
- Diminished ability to concentrate.
- Difficulty in reasoning and judgment.

HOW TO IMPROVE OXYGEN FLOW TO THE BRAIN

- Breathe in fresh air: Air from a place where there is smoking, a closed room, or from a place where there is a low flame burning (like a grill) contains increased levels of carbon monoxide (chemical formula: CO). This odorless, colorless gas keeps the blood from transporting oxygen, and causes silent chemical asphyxiation. In low doses, carbon monoxide causes confusion and drowsiness; in high doses, it results in death from asphyxiation.
- Perform a series of deep breathing exercises, especially if the job requires little physical activity.
- Get regular aerobic exercise, such as brisk walking.
- Keep lungs healthy (see Chapter 13).
- Follow a diet low in saturated fat and cholesterol that is also rich in antioxidants. This improves arterial health and prevents blockage from athersclerosis.

Energy Consumed by the Human Brain

The brain itself uses about a fifth of the oxygen that we breathe in and the energy that we consume each day from food.

The majority of this energy is used to generate the electrical impulses transmitted over the synapses (connections between neurons).

	Glucose Usage	Equivalence in Calories
Per Minute	80 mg	0.32 kcal
Per Hour	4.8 g	19.2 kcal
Per Day (24 hrs)	115.2 g	460 kcal

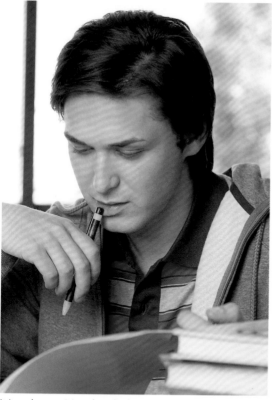

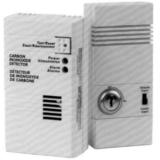

Installing a carbon monoxide detector is very useful for checking the indoor air quality.

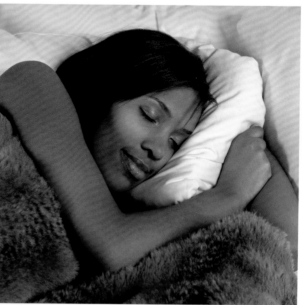

It is truly surprising that the brain requires so little to do so much work and perform its numerous and complex functions: Basically, a continuous supply of oxygen and glucose.

The Brain Compared to Rest of the Body

After the liver, the brain is the organ with the highest metabolic rate. With a weight of only 2% of the total body weight, it receives 15% of the blood flow and 20% of the oxygen breathed. It is therefore important for the brain to receive an adequate supply of oxygen and glucose for proper functioning.

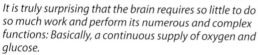

50 ml per minute

20%

750 ml per minute

15%

1.4 kg

2%

Weight

Blood Flow

Oxygen Usage

Percentage as compared with the rest of the body

BASIC NEEDS
OF THE BRAIN - 2

GLUCOSE

*In addition to oxygen, glucose is the most important need
of the brain. But not just any source of glucose is healthy;
it has to come from foods rich in vegetable fiber.*

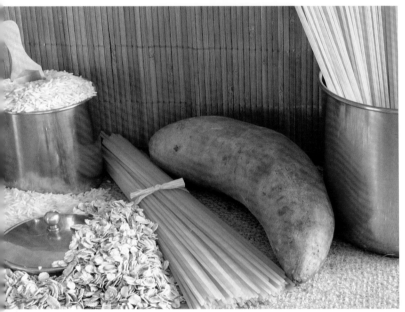

Glucose comes from the digestion of food, and from stocks in the liver in the form of glucogen.

With the exception of neurons, all of the body's cells need insulin in order to transport glucose from the bloodstream into the cell. Neurons do not need insulin in order to obtain glucose, which is the reason that in insulin-deficient diabetes, neurons continue receiving their supply of glucose as long as the blood contains at least 80 mg of glucose per 100 milliliters.

HOW MUCH GLUCOSE?

Not too much, not too little; in order to function correctly, the brain requires that the blood flowing through it maintain a consistent glucose level between these two limits:

- **Lower Limit**: 80 mg of glucose for every 100 ml of blood (= 0.8 grams per liter). When the glucose level falls below this 80 mg/100 ml of blood, brain performance starts to decrease (see table on facing page "Blood Glucose Level and Brain Function").

- **Upper Limit**: Around 180/100 ml. Diabetics well know that when their blood glucose level increases too much due to poor control, they feel uncomfortable and irritable. When the glucose level goes above 400 mg per 100 ml of blood, the brain can barely function, and coma ensues.

Drastic decreases and fluctuations in glucose levels due to a diet high in refined sugar affect brain function and weaken the mind.

Glucose is the primary fuel for neurons. Without glucose, the brain cannot work, since this sugar that is so abundant in nature, is responsible for nourishing the electrical mini-command center present in each neuron. All of the complex chemical reactions happening inside of the brain require the presence of glucose.

As shown on the table on the previous page, "Energy Consumed by the Human Brain", the brain alone consumes 460 kcal in 24 hours, a fifth of the 2 300 kcal that the average adult consumes.

A SURE SUPPLY

Neurons cannot store up glucose, and therefore they must continually receive it from the blood.

SOURCES OF GLUCOSE

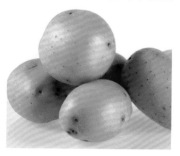

All starches and sugars from food are eventually converted to glucose during digestion. However, glucose coming from healthy sources, such as whole grains, tubers or fruits that are high in fiber, is not the same as when it comes from refined sweets or candy.

According to a study by the University of Toronto (Canada), the favorable effect on brain function and memory was shown to be better after consuming 50 g of carbohydrates in the form of potatoes or barley, than after consuming 50 g of refined sugar (pure glucose).[a]

The positive effect that the potato, barley and other tubers and grains have on brain function may be due to the fact that their digestion provides a constant glucose supply for hours, while the digestion of refined sugar causes surges in glucose levels, only to then decrease.

HOW TO IMPROVE GLUCOSE SUPPLY TO THE BRAIN

Have a Hearty Breakfast

Breakfast including preferably whole grains , tubers (potato, cassava and the like) or legumes like in Mexico (where a bean-based breakfast is so popular) guarantees the glucose supply to the brain for the whole morning, and improves school and work performance.

Eat Whole Grains

Whole grains are rich in vegetable fiber, which regulates the release of glucose during digestion and allows its level to remain suitable in the blood. All of these foods have a low glycemic index, which means that they do not raise the blood sugar very much after being consumed.

A study by the University of Northumbria (Newcastle, United Kingdom) shows that a breakfast including whole grains with a low glycemic index (such as muesli) significantly improves attention and memory in school-aged children.[b]

Reduce or Eliminate Consumption of Products Low in Fiber

Products made with white sugar and refined flour such as breads, cakes and candies are low in fiber, and have a high glycemic index (they cause a significant increase in glucose levels after being consumed). Eating these products causes surges spikes in blood glucose levels, and does not help keep the constant level that the brain requires.

Eat on a Regular Schedule

Eating on a regular schedule helps maintain suitable blood glucose levels, which promotes good brain function. This also allows for biological rhythms and gives the digestive organs needed resting periods.

b. A low glycaemic index breakfast cereal preferentially prevents children's cognitive performance from declining throughout the morning. Ingwersen J, Defeyter MA, Kennedy DO, Wesnes KA, Scholey AB. Appetite. 2007 Jul;49(1):240-4. Epub 2007 Jan 16. PMID: 17224202

Blood Glucose Level and Brain Function

Mg of Glucose per 100 ml of Blood	Brain Function
Over 400	Comatose.
180-400	Uncomfortable.
80-180	Normal.
60-80	Diminished concentration, memory and irritability.
50	Difficulty with word pronunciation.
40	Uncoordinated movements.
30	Comatose.
20	Seizures.
10	Brain death.

a. Cognitive performance is associated with glucose regulation in healthy elderly persons and can be enhanced with glucose and dietary carbohydrates. Kaplan RJ, Greenwood CE, Winocur G, Wolever TM. Am J Clin Nutr. 2000 Sep;72(3):825-36. PMID: 10966906

HEALTHY HABITS FOR THE BRAIN

Habits of daily living influence the good condition of the brain, especially good hydration, rest, physical activity and breathing fresh air.

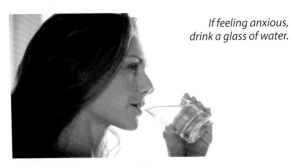

If feeling anxious, drink a glass of water.

DRINK ENOUGH WATER

The brain contains a higher proportion of water than any other organ. Water is where many chemical reactions occur in the nerve tissue.

Poor hydration causes lack of concentration and irritability, sometimes without even realizing it.

GET ENOUGH SLEEP

It is said that sleep is food for the brain. While resting (specifically during sleep,) neurons are freed from free radicals and other waste products that have accumulated during active periods. Without sufficient and regular sleep, brain function decreases, and brainpower and willpower are lost. According to a study at the University of Pensylvania (United States), the following are some of the effects that lack of sleep has on the mind:[a]

• Attention lapses.

• Memory lapses.

• Depressed mood.

• Decrease in cognitive functions (alertness).

Tips for Sleeping Well

• Have a small dinner, no later than two hours before bedtime.

• For adult males, do not drink water later than 4 hours before bedtime, to avoid having to get up to urinate due to an enlarged prostate.

• Always go to bed at the same time.

• Avoid long naps.

• Reduce or eliminate coffee, tea, and caffeinated beverages.

• Drink a soothing herbal hot tea.

• Take a warm bath or shower before bedtime.

GET PHYSICAL ACTIVITY

It is known that people who stay physically active between the ages of 20 and 60 have less risk of suffering from Alzheimer's in the late stages of life.[b]

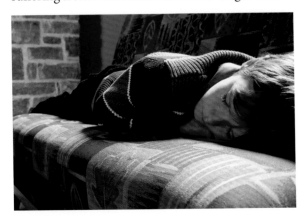

Sleep feeds the brain.

Regular physical activity protects against mental deterioration and memory loss, by way of the following mechanisms:

• It can regenerate neurons: Studies done with laboratory animals show that regular physical activity causes new neurons to develop in the hippocampus, the part of the brain where memory resides.[c] The time-honored belief that neurons cannot regenerate in the adult brain is being revised as a result of recent studies.

a. Behavioral and physiological consequences of sleep restriction. Banks S, Dinges DF. J Clin Sleep Med. 2007 Aug 15;3(5):519-28. PMID: 17803017

b. Patients with Alzheimer's disease have reduced activities in midlife compared with healthy control-group members. Friedland RP, Fritsch T, Smyth KA, Koss E, Lerner AJ, Chen CH, Petot GJ, Debanne SM. Proc Natl Acad Sci U S A. 2001 Mar 13;98(6):3440-5. Epub 2001 Mar 6. PMID: 11248097

c. What we need to know about age related memory loss. Small GW. BMJ. 2002 Jun 22;324(7352):1502-5. Review. PMID: 12077041

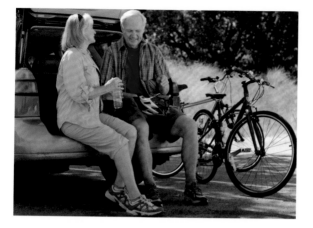

One of the factors that promotes neuron regeneration is, specifically, physical activity.

- It increases blood flow to the brain and, with it, the supply of oxygen to neurons. Poor oxygenation of the neurons due to an inactive lifestyle decreases memory capacity.

GET FRESH AIR

Breathing supplies oxygen to the blood, which in turn transports it to the organ that needs it the most: the brain.

Breathing correctly is not the only important step to have a well-oxygenated blood. In addition, the air entering the lungs should be as free from smoke and chemical pollutants. as possible Many of these, such as tobacco smoke and heavy metals like lead, are present in polluted air. These pollutants impair brain development, especially in children.

TAKE WALKS IN THE COUNTRYSIDE

A brisk walk through the park or in the countryside is one of the best exercises for good brain oxygenation. It also relaxes agitated nerves after a day's hustle and bustle.

KEEP THE BLOOD CLEAN

The popular expression "clean blood" applies to the need that the brain has for blood to be free of drugs, toxic substances or an increased level of waste products.

The brain receives 15% of the body's blood flow. That is, 15% of all of the blood that comes out of the heart passes through the brain.

Each minute that goes by, 750 ml of blood passes through the brain, which is equivalent to 45 liters per hour. This means that every hour, all of the body's blood (about 6.5 liters) passes through the brain 7 times.

In addition to oxygen and glucose, blood supplies the neurons with other substances that are also needed for good function: essential fatty acids, proteins, B-group vitamins (including B_9 or folic acid), minerals and hormones.

Ways to Keep the Blood Clean

- Avoid the use of alcohol, tobacco and other drugs.
- Drink enough water every day, in order to promote the kidneys' elimination function.
- Reduce or eliminate meat from the diet, as it generates waste products such as urea and uric acid, which slow brain function. Proteins from legumes also produce urea and uric acid, but due to the alkalinization effect of vegetable proteins, they promote the elimination of waste products.
- Increase intake of depurative fruits and vegetables such as lemon, onion and celery, which promote elimination of toxins from the bloodstream.

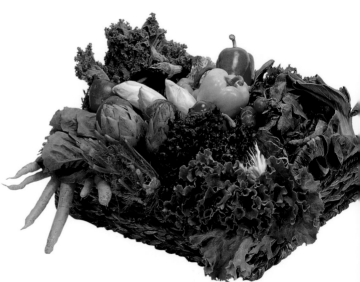

PHYSICAL PROTECTION FOR THE BRAIN

MECHANICAL AND ELECTROMAGNETIC AGENTS

The nerve tissue that makes up the brain is very sensitive to physical agents, whether mechanical or electromagnetic. Despite being better protected than any other organ in the body, the brain needs physical protection.

AVOID BLOWS TO THE HEAD

Head trauma, especially repeated head trauma, can cause brain damage.

People who have suffered a blow to the head with loss of consciousness that lasted an hour or longer are at greater risk of suffering age-related memory loss.[a]

An interesting study demonstrated that swimmers and runners have better memories than soccer players at the same age.[b] This difference is attributed to the greater frequency with which the soccer players suffer head trauma.

Practice of violent sports that involve blows to the head, such as boxing, is associated with a decrease in brain function.

AVOID TIME NEAR POWER LINES

A study done in Denmark demonstrated that power company workers who are exposed to low-frequency electromagnetic fields (50 Hz) are at greater risk of suffering senile dementia and amyotrophic lateral sclerosis.[c] A prior study done at the University of North Carolina (United States) demonstrated similar results.[d]

So it is prudent to avoid spending time near power lines, transformers, motors and any device that produces 50 Hz electromagnetic fields.

BE CAREFUL WITH MOBILE PHONES

The relationship between the use of mobile phones and the development of brain tumors is a subject of controversy. Although there are several studies that rule out a possible carcinogenic effect with these devices, it is wise to avoid abusing them.

The recommendation to avoid spending too much time talking on a mobile phone is directed especially to children, since their brain tissue is more sensitive to radiation.

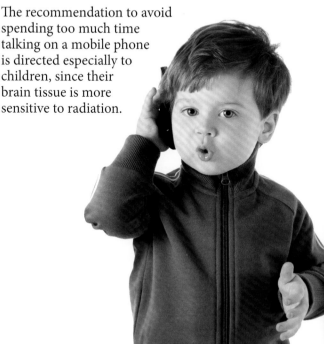

a. What we need to know about age related memory loss. Small GW. BMJ. 2002 Jun 22;324(7352):1502-5. Review. PMID: 12077041
b. Neuropsychological impairment in amateur soccer players. Matser EJ, Kessels AG, Lezak MD, Jordan BD, Troost J. JAMA. 1999 Sep 8;282(10):971-3. PMID: 10485683
c. Exposure to electromagnetic fields and risk of central nervous system disease in utility workers. Johansen C. Epidemiology. 2000 Sep;11(5):539-43. PMID: 10955406
d. Electrical occupations and neurodegenerative disease: analysis of U.S. mortality data. Savitz DA, Loomis DP, Tse CK. Arch Environ Health. 1998 Jan-Feb;53(1):71-4. PMID: 9570311

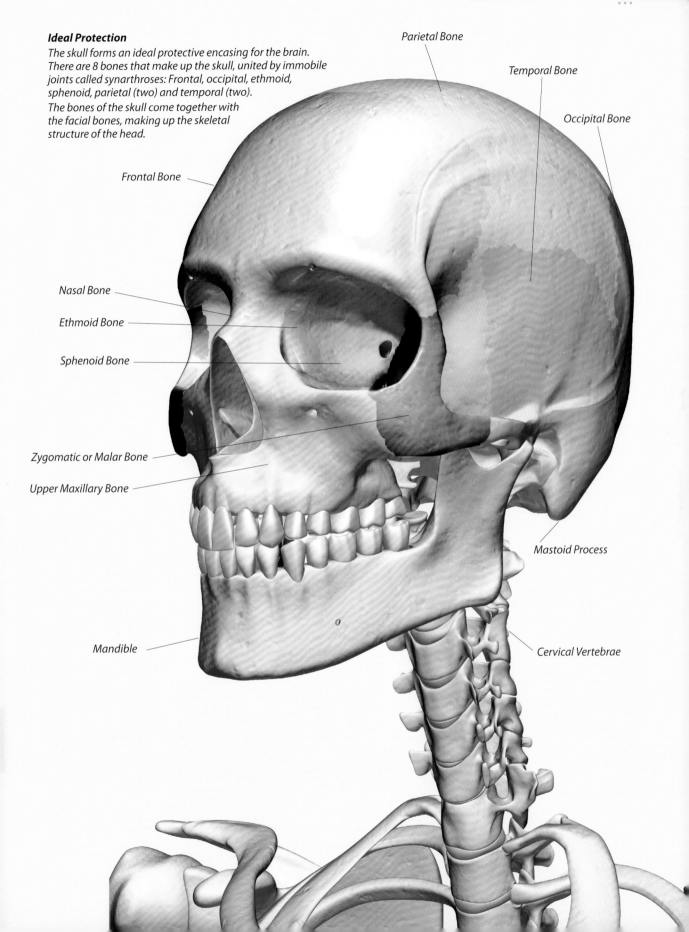

Ideal Protection

The skull forms an ideal protective encasing for the brain.
There are 8 bones that make up the skull, united by immobile
joints called synarthroses: Frontal, occipital, ethmoid,
sphenoid, parietal (two) and temporal (two).

The bones of the skull come together with
the facial bones, making up the skeletal
structure of the head.

Parietal Bone

Temporal Bone

Occipital Bone

Frontal Bone

Nasal Bone

Ethmoid Bone

Sphenoid Bone

Zygomatic or Malar Bone

Upper Maxillary Bone

Mastoid Process

Mandible

Cervical Vertebrae

CHEMICAL PROTECTION FOR THE BRAIN - 1

AVOID PSYCHOACTIVE DRUGS

In contrast to the strong physical protection that the brain has been endowed with, it is very vulnerable to certain chemical substances that can get to it through the bloodstream by crossing the hematoencephalic barrier, such as ethylic alcohol and other addictive drugs.

AVOID ALCOHOL

Experimental research has definitely shown that alcohol consumption causes neuron death, even in moderate doses.[a] Each drink of alcohol causes irreversible damage in the brain, which is even worse in higher amounts. These days, alcohol consumption is one of the primary causes of neuron deterioration.

Alcoholic beverages can be especially harmful to the brains of children and adolescents, primarily due to the following two reasons:

- Greater sensitivity of the developing brain to neuron toxins like alcohol.
- Difficulty of most young people, especially females, in eliminating alcohol from the bloodstream, due to immaturity of the liver's detoxification systems. Because it takes longer to eliminate it, alcohol continues to cause damage over a longer period of time.

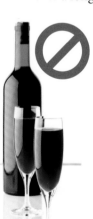

For this reason, the European Charter on Alcohol, adopted by the WHO (World Health Organization) in 2001, says in its third paragraph:

"All children and adolescents have the right to grow up in an environment protected against the negative consequences associated with alcohol consumption and, to the extent possible, from the promotion of alcoholic beverages."[b]

ABSTAIN FROM TOBACCO

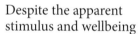

The nicotine in tobacco causes vasoconstriction (narrowing) of the cerebral arteries, which limits blood flow to the brain and the oxygen supply to neurons.

Despite the apparent stimulus and wellbeing produced by tobacco, its true effect on the brain is like a slow, neuron-destroying poison.

Tobacco is a source of free radicals that oxidize and deteriorate neurons. This may be why smokers are more likely to suffer from Alzheimer's disease and other forms of dementia.

ABSTAIN FROM DRUGS

In addition to the legal drugs mentioned, such as alcohol and tobacco, all other drugs also damage the brain. Cocaine, heroin, amphetamines, hash or marijuana, and designer drugs attack neurons directly, and their habitual use causes mental deterioration and dementia.

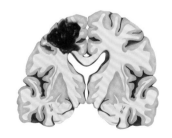

Cocaine Destroys the Brain
Brain bleed caused by cocaine use.

a. Moderate alcohol consumption and loss of cerebellar Purkinje cells. Karhunen PJ, Erkinjuntti T, Laippala P. BMJ. 1994 Jun 25;308(6945):1663-7. PMID: 8025457

b. http://www.msc.es/ciudadanos/proteccionSalud/adolescencia/alcohol/declaEsto.htm

Avoid Coffee and Other Caffeinated Beverages

Although in low doses caffeine seems to improve attention and fight feelings of fatigue, it causes nervousness and anxiety in higher doses. Caffeine induces the release of adrenaline at nerve endings between neurons (synapses). The repeated stimulus caused by adrenaline overloads the nervous system and weakens its reaction to stress.

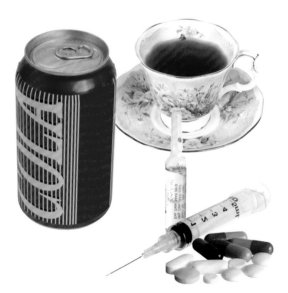

Careful with Hidden Caffeine
Soft drinks, some weight-loss products, tea (primarily black tea) and some medications can contain significant amounts of caffeine.

Unwanted Effects on the Brain from Habitual Use of Caffeine:

- Addiction: Caffeine is really an addictive and psychoactive drug that alters normal brain function. Stopping its use causes true withdrawal symptoms similar to those caused by nicotine or other drugs.

- It narrows the arteries of the brain (vasoconstrictive effect), which reduces blood flow and oxygen supply to neurons. The consequence of this is reduced oxygenation of the brain and reduced intellectual performance, despite the subjective sensation of greater activity.

- Promotes insomnia.[c]

- Promotes hyperactivity and restlessness in children.

- It causes a predisposition to depression, panic attacks and other psychiatric disorders.[d,e] Caffeine intake is especially harmful for psychiatric patients.[f]

Potentially Beneficial Effects of Coffee on the Brain:

A study done with laboratory mice has shown that moderate quantities of coffee over the years can help prevent Alzheimer's disease.[g] Others discuss a protective effect against Parkinson's disease, although reality demonstrates that when a Parkinson's patient drinks coffee, trembling and balance become worse.

The possible neuroprotective effects of coffee only apply to Alzheimer's and Parkinson's diseases in research animals. Despite this, there is controversy over its practical validity, and the researchers themselves advise caution when recommending coffee for prevention of these two diseases.[h]

On the other hand, the human experience shows that coffee intake changes circulation in cerebral arteries, in addition to causing other negative effects for the heart, pancreas, bones and other body parts. For example, people with high blood pressure who drink 3 or more cups of coffee per day have over twice the risk of suffering cerebral thrombosis or embolism.[i]

Due to all of this, the potential neuroprotective benefits of coffee do not make up for its negative effects in no way justify recommendation of their use.

c. A translational, caffeine-induced model of onset insomnia in rats and healthy volunteers. Paterson LM, Wilson SJ, Nutt DJ, Hutson PH, Ivarsson M. Psychopharmacology (Berl). 2007 May;191(4):943-50. Epub 2007 Jan 16. PMID: 17225163

d. Caffeine intake, toxicity and dependence and lifetime risk for psychiatric and substance use disorders: an epidemiologic and co-twin control analysis. Kendler KS, Myers J, O Gardner C. Psychol Med. 2006 Dec;36(12):1717-25. Epub 2006 Aug 8. PMID: 16893482

e. Caffeine challenge in patients with panic disorder: baseline differences between those who panic and those who do not. Masdrakis VG, Papakostas YG, Vaidakis N, Papageorgiou C, Pehlivanidis A. Depress Anxiety. 2007 Apr 10; [Epub ahead of print] PMID: 17427182

f. Caffeine and its effect on persons with mental disorders. Simmons DH. Arch Psychiatr Nurs. 1996 Apr;10(2):116-22. Review. PMID: 8935988

g. Caffeine protects Alzheimer's mice against cognitive impairment and reduces brain beta-amyloid production. Arendash GW, Schleif W, Rezai-Zadeh K, Jackson EK, Zacharia LC, Cracchiolo JR, Shippy D, Tan J. Neuroscience. 2006 Nov 3;142(4):941-52. Epub 2006 Aug 28. PMID: 16938404

h. The neuroprotective effects of caffeine: a prospective population study (the Three City Study). Ritchie K, Carriere I, de Mendonca A, Portet F, Dartigues JF, Rouaud O, Barberger-Gateau P, Ancelin ML. Neurology. 2007 Aug 7;69(6):536-45. PMID: 17679672

i. Coffee consumption in hypertensive men in older middle-age and the risk of stroke: the Honolulu Heart Program. Hakim AA, Ross GW, Curb JD, Rodriguez BL, Burchfiel CM, Sharp DS, Yano K, Abbott RD. J Clin Epidemiol. 1998 Jun;51(6):487-94. PMID: 9635997

CHEMICAL PROTECTION FOR THE BRAIN - 2

AVOID NEUROTOXIC PLANTS

There are plants used as food in different parts of the world that can be toxic to the brain.

Habitual consumption of certain plant foods can damage neurons and cause serious brain injury, leading to paralysis or intellectual deterioration. This is because these plants contain neurotoxins.

In some cases, proper processing of these plants allows elimination of their neurotoxins, but this does not always happen in developing countries.

GRASS PEA (*LATHYRUS SATIVUS*)

A seed that is similar to peas, used in Africa and Asia for its nutritional value. In southern Europe, it was used during times of famine. In its raw state, it contains a neurotoxin that causes paralysis and several nerve disorders. Soaking and proper cooking destroy this toxin. Therefore, well soaked and cooked, it's no problem to use grass peas.

CASSAVA OR MANIOC (*MANIHOT ESCULENTA*)

Cassava is more drought-resistant than the sweet variety that is usually grown, but it contains much more cyanide. This toxin degenerates the brain's motor neurons. To eliminate cyanide, cassava must be properly processed by soaking and toasting.

Habitual consumption of improperly processed cassava or manioc causes an incurable leg paralysis called "konzo" in the Congo.

QUEEN SAGO (*CYCAS CIRCINALIS*)

The seeds from this palm-like tree are used for flour on the islands of Guam, Rota and Marianas in the western Pacific. However, they contain a neurotoxin that causes motor neuron degeneration of the brain and of the spinal cord. This degeneration can manifest in one of the following ways:

- As amyotrophic lateral sclerosis (generalized muscle weakness).[a]
- As Parkinson's disease accompanied by dementia.

It is known that Chamorro natives of the western Pacific often suffer from these neurodegenerative diseases, traditionally attributed to the consumption of the flour of the queen sago. However, research by the National Institute of Neurological Disorders (Maryland, United States) has shown that the manner in which Chamorro women prepare the queen sago seed flour by washing it with water eliminates 87% of the toxin. This makes it unlikely that the degenerative diseases of the Chamorro are due to the consumption of queen sago flour.

It is currently thought that the cause of degenerative disease on the Pacific islands is the consumption of little red flying foxes (*Pteropus scapulatus*). These animals are a kind of fruit-feeding bats that eat queen sago seeds, and concentrate the neurotoxin in their flesh.

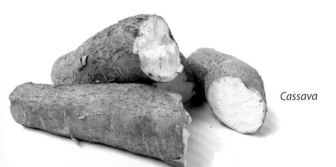

Cassava

---

a. Guam amyotrophic lateral sclerosis-parkinsonism-dementia linked to a plant excitant neurotoxin. Spencer PS, Nunn PB, Hugon J, Ludolph AC, Ross SM, Roy DN, Robertson RC. Science. 1987 Jul 31;237(4814):517-22. PMID: 3603037

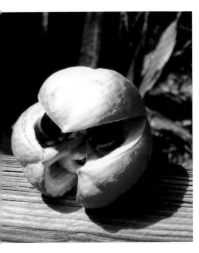

**Ripe,
Opened Ackee Fruit**
Ackee is the national tree of Jamaica. Its ripe and opened fruit is used in traditional dishes, but the unripened fruits (unopened) are toxic to the brain.

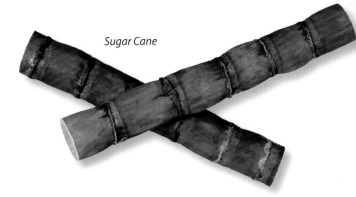

Sugar Cane

UNRIPENED ACKEE FRUIT (BLIGHIA SAPIDA)

Ackee is the national fruit of Jamaica. Its edible part is the aril or fleshy area surrounding its seeds. Ripe ackee is a good source of vitamins and antioxidants.

However, when the fruit is unripened and still closed, all of it, including the aril, contains toxins. Upon ripening, the fruit opens spontaneously and these toxins disappear. Then, the aril acquires the consistency of a fried egg, and can now be eaten. Several typical Jamaican dishes as well as a very nutritious oil are made with it.

Eating unripened (unopened) ackee fruits, also called vegetable brains, cause the Jamaican vomiting sickness. These unripened or closed fruits are flavorful, but contain a toxic amino acid that causes vomiting, extreme thirst, altered mental state, and seizures. Eating unopened ackee fruit can cause coma and even death.

First Aid in Case of Accidental Poisoning from Unripened Ackee Fruit:

Vegetable carbon is the best remedy for poisoning from unripened ackee fruit, since it keeps the poison in the digestive tract without allowing it to get into the bloodstream. It is best to use it within 30 minutes of eating the fruit. The recommended dosage for adults is 50-100 g (15-30 g for children).

MOLDY SUGAR CANE

The fungus *Arthrinium,* responsible for the production of mold on sugar cane, produces nitropropionic acid, a neurotoxic mycotoxin. Eating moldy sugar cane causes a comatose state that could last from 7-40 days. The coma resolves spontaneously, but leaves permanent effects, such as spasmodic movements in the limbs.

GUANABANA LEAVES (ANNONA MURICATA)

Several decades ago, researchers noticed an increased number of Parkinson's-like cases among the inhabitants of the island of Guadalupe, in the Antilles. It was suspected that this special type of Parkinson's, called Guadeloupean parkinsonism, must be caused by a habit that was particular to the inhabitants of the island, and it has been proven that it is the consumption of guanabana leaf infusions and infusions from other plants of the *Annonaceae* family.

These leaves contain annonacin, a neurotoxic alkaloid that causes degeneration of the neurons in dark matter and of other basal ganglia in the brain. It seems there is a hereditary predisposition to suffer this brain degeneration. After stopping consumption of guanabana leaf infusions, there is some improvement.

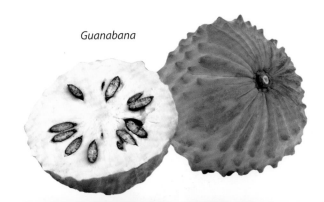

Guanabana

CHEMICAL PROTECTION FOR THE BRAIN - 3

AVOID FREE RADICALS

Free radicals are the primary chemical threat to the brain. Alzheimer's disease, premature aging, and other forms of brain degeneration are caused by these aggressive molecules.

Free radicals are oxidizing molecules that lack electrons. In order to become stable, free radicals steal electrons from other molecules, causing their oxidation.

Free radicals can also be called waste products or toxins. Many of them are produced in the body itself, especially in the brain, causing oxidation and deterioration of many molecules that are important to cells, such as proteins, the lipids that make up the cell membrane and DNA itself (deoxyribonucleic acid, the backbone of heredity).

HOW FREE RADICALS ARE PRODUCED

Free radicals are produced as a result of several circumstances –some avoidable, others unavoidable:

- **Unavoidable Circumstances**:
  – The metabolic activity of the cells themselves, and particularly of the neurons, the cells that consume the most oxygen out of the entire body, along with those of the liver. As a result of the intense chemical and electrical work of the brain, aggressive and unstable molecules are produced, e.g., free radicals

- **Avoidable Circumstances**: Abnormal situations that increase the production of free radicals in the brain.
  – Poor blood supply due to partial, or sometimes total, blockage of cerebral arteries.
  – Consumption of toxic substances such as alcohol, tobacco and other drugs.
  – Consumption of chemical pollutants in air, water, and food.
  – Infections in any part of the body.
  – Exposure to ionizing radiation.

EFFECTS OF FREE RADICALS

Generally, throughout the body

- Functional deterioration.
- Premature aging.
- Cancerous mutations.

On the brain

The brain is the organ in the body where the most oxidation occurs, and where the most free radicals are produced.

In addition, the brain is the organ where free radicals cause the most damage:

- Deterioration of intellectual and motor functions.
- Premature aging.
- Neurodegenerative diseases such as Alzheimer's and Parkinson's.

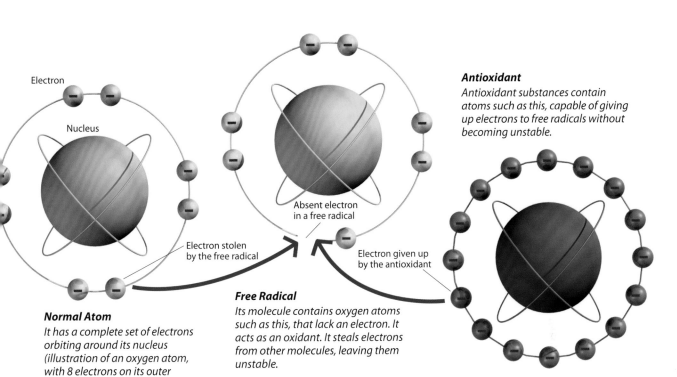

Electron

Nucleus

Antioxidant
Antioxidant substances contain atoms such as this, capable of giving up electrons to free radicals without becoming unstable.

Electron stolen by the free radical

Absent electron in a free radical

Electron given up by the antioxidant

Normal Atom
It has a complete set of electrons orbiting around its nucleus (illustration of an oxygen atom, with 8 electrons on its outer layer).

Free Radical
Its molecule contains oxygen atoms such as this, that lack an electron. It acts as an oxidant. It steals electrons from other molecules, leaving them unstable.

Heavy Metals that Affect the Brain

Heavy metals act as free radicals and build up in the body, especially in the brain, causing neuron degeneration and altered mental functions.[a] Avoiding becoming contaminated by these metals is essential to good brain function.

Neurotoxic Heavy Metal	Effects	Foods or Products with the Highest Amount
Lead	• Children under 2 who suffer from lead poisoning lose 5-7 IQ points. • Lead causes irreversible mental retardation and behavioral disorders. • In adults, it is associated with Parkinson's disease and amyotrophic lateral sclerosis.	• Chemical products used in the glass, paint, welding, and ceramics industries. • Glazed clay dishes (do not use for cooking). • Vegetables grown near roadways and exposed to exhaust vapors.
Mercury (in the form of metylmercury, the most toxic)	• Prenatal exposure, even low doses, causes irreversible brain damage in the fetus. • In adults, it is associated with neurodegenerative diseases, such as Parkinson's and amyotrophic lateral sclerosis.	• Large predatory fish, such as swordfish and tuna. • Shellfish.
Aluminum	• Consumption is associated with Alzheimer's disease and other forms of dementia.	• Tap water in certain geographic areas. • Home kidney dialysis machines. • Certain antiperspirants and deodorants.

a. Effects of metals on the nervous system of humans and animals. Carpenter DO. Int J Occup Med Environ Health. 2001;14(3):209-18. PMID: 11834461

CHEMICAL PROTECTION FOR THE BRAIN - 4

ANTIOXIDANTS AGAINST FREE RADICALS

Toxic free radicals that cause brain damage can easily be neutralized with the antioxidants present in plants.

PROTECTION AGAINST FREE RADICALS

Antioxidants are molecules that are capable of neutralizing free radicals, giving them the electrons that they demand. When they give up electrons, antioxidants go through a process of oxidation.

Unlike other molecules, antioxidants do not become unstable from oxidation and giving up electrons. However, they lose the ability to neutralize more free radicals, which is the reason they must be replaced. This is one of the reasons we should consume antioxidants every day.

Endogenous Antioxidants

The brain has been given a natural system of protection against free radicals. This physiological defense is made up of endogenous antioxidants produced by the neurons themselves. Were it not for them, neurons would become old in just a few years.

The main endogenous antioxidants produced by neurons and other cells are:

• Glutathione.
• Certain enzymes such as catalase and the superoxide dismutase.

Exogeneous Antioxidants

Exogeneous antioxidants are obtained from foods and medicinal herbs. They must be consumed daily, since antioxidants produced by the cells themselves are not enough to neutralize all of the free radicals produced.

The main exogenous antioxidants are:

• Vitamin C.
• Vitamin E.
• Flavonoids.
• Carotenoids, like beta carotene (provitamin A).
• Garlic allicin.
• Other phytochemicals produced by vegetable foods and medicinal herbs.

Fortunately, fruits and vegetables, as well as legumes, grains, nuts, seeds, and certain medicinal herbs provide the antioxidants needed by the brain.

BALANCE BETWEEN FREE RADICALS AND ANTIOXIDANTS

When the number of free radicals is greater than the number of antioxidants, neurons are subjected to an oxidative stress due to excess oxidation.

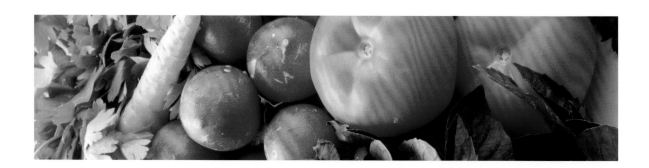

In this situation, neurons can degenerate, giving rise to a loss of intellectual power, cognitive deterioration and diseases such as Alzheimer's or Parkinson's.

The conditions of modern life, worsened by artificial foods and chemical contamination, promote imbalance in favor of free radicals.

Foods and supplements high in antioxidants can help restore the needed balance in the brain, before it is too late and the neurons go through degenerative processes such as those occuring with Alzheimer's and Parkinson's.

VITAMIN C: THE MAIN ANTIOXIDANT FOR THE BRAIN

Vitamin C, which humans can only get naturally through foods (other animals can synthesize it in their bodies), is the main antioxidant for the brain.

It has been shown that the nerve tissue has a greater concentration of vitamin C than all of the other body tissues. That is, a good amount of the vitamin C consumed each day goes to the brain to protect neurons against free radicals.

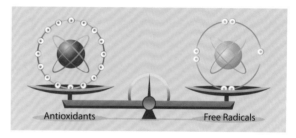

Balance
There are enough antioxidants to neutralize the free radicals.

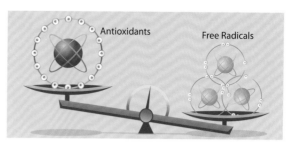

Oxidative Stress
Free radicals are predominant, due to insufficient numbers of antioxidants. As a result, degenerative diseases, premature aging and cancer ensue.

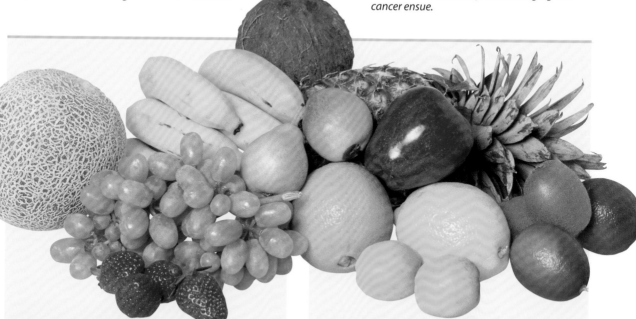

How to Get Antioxidants

Colored fruits and vegetables are the best dietary source of antioxidants. The more intense the color, the greater the antioxidant effect.

The Brain: Threatened

More than any other organ in the body, the brain is threatened by the oxidant effect of free radicals. And more than any other organ, it needs to be protected by consuming antioxidants.

MICROBIOLOGICAL PROTECTION FOR THE BRAIN - 1

MENINGITIS PREVENTION

Meningitis is inflammation of the meninges, coverings surrounding the brain. It may be caused by viruses, bacteria or fungi. Prevention is based on basic standards of hygiene.

Viral meningitis usually resolves without consequences to the brain.

Bacterial meningitis can cause permanent brain damage, and even death, so it is very important to know how it can be prevented. The most frequent repercussions of bacterial meningitis are:

- Neurological disability, which can range from learning difficulties to mental retardation.
- Movement disorders in the arms and legs.
- Vision and hearing disorders.

Meningitis, whether caused by viruses or bacteria, is transmitted primarily through saliva.

Meningitis prevention includes reinforcing basic standards of hygiene, especially among children and adolescents.

Healthy Carriers

Meningococci may be present in the throat or nose of many people, without causing any symptoms. It is estimated that 20% of the population in countries where meningococcal infections are common, are healthy carriers of meningococci.

Meningococci carriers are immune to those germs, but people who come into contact with them are not, especially children and adolescents.

FREQUENT HANDWASHING

The hands are the primary vehicle for spreading germs. The most significant and effective hygiene measure for a meningitis outbreak is simply handwashing.

AVOID THE EXCHANGE OF SALIVA

To prevent meningitis and other infectious diseases, children especially must be taught to avoid gestures or actions involving an exchange of saliva with others, for example: sharing cups, bottles, cutlery, drinking straws, toothbrushes, lipsticks or wind musical instruments.

AVOID CROWDS

Avoid crowds such as those common to public transportation, parties and nightclubs.

AVOID NIGHTCLUBS

Nightclubs are places where the risk of transmission is high, because of their many risk factors, such as shown in the attached illustration.

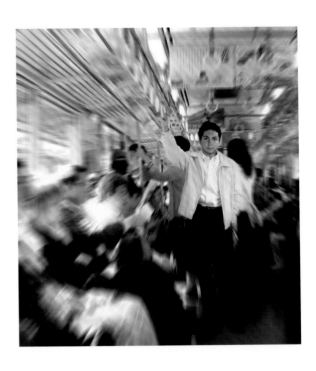

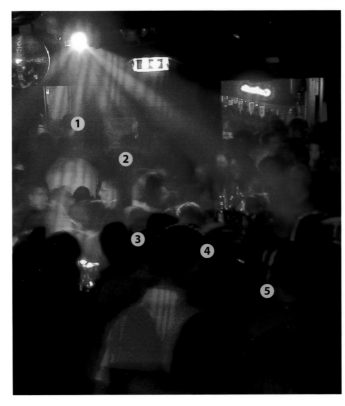

Nightclub Risk Factors

(1) Tobacco smoke irritates the mucosa of the throat and nose, making them more sensitive to bacteria such as the meningococci.

(2) Loud music and environmental noise force loud speaking, thereby increasing the release of potentially contaminated saliva droplets.

(3) Close contact among large numbers of people increases the likelihood of transmission.

(4) Mouth-kissing is a very efficient way to transmit the meningococci and other infectious agents.

(4) Mouth-kissing is a very efficient way to transmit the meningococci and other infectious agents.

ANTIMICROBIAL PROPHYLAXIS

When a child is sick with bacterial meningitis, antibiotics should be given (rifampicin, cephalosporins or ciprofloxacin) to all contacts over the last 7 days, primarily:

- Classmates, especially if they are preschool children in childcare facilities.
- Family members and caregivers of the sick child who could likely be in contact with his saliva.

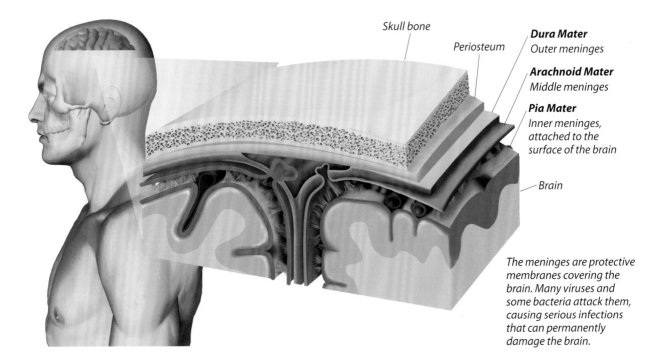

Skull bone

Periosteum

Dura Mater
Outer meninges

Arachnoid Mater
Middle meninges

Pia Mater
Inner meninges, attached to the surface of the brain

Brain

The meninges are protective membranes covering the brain. Many viruses and some bacteria attack them, causing serious infections that can permanently damage the brain.

MICROBIOLOGICAL PROTECTION FOR THE BRAIN - 2

ENCEPHALITIS PREVENTION

Encephalitis is the inflammation of the encephalus, the main part of the brain. Prevention includes avoiding bites from animals, mosquitoes and ticks.

AVOID CONTACT WITH WILD ANIMALS

Currently, most cases of rabies in humans occur due to a bite or even contact with wild animals.

All wild mammals, especially skunks, raccoons, foxes, coyotes and bats, can be carriers of the rabies virus. The symptoms occur 10-40 days after the bite or contact.

A rabies vaccine given to the person who has been bitten is effective if administered within 48 hours after it occurs. It must be given to any person who has suffered any of the following by an animal not vaccinated against rabies, even if it appears healthy:

• Bite
• Scratch or swipe
• Licking of an open wound that was already present.

If a pet or domestic animal that is not vaccinated against rabies is bitten by a wild animal, it is recommended that it be euthanized immediately in a veterinary office.

AVOID MOSQUITO AND TICK BITES

Throughout the world, mosquitoes and ticks are the primary transmitters of encephalitis. See how to protect against them in the next unit.

Encephalitis

Encephalitis is a serious inflammation of the brain, often caused by viruses or protozoa. It manifests itself through fevers, severe headaches, seizures, and mental confusion that can even lead to coma.

In most cases, encephalitis resolves satisfactorily, although full recovery is slow (up to several months). However, in children and people who are weak, it can leave permanent effects of delay or mental slowness and paralysis.

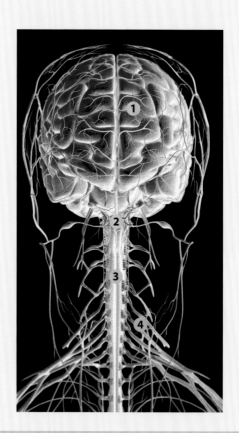

(1) Encephalus
(2) Brainstem
(3) Spinal Cord
(4) Spinal Nerves

Main Types of Encephalitis

Infectious Agent	Manner of Transmission	Type of Encephalitis	Areas of the World Affected	Symptoms
Virus	Mammal bites	Rabies	Cold and mild regions worldwide	Fever, headache, paralysis, and muscle spasms, difficulty swallowing.
	Mosquito bites	Japanese encephalitis	Japan and Southeast Asia	Fever, headache, seizures and confusion. In adults, it usually resolves without consequences for the brain.
		Equine encephalitis, St. Louis encephalitis and California encephalitis	North America	
		Venezuelan equine encephalitis	Central and South America, especially during the rainy season	
		Rocio virus encephalitis	Brazil	
		West Nile Virus and Rift valley fever.	Africa and the Middle East	
		Australian encephalitis	Australia and New Guinea	
	Tick bites	Russian spring-summer encephalitis or Taiga encephalitis	Russia and Siberia	
		Central European encephalitis	Central Europe	
Protozoa	Mosquito bites	Cerebral malaria	Tropical and subtropical areas of Central and South America, Africa, the Middle East, Southern Asia and Oceania.	Severe form of malaria caused by the protozoa Plasmodium falciparum. Attacks the brain and can be deadly.
		African trypanosomiasis or sleeping sickness	Savannas of Uganda, Kenya and Tanzania.	Brain damage occurs between one month and one year after the mosquito bite.

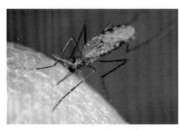

Mosquito "Anopheles gambiae", which most frequently transmits malaria.

The rabies virus climbs via the peripheral nerves from the place of the bite to the brain, where it causes severe encephalitis which destroys neurons.
Rabies transmitted by wild animals continues to be a threat to the integrity of the brain in rural areas of warm and cold regions around the world.

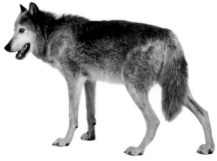

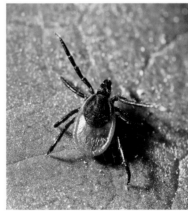

The tick "Ixodes ricinus", which causes Central European encephalitis.

MICROBIOLOGICAL PROTECTION FOR THE BRAIN - 3

AVOID MOSQUITOES AND TICKS

Mosquitoes and ticks are the primary transmitters of viruses and protozoa that are harmful to the brain.

A simple mosquito or tick bite, especially in certain areas of the world, can transmit viruses or protozoa that are harmful to the brain. Many kinds of encephalitis (inflammation of the brain) are the result of a mosquito or tick bite.

Encephalitis symptoms usually appear between 3 and 15 days after a mosquito or tick bite.

Travelers in tropical or subtropical areas inhabited by mosquitoes are at a greater risk of encephalitis than the native population, because they usually lack defenses against the viruses and protozoa that cause encephalitis. Therefore, they must take strict precautions against mosquitoes and ticks.

PROTECTION AGAINST MOSQUITOES

- Do not go out at night.
- Do not stay outdoors between dusk and dawn, which is when mosquitoes are most active.
- Wear appropriate clothing.
- When outdoors, wear clothing that covers the most skin possible, wearing long sleeves and pants, as well as a hat or cap.
- Use mosquito nets.
- Place a mosquito net on baby strollers.
- Place mosquito nets on the windows and doors of the house.
- Spray clothing with insect repellent.
  - It is important to apply repellents like permethrin on clothing, since mosquitoes can bite through woven fabrics.

- Spray especially under the openings of shirtsleeves and pant legs, since this is where insects try to enter.
- Use insect repellents on exposed skin: Skin not covered by clothing, such as the face and hands, should be sprayed with insect repellent.

HERBAL INSECT REPELLENT FOR EXTERNAL USE

These herbal repellents can be used on clothing or on the skin.

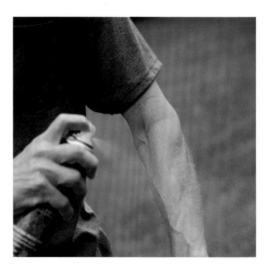

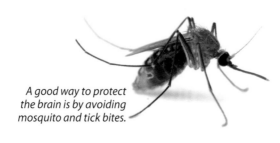

A good way to protect the brain is by avoiding mosquito and tick bites.

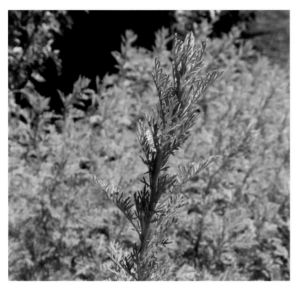

Ajenjo

- Citronella grass oil (*Cymbopogon nardus*), a plant native to Sri Lanka, India, and Indonesia, extending to tropical regions of Asia and Africa.
- Tea tree oil (*Melaleuca alternifolia*), which is also antimicrobial and soothing to the skin.
- Clove essential oil (*Eugenia caryophyllata*).
- Infusion with 10-20 g of Wormwood leaves (*Artemisia absinthium*) per liter of water.
- Chinaberry (*Melia azedarach*): A tree native to India. Its seeds, bark and leaves are an effective insecticide, pesticide, insect repellent, and antiparasitic.

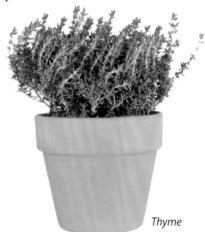

- Pyretrines extracted from the Chrysanthemum (*Chrysanthemum cinerariaefolium*).
- Orange, lemon, or other citrus peel extracts.
- Essences from aromatic herbs such as common thyme (*Thymus vulgaris*), Pennyroyal (*Mentha pulegium*) or lemon balm (*Melissa officinalis*). The essence of eucalyptus (*Eucalyptus globulus*) is also a good repellent.

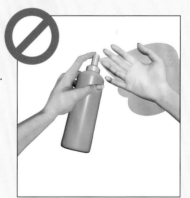

Thyme

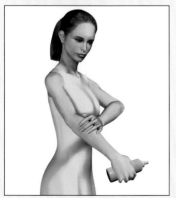

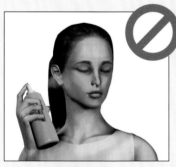

Chemical Repellent DEET

DEET (N, N-Diethyl-3-methylbenzamide, formerly called diethyl-methyl-toluamide) is one of the safest repellents. Even so, certain precautions must be taken:

- It can cause an allergic reaction in sensitive people.
- Do not apply to wounds or irritated areas of the skin, as it can get into the bloodstream and be toxic to the nervous system.
- Avoid contact with the eyes, lips, anus and the mucosa of the genitals, as it causes irritation.
- Do not apply on children's hands, so they do not later touch their eyes or mouth.
- Wash hands after applying.

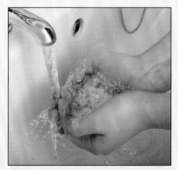

FOOD FOR THE BRAIN

The quality as well as the quantity of food eaten have a decisive influence on brain function.

DIET RICH IN ANTIOXIDANTS

Due to its high oxygen consumption and the hard work it carries out, free radicals accumulate in the brain's neurons. If these free radicals not are properly neutralized with antioxidants, degenerative diseases such as Alzheimer's or Parkinson's occur.

Beta-carotene, vitamins C and E, and plant pigments such as anthocyanins and chlorophyll are powerful antioxidants that protect neurons, neutralizing the free radicals that damage them (see "Chemical Protection for the Brain - 4").

It has been shown that the more antioxidants in the blood, the better the memory. (see " Memory Improvement").

Blueberries, blackberries, black currants, strawberries, and black olives are rich in anthocyanins, plant pigments that have an antioxidant action.

The foods and plants shown on the following pages should not be missing from the diet of those wishing to take great care of the brain.

The antioxidants that protect the brain are mainly found in fresh fruits and vegetables, as well as in seeds and nuts.

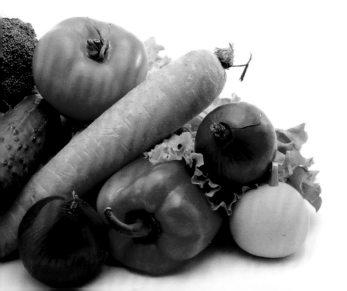

AVOID OVEREATING

Overeating attracts blood to the stomach and other digestive organs, reducing the blood supply available to the brain. After a large meal, brain performance decreases.

EAT HEALTHY FATS

The brain needs healthy fats, as it has a high proportion of this nutrient, greater than that of any other organ. The following foods are good sources of healthy fat for the brain:

- **Virgin Olive Oil**: Regular consumption protects against deterioration of the memory and other cognitive functions.[a]

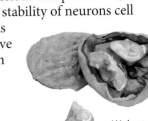

Olive oil

- **Walnuts**: A good source of alpha-linolenic acid or ALA (an essential omega-3 fatty acid, precursor to long-chain fatty acids such as in fish), phosphorus, lecithin, vitamins B_1 and B_6, as well as trace elements. This makes walnuts an ideal food to promote proper neuron function, and thereby strengthen the memory.

- **Almonds**: Rich in vitamin E, phospholipids and calcium, magnesium and potassium, which promote the stability of neurons cell membranes. Thanks to this, almonds have a favorable effect on memory.

Walnut

---

a. High monounsaturated fatty acids intake protects against age-related cognitive decline. V. Solfrizzi, MD, F. Panza, MD, F. Torres, MD, F. Mastroianni, MD, A. Del Parigi, MD, A. Venezia, MD and A. Capurso, MD Neurology 1999;52:1563. PMID: 10331679

- **Flaxseed**: Very rich in alpha-linolenic acid (ALA), necessary for brain development, especially in children.

Conversely, animal fats promote deposits of fats and cholesterol in cerebral arteries. Habitual consumption is a risk factor for age-related memory loss, vascular dementia and Alzheimer's disease.

AVOID CERTAIN FOOD ADDITIVES

There are certain additives, especially artificial dyes and sweeteners, that can alter brain function in sensitive people. See "Mind and Behavior-Altering Products".

BE SURE TO GET ENOUGH IODINE

Iodine is a necessary mineral for brain development during childhood. Children with a diet low in iodine have a low IQ.

It has been shown that pregnant women who consume low amounts of iodine give birth to babies with decreased brain development.

Iodine content in food varies widely and depends on the area where it is produced. It is generally low in the inland regions and higher on the coast.

In reality, iodine is necessary for the brain, even before birth.

Safe Ways to Increase Iodine Intake

- Consume iodized salt or unrefined sea salt.
- Take a daily supplement of 200 µg (micrograms) of iodine in the form of potassium iodide tablets. This is recommended for all pregnant women living in inland areas, where there may be a lack of iodine in food.

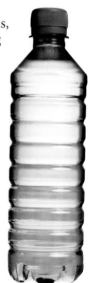

Salt

- Eat edible seaweed such as kelp.
- Fish from the ocean are also a good source of iodine. However, due to their high mercury content as a result of increasing sea pollution in recent decades, health authorities in many countries recommend that pregnant women limit fish consumption. Mercury is toxic to the brain of the fetus and the child, and counteracts the positive effects of iodine from fish.

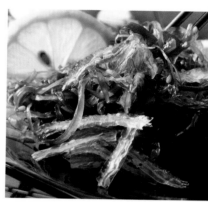

Seaweed

DRINK DISTILLED WATER

A study done in Germany shows that drinking water can contain a high aluminum concentration due to the acid rain effect and treatment of water with aluminum salts.[b]

In places where water contains more aluminum and other metals, there is a greater risk of suffering such neurodegenerative diseases as Alzheimer's, Parkinson's and amyotrophic lateral sclerosis.

Water distillation through evaporation and, later, condensation, eliminates the metals and pesticides that it may contain.

Drinking distilled water promotes the elimination of aluminum and other toxic metals in our blood and tissues.

b. High aluminum concentrations in well water of southern Lower Saxony sandy soil areas caused by acid precipitation: evaluation from the public health and ecologic viewpoint. Muhlenberg, W. Offentliche Gesundheitswesen, 1990; 52:1-8. PMID: 2138268

NEUROPROTECTORS

Neuroprotectors are antioxidant substances that protect the brain and the rest of the nervous system from the wear and tear that it is continuously subjected to as a result of its intense metabolic activity.

Taking good care of the brain today is more possible than ever, thanks to neuroprotective foods and plants confirmed by science. The best source of Neuroprotectors are plant foods in their natural state or minimally processed, and certain medicinal herbs such as *Ginkgo biloba*.

Recent research confirms that neuroprotective foods and plants are good for:

• Preventing the development of degenerative brain diseases such as Parkinson's, Alzheimer's, multiple sclerosis and dementia.

• Improving intellectual performance and mental stability.

• Stopping the aging of the brain.

The foods and plants with the best neuroprotective effect on the following pages have been the subject of scientific research. It is very likely that there are other neuroprotective foods and plants, but these are only the most effective among them, according to the latest research.

STOP THE AGING OF THE BRAIN

Throughout life, the brain accumulates "insults" or attacks caused by free radicals against their precious cells, the neurons. Some of these attacks are voluntary, and therefore, preventable. However, others come with age, and are inevitable.

Unlike most of the body's cells, neurons cannot reproduce like can, for example, skin after a wound or injury. In other words, when a neuron becomes degenerated or damaged, there is no replacement for it. Therefore, each neuron lost results in a small decrease in a person's cognitive (alertness), intellectual, sensory or motor functions.

It is estimated that each day, adults lose a few thousand neurons, which will never be replaced. This amount is normal, falling within physiological

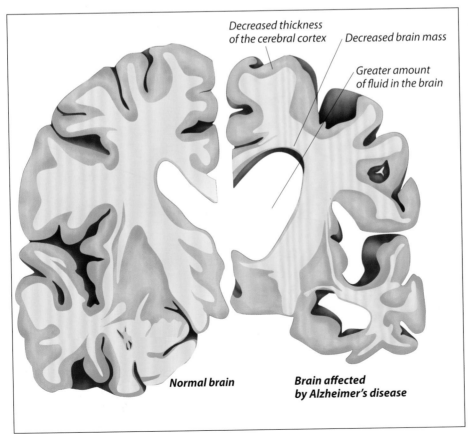

Decreased thickness of the cerebral cortex

Decreased brain mass

Greater amount of fluid in the brain

Normal brain

Brain affected by Alzheimer's disease

limits, and relatively small as compared to the 20 billion neurons making up the brain.

However, alcohol, psychoactive drugs, mercury, and other heavy metal contaminants, poor nutrition, and circulatory disorders, cause the loss of very high numbers of neurons, in the millions or even billions.

Fortunately, neuroprotective foods and plants are able to:

- Protect the brain's neurons against the attacks they suffer throughout life.
- Minimize the consequences of acute attacks, such as lack of blood supply due to blockage of a cerebral artery (cerebral thrombosis and embolism).
- Reduce the number of neurons lost each day.
- Stop the aging of the brain.

Pioneers of the Neuroprotective Effect of Plants

IN THE 6TH CENTURY, B.C.

Taking a closer look at the neuroprotective and antioxidant effect of flavonoids and other plant pigments that give color to fruits and vegetables; seeing that that the tocotrienols in vegetable oils and whole grains protect neurons against toxins; or knowing the beneficial effects of plant foods on brain function and intellectual performance, the experience of 4 young Hebrews in the 6th Century B.C. comes to mind, as told in the Book of Daniel.[a] Those young men were found to be the most intelligent in the Kingdom, after having chosen a diet without meat or wine.

One might say that the story of Daniel and his three companions was the first experiment about the neuroprotective effect of plants. Over 2,500 years ago, in the Court of the King of Babylon, it was shown a diet based on plants and water, promotes proper brain function.

IN THE 19TH CENTURY

In the second half of the 19th Century, when scientists did not discuss free radicals or antioxidants, and when the effect of flavonoids on neurons was unknown, a health food pioneer mentioned the beneficial effect of plants on intellectual functions residing in the brain: "Grains, fruits, nuts, and vegetables constitute the diet chosen for us by our Creator. These foods, prepared in as simple and natural a manner as possible, are the most healthful and nourishing. They impart strength, a power of endurance, and vigor of intellect that are not afforded by a more complex and stimulating diet."[b]

Modern science confirms the boldness of these pioneers of healthy eating who, without the benefit of scientific data, dared to affirm neuroprotective effect of fruits, vegetables and other plants.

---

b. White, Ellen. *The Ministry of Healing*, p. 296. PPPA.

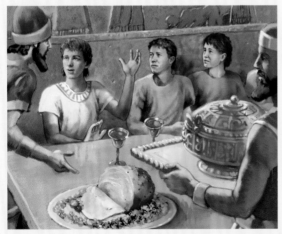

Daniel and his three companions in Babylon.

---

a. Daniel 1:8-20

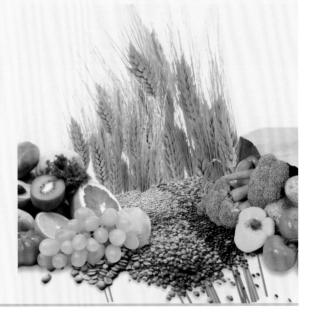

NEUROPROTECTIVE FOODS AND PLANTS - 1

*Garlic, berries such as blueberries and other woodland fruits
and seeds like sesame are effective neuroprotectors.*

GARLIC

Studies with aged garlic extrac (Kyolic®), which has even greater antioxidant power than raw garlic, have shown that consuming it on a regular basis reduces the risk of dementia and stops cognitive or intellectual deterioration that comes with aging.[a]

This favorable effect of garlic on brain function is explained by the following effects of garlic:

- It improves cerebral circulation, increasing blood flow to the brain.

- It reduces the level of cholesterol and prevents its oxidation and deposit on arterial walls.

- It increases the level of natural antioxidants in the cells, such as the superoxide dismutase, catalase and glutathione.

- It protects neurons from oxidative stress and inflammation, destroying free radicals (aggressive molecules).

- It stops cell aging, thanks to its powerful antioxidant action.

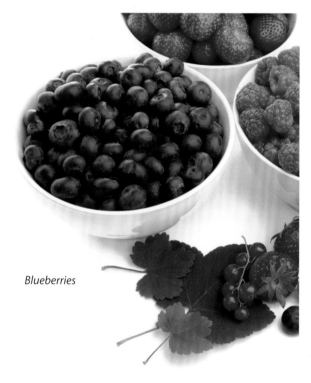

Blueberries

To keep the brain young and intellectually in shape, eat garlic each day in the form of extracts such as Kyolic® (aged garlic extract), or have it raw.

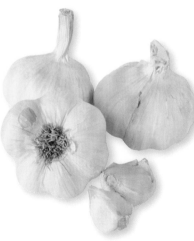

BLUEBERRIES

Blueberries owe their intense bluish color to a high concentration of anthocyanidins, a type of flavonoid.

Among all fruits with flavonoids, all of which have an antioxidant and neuroprotective effect, blueberries are studied the most. According to the research available to date, blueberries are the fruit that most protect neurons. It has been shown that research animals (mice) fed with a blueberry-rich diet:

- Were better able to withstand the effects of stress on neurons, after 10 weeks of adding blueberries to their diet.[b]

a. Garlic reduces dementia and heart-disease risk. Borek C. J Nutr. 2006 Mar;136(3 Suppl):810S-812S. Review. PMID: 16484570

b. Blueberry supplemented diet reverses age-related decline in hippocampal HSP70 neuroprotection. Galli RL, Bielinski DF, Szprengiel A, Shukitt-Hale B, Joseph JA. Neurobiol Aging. 2006 Feb;27(2):344-50. PMID: 15869824

- Were better able to withstand the loss of blood flow to the brain: The animals that consumed a diet supplemented with blueberries for 6 weeks lost 17% of their neurons after obstruction of a cerebral artery, while those who ate a normal diet, lost 40%, according to a study conducted by Prince Edward Island University in Canada.[c]

A study by Tufts University in Boston (United States), showed that regular consumption of blueberries and other deep-colored fruits rich in flavonoids, has the following benefits:

- Protects neurons against the decline in cognitive and motor functions that come with aging.
- Improves intellectual or cognitive function.
- Reduces the negative consequences of Parkinson's, Alzheimer's and other degenerative diseases on brain function.

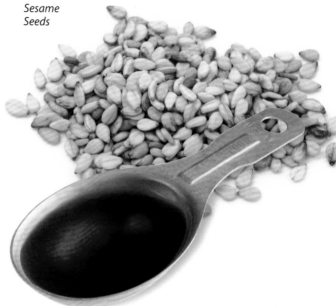

Sesame Seeds

These beneficial effects of blueberries are due to the antioxidant, anti-inflammatory and neuroprotective effects of the flavonoids that give them their typical bluish color.

SESAME SEED OIL

Sesame is an effective neuroprotector and antioxidant, as well as an excellent source of iron, calcium, and other minerals.

Experiments with laboratory mice show that sesame seed oil accelerates the recovery of damaged parts of the brain having suffered ischemia (lack of blood) due to artery blockage.[d]

Therefore, sesame seeds and their oil are good for those who suffer from poor blood flow to the brain, which usually presents as intellectual impairment and memory loss.

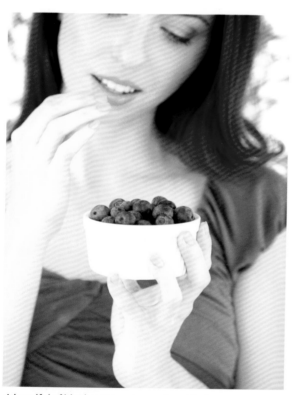

A handful of blueberries or deep colored fruits every day protects the brain and improves intellectual performance.

c. Feeding rats diets enriched in lowbush blueberries for six weeks decreases ischemia-induced brain damage. Sweeney MI, Kalt W, MacKinnon SL, Ashby J, Gottschall-Pass KT. Nutr Neurosci. 2002 Dec;5(6):427-31. PMID: 12509072

d. Effect of dietary sesame oil as antioxidant on brain hippocampus of rat in focal cerebral ischemia. Ahmad S, Yousuf S, Ishrat T, Khan MB, Bhatia K, Fazli IS, Khan JS, Ansari NH, Islam F. Life Sci. 2006 Oct 12;79(20):1921-8. Epub 2006 Jun 17. PMID: 16822528

NEUROPROTECTIVE FOODS AND PLANTS- 2

Regular consumption of deep-colored fruits and vegetables,
such as pomegranate, help prevent Alzheimer's disease.

FRUITS AND VEGETABLES RICH IN FLAVONOIDS

Flavonoids or bioflavonoides are one of the natural pigments present in flowers and fruit, which give them an orange, red, or purple hue. They are also found in a smaller proportion in leaves and seeds. More than 6,000 different types of flavonoids have been identified, all belonging to the chemical family of polyphenols.

Flavonoids are one of the many non-nutritive components of food, called phytochemicals.

Until recently it was thought that flavonoids served only to give plants their hue and make them more attractive to for us and for pollinating insects, which in itself is already very beneficial to health and the balance of nature.

However, in recent decades there has been a flood of research on the healthy properties of flavonoids (antioxidant, anti-inflammatory, anticancer, etc.). These natural pigments have been put in plants for much more than to just attract with their colors.

But polyphenolic flavonoids in fruits and vegetables still have more pleasant surprises in store for us. The most recent to be discovered has been their notable neuroprotective effect.[a] Flavonoids could be called a close friend to neurons, because they protect them from oxidative deterioration caused by their intense metabolic activity, and the free radicals that reach the brain.[b]

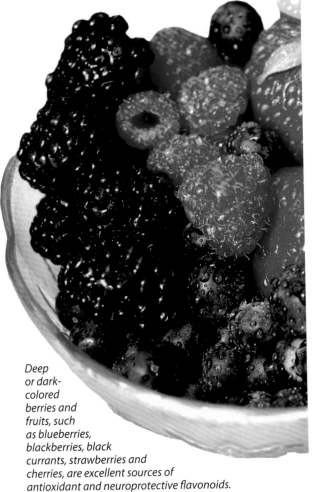

Deep or dark-colored berries and fruits, such as blueberries, blackberries, black currants, strawberries and cherries, are excellent sources of antioxidant and neuroprotective flavonoids.

Organic Is Best

Wild and organically-grown fruits and berries contain up to 30% more antioxidants than from traditional growing, according to the Organic Consumers Association in the United States.[a]

a. http://www.organicconsumers.org/organic/antioxi20205.cfm

a. The beneficial effects of fruit polyphenols on brain aging. Lau FC, Shukitt-Hale B, Joseph JA. Neurobiol Aging. 2005 Dec;26 Suppl 1:128-32. Epub 2005 Sep 27. PMID: 16194581
b. Flavonoids and the aging brain. Schmitt-Schillig S, Schaffer S, Weber CC, Eckert GP, Muller WE. J Physiol Pharmacol. 2005 Mar;56 Suppl 1:23-36. PMID: 15800383 [PubMed - in process]

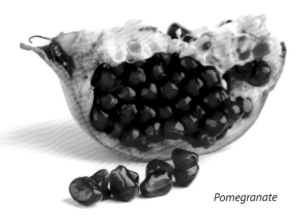

Pomegranate

POMEGRANATE JUICE

Pomegranates (*Punica granatum*) are one of the fruit richest in flavonoids and other antioxidant polyphenols, capable of neutralizing the harmful effects of free radicals. Until now, only the cardioprotective and anticancer effects of the pomegranate were known, but a study at Loma Linda University (California, United States) has shown that the pomegranate is also a powerful neuroprotector.[c] There are three notable effects of pomegranate juice:

• Improves cognitive functions of the brain and learning ability.

• Reduces by half the amount of beta-amyloid, the toxic substance that accumulates in the neurons in Alzheimer's disease.

• Protects the newborn's brain against the lack of oxygen, which can occur in difficult births, resulting in serious neurological repercussions for life. This neuroprotective effect for newborns is achieved when pregnant women drink pomegranate juice during the last trimester of pregnancy. Animal experiments at the University of Washington, (Seattle, United States), confirm this neuroprotective effect.[d]

How to Use

Drink a glass of pomegranate juice each day to stop aging of the brain and reduce the risk of developing Alzheimer's disease.

Pregnant women can drink between a half and a full glass of pomegranate juice to protect her future newborn's brain, especially during the third trimester of pregnancy.

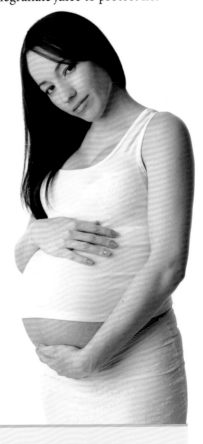

c. Hartman RE, Shah A, Fagan AM, Schwetye KE, Parsadanian M, Schulman RN, Finn MB, Holtzman DM. Pomegranate juice decreases amyloid load and improves behavior in a mouse model of Alzheimer's disease. Neurobiol Dis. 2006 Dec;24(3):506-15. Epub 2006 Sep 28. PMID: 17010630

d. Maternal dietary supplementation with pomegranate juice is neuroprotective in an animal model of neonatal hypoxic-ischemic brain injury. Loren DJ, Seeram NP, Schulman RN, Holtzman DM. Pediatr Res. 2005 Jun;57(6):858-64. Epub 2005 Mar 17. PMID: 15774834

Pomegranate Juice to Fight Alzheimer's

Pomegranate juice not only protects the adult brain against the deterioration associated with aging and against Alzheimer's disease, but it also protects the newborn brain when taken by pregnant women.

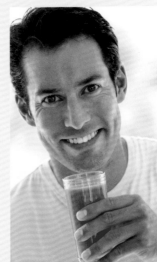

NEUROPROTECTIVE FOODS AND PLANTS - 3

*Grape seeds increase production of antioxidants in neurons,
and the leaves of the Ginkgo biloba tree improve blood flow to the brain.*

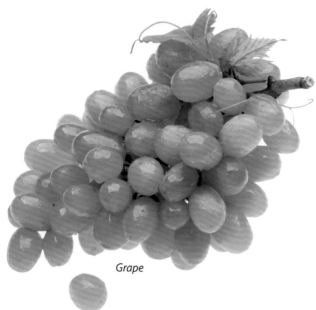

Grape

GRAPE SEED EXTRACT

Grape seeds (*Vitis vinifera*), especially the red or black varieties, have a high concentration of antioxidant substances. The most notable, due to the many studies that have been done on them, are the Oligomeric proanthocyanidins, or OPCs, which come from the chemical family of polyphenolic flavonoids.

Research done especially at the University of Madras (India) with research animals, have shown the ability of grape seed extract to increase the level of antioxidant enzymes occurring naturally in neurons, such as superoxide dismutase, catalase and glutathione peroxidase, and the level of other non-enzymatic antioxidants such as Vitamins C and E.[a]

An elevated level of antioxidants in neurons protects against deterioration caused by stress and aging. The action of grape seed extract on neurons is known by researchers as antioxidant rejuvenation.

How to Use
Take 50-200 mg daily in tablets or drops.

GINKGO: A FRIEND TO THE BRAIN

The Ginkgo tree (*Ginkgo biloba*) is a friend to circulation and the brain. It is well known for its ability to promote oxygen and glucose transport to neurons. In this way, ginkgo protects neurons, since, in order to perform their gigantic chemical and electrical work, nerve cells need a constant supply of oxygen and glucose.

Studies done at the State University of Maringa, (Parana, Brazil) show that research animals that suffer a stroke are better at regaining their cognitive functions (alertness) and memory if they receive ginkgo extract after having the stroke.[b]

But ginkgo not only helps when taken after a brain injury in order to minimize its effects, but it also acts as a preventive measure. At the Safarik University in Kosice (Slovak Republic) it was shown that research animals treated for 7 days with ginkgo extract are much better able to withstand ischemia (lack of blood) in the brain, than those left untreated.[c]

These experiments confirm the neuroprotective effect of ginkgo, and support its use both before and after the brain suffers an attack due to a lack of blood flow, neuron degeneration, or some other cause.

a. Rejuvenation of antioxidant system in central nervous system of aged rats by grape seed extract. Balu M, Sangeetha P, Haripriya D, Panneerselvam C. Neurosci Lett. 2005 Aug 5;383(3):295-300. PMID: 15955424

b. Sustained neuroprotection and facilitation of behavioral recovery by the Ginkgo biloba extract, EGb 761, after transient forebrain ischemia in rats. Paganelli RA, Benetoli A, Milani H. Behav Brain Res. 2006 Nov 1;174(1):70-7. Epub 2006 Aug 24. PMID: 16934342

c. Mapping of rat hippocampal neurons with NeuN after ischemia/ reperfusion and Ginkgo biloba extract (EGb 761) pretreatment. Domorakova I, Burda J, Mechirova E, Ferikova M. Cell Mol Neurobiol. 2006 Oct-Nov;26(7-8):1193-204. Epub 2006 Jun 7. PMID: 16758319

OTHER NEUROPROTECTORS

- **Spinach and Spirulina**: Along with blueberries, they promote recovery of the damaged parts of the brain in research animals.[d]

- **Grapes**, including the peel: Protect neurons against lack of blood supply.[e]

- **Mangosteen** *(Garcinia mangostana)*: From the bark of this Asian fruit comes a watery extract that has a neuroprotective effect against the oxidative deterioration of neurons, according to what was shown in research animals at the University of Silpakorn (Thailand).[f]

- **White Mulberry Leaves** *(Morus alba)*: In China and Korea, this infusion is used for its antidiabetic and antioxidant effects. White mulberry leaves are the preferred food for silkworms, but they are also nutritious and medicinal for humans. A study by the University of Kyunghee (South Korea) showed that white mulberry leaves protect neurons against ischemia (lack of blood supply) in the brain.[g]

- **Mango Leaves and Bark** *(Mangifera indica)*: From these comes mangiferin, a polyphenolic flavonoid that has a strong antioxidant and neuroprotective effect.[h] In Cuba, an antioxidant extract called Vimang is produced from mango bark.

Ginkgo biloba

d. Dietary supplementation with blueberries, spinach, or spirulina reduces ischemic brain damage. Wang Y, Chang CF, Chou J, Chen HL, Deng X, Harvey BK, Cadet JL, Bickford PC. Exp Neurol. 2005 May;193(1):75-84. PMID: 15817266

e. Dietary grape supplement ameliorates cerebral ischemia-induced neuronal death in gerbils. Wang Q, Simonyi A, Li W, Sisk BA, Miller RL, Macdonald RS, Lubahn DE, Sun GY, Sun AY. Mol Nutr Food Res. 2005 May;49(5):443-51. PMID: 15830335

f. Antioxidative and neuroprotective activities of extracts from the fruit hull of mangosteen (Garcinia mangostana Linn.). Weecharangsan W, Opanasopit P, Sukma M, Ngawhirunpat T, Sotanaphun U, Siripong P. Med Princ Pract. 2006;15(4):281-7. PMID: 16763395

g. Enhancement of neuroprotection of mulberry leaves (Morus alba L.) prepared by the anaerobic treatment against ischemic damage. Kang TH, Oh HR, Jung SM, Ryu JH, Park MW, Park YK, Kim SY. Biol Pharm Bull. 2006 Feb;29(2):270-4. PMID: 16462030

h. Neuroprotection by two polyphenols following excitotoxicity and experimental ischemia. Gottlieb M, Leal-Campanario R, Campos-Esparza MR, Sánchez-Gómez MV, Alberdi E, Arranz A, Delgado-García JM, Gruart A, Matute C. Neurobiol Dis. 2006 Aug;23(2):374-86. Epub 2006 Jun 27. PMID: 16806951

NEUROPROTECTIVE FOODS AND PLANTS - 4

Palm and coconut oils have been called unhealthy due to their high proportion of saturated fat acids. However, along with the bran from grains, they are one of the primary sources of tocotrienol, a form of vitamin E, a powerful antioxidant and neuroprotector.

OILS RICH IN TOCOTRIENOL, THE NEW VITAMIN E

Recent studies have found a new form of vitamin E, called tocotrienol, in certain foods. Chemically, it is an unsaturated vitamin E, with four known varieties: alpha, beta, gamma and delta tocotrienol.

All of the varieties of vitamin E are essential to brain function. The best known variety, called alpha-tocopherol, is found in oleosome seeds and fruits, such as soy, corn, olive, avocado, and almond. But tocotrienol is found in other foods, such as palm oil, coconuts, and the bran in grains. Studies at Ohio State University Medical Center (Ohio, United States) have shown the antioxidant and neuroprotective effects of tocotrienol, which is able to protect neurons against a variety of toxins, that is much greater than the effect of the known varieties of vitamin E, such as tocopherols.[a]

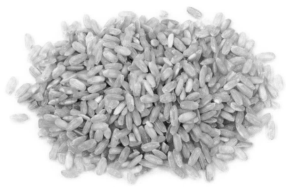

Palm Oil

Coconut Oil

a. Tocotrienol: the natural vitamin E to defend the nervous system? Sen CK, Khanna S, Roy S. Ann N Y Acad Sci. 2004 Dec;1031:127-42. Review. PMID: 15753140

After a stroke in a research animal, the administration of tocotrienol reduces brain damage and protects neurons against oxygen deficiency.[b]

Products Rich in Tocotrienol

- Palm Oil: This oil has lost favor due to its high percentage of saturated fatty acids –the highest of all vegetable oils. However, it is rich in tocotrienol, the neuron protector vitamin E, which makes moderate consumption the most recommended.

- Coconut and coconut oil, have also lost favor due to their saturated fatty acid content. However, it has been shown that the fatty acids in coconut are of a medium-chain type, and do not promote arteriosclerosis, unlike the saturated long-chain fatty acids in meat; plus, coconut contains the neuroprotector tocotrienol.

b. Vitamin E isoforms alpha-tocotrienol and gamma-tocopherol prevent cerebral infarction in mice. Mishima K, Tanaka T, Pu F, Egashira N, Iwasaki K, Hidaka R, Matsunaga K, Takata J, Karube Y, Fujiwara M. Neurosci Lett. 2003 Jan 30;337(1):56-60. PMID: 12524170

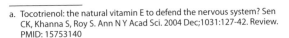

Rice

- Grains such as rice, wheat, barley and oats. The highest content of tocotrienol is in their bran, one reason to prefer whole grains. Tocopherol, the most well-known form of vitamin E, is concentrated in the germ.
- Supplements: The recommended dose is 50-100 mg of tocotrienol per day.

Soy

A study done at the La Fe University Hospital in Valencia (Spain) has shown that with a diet rich in soy, research animals are much better at withstanding the obstruction of a cerebral artery, and their brains are less damaged.[c] This neuroprotective effect of soy is attributed to its isoflavone content. Similar results have been achieved in other studies.

It can be expected that people who consume soy products rich in isoflavones (primarily milk and tofu, but not texturized soy protein) are better prepared to face a reduction in blood flow to the brain. Cerebrovascular accidents (cerebral thrombosis and embolism), and age-related arteriosclerosis, are the primary causes of a reduction in blood flow to the brain.

c. Dietary phytoestrogens improve stroke outcome after transient focal cerebral ischemia in rats. Burguete MC, Torregrosa G, Perez-Asensio FJ, Castello-Ruiz M, Salom JB, Gil JV, Alborch E. Eur J Neurosci. 2006 Feb;23(3):703-10. PMID: 16487152

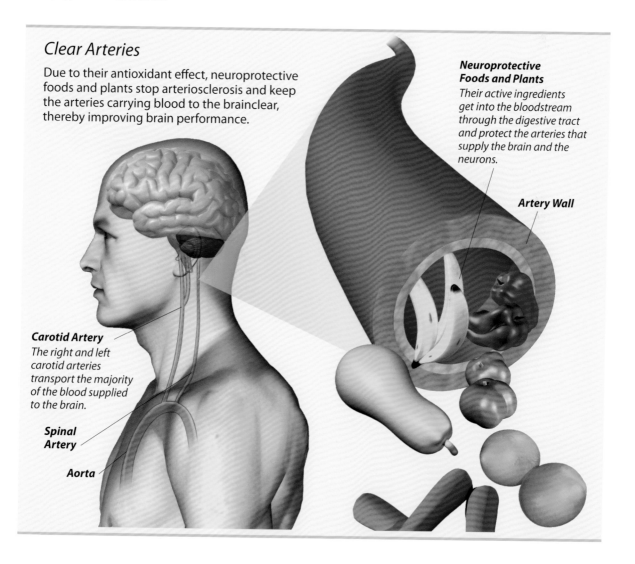

Clear Arteries

Due to their antioxidant effect, neuroprotective foods and plants stop arteriosclerosis and keep the arteries carrying blood to the brainclear, thereby improving brain performance.

Neuroprotective Foods and Plants
Their active ingredients get into the bloodstream through the digestive tract and protect the arteries that supply the brain and the neurons.

Artery Wall

Carotid Artery
The right and left carotid arteries transport the majority of the blood supplied to the brain.

Spinal Artery

Aorta

PSYCHOLOGICAL AND SPIRITUAL CARE FOR THE BRAIN

Complete health also includes psychological and spiritual wellbeing. In order to take good care of the brain, intellectual functions, feelings and spirituality must be nurtured.

AVOID STRESS

In research involving humans, it has been seen that high doses of cortisol can damage the brain and cause deterioration of the memory and other cognitive functions.[a] Cortisol is a hormone produced by the adrenal gland that increases in situations of sustained stress.

To avoid stress and deterioration of brain function, it helps to:

• Live in a calm environment, with little noise.

• Avoid doing too many things at once (for example, watch TV. while eating or holding a conversation).

• Set realistic goals.

KEEP ACTIVE INTELLECTUALLY

It has been shown that people with greater intellectual activity have a greater number of synapses (neuron connections), which helps compensate partially for the cerebral decline that comes with age.

In addition, with greater intellectual activity and level of education, there is less risk of Alzheimer's.

CONTROL WHAT ENTERS THROUGH THE SENSES

The brain continually receives enormous amounts of information by way of the senses –primarily the senses of sight and hearing. All of that information in the form of images and sounds must be processed and made sense of in the brain, leaving a certain mark on the brain, in the form of subtle chemical reactions in the neurons.

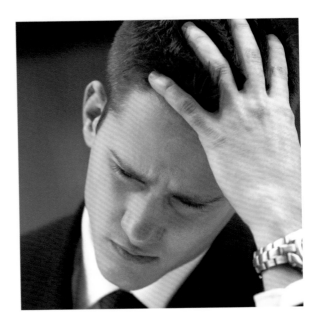

The expression *Garbage in, garbage out* used in reference to computers to explain that when fed incorrect data, they produce incorrect results, can also be applied to the brain. If poor-quality information enters the brain through the senses, it will also produce poor results.

It is known that viewing images of moral depravation and violent scenes cause some type of alteration in the brain, promoting aggressiveness. On the other hand, when the sight spends time viewing positive images, the neurons function better and the mind reaches greater heights.

It is not easy to control the effect produced in the brain by information that comes in through the senses; however, it is possible, and necessary, to control what we allow to come in through our vision, our hearing and through the other senses.

a. Decreased memory performance in healthy humans induced by stress-level cortisol treatment. Newcomer JW, Selke G, Melson AK, Hershey T, Craft S, Richards K, Alderson AL. Arch Gen Psychiatry. 1999 Jun;56(6):527-33. PMID: 10359467

Myelin Sheath
This is an electrical insulator to
the axon. When it deteriorates,
such as in the case of multiple
sclerosis, the transmission of
nerve impulses is much slower.

*Soma
or cell body*

Nucleus

Dendrites
These pick up nerve impulses and
transmit them toward the cell
body, where they are processed
and amplified.

Axon
Transmits nerve impulses,
normally from the cell body to
other neurons.

The Neuron
*The most important type of cell in
the nervous system.*

TAKE CARE OF FEELINGS

Feelings are an important ability of the mind, located in some part of the brain. Every human needs to receive affection as well as give affection, and in doing so, both intellectual and brain performance are improved.

Taking care of affections and correctly directing them is also a way to take care of the brain. The delicate balance of the brain chemistry is altered when affections go unattended or are out of control.

TRUST AND HOPE

Trust and hope stop the decline of cognitive functions of the brain. In some way that science has not yet identified, positive trust and hope strengthen the brain and improve its function. The brain needs to believe and trust, almost as much as it needs oxygen and glucose.

Believers who have an active spiritual life have more opportunities to exercise trust and hope. And their cognitive functions are better preserved than those of non-believers. This is the conclusion of a study done by the University of Texas (United States).[b]

Nurture Spirituality

All humans, whether believers or not, have a spiritual dimension to their lives. Nurturing it is also a way to take care of the brain. Many believers say that studying the sacred texts and meditating on their deep thoughts help keep the mind agile and alert.

b. Religious attendance and cognitive functioning among older Mexican Americans. Hill TD, Burdette AM, Angel JL, Angel RJ. J Gerontol B Psychol Sci Soc Sci. 2006 Jan;61(1):P3-9. PMID: 16399939

NATURAL TREATMENTS FOR THE BRAIN - 1

The brain seems inaccessible, locked in a safe made up of the hard bones of the skull. Nevertheless, it is very sensitive to physical stimuli on the skin, such as heat, cold or pressure.

COMPLETE ROOM TEMPERATURE OR WARM BATH

This is a room temperature or slightly warm bath of the whole body, except the head.

The stimulus of the water on the skin gets to the brain, producing sedation and muscle relaxation.

The sedating effect is greater when the water is room temperature or lukewarm, as compared to when it is very hot.

Effects
• Sedation of the entire nervous system.
• Decrease in muscle tone, relaxation.

Indications
• Insomnia.
• Anxiety.
• Parkinson's disease.
• Brain-based movement disorders (twitches, chorea, ataxia, etc.)
• Paralysis with stiffness or spasticity.

Contraindications
• Cardiac or respiratory failure, because of the overload that hot water produces for the heart and respiratory function.

• Pregnancy, especially during the first trimester, due to the harmful effect of high temperatures for the fetus.

Variations
• In order to increase the sedative effect, add one or two liters of infusion or preparation of one of these plants to the bath:
  – Chamomile (*Matricaria chamomilla*).
  – Lemon balm (*Melissa officinalis*).
  – Lavender (*Lavandula angustifolia*).
  – Valerian Root (*Valeriana officinalis*).
  – You can also add 10-15 drops of essence of lavender or lemon balm.
• Hubbard Tank: This is a bath designed especially for making whole body immersion more comfortable, and is used in hydrotherapy centers. It has a turbine that agitates the water and keeps it at an even temperature.

Water temperature: 34-37ºC (94-98ºF).

Duration: 10-15 minutes.

Afterward: Rub your skin with a cold cloth. Then, rest for half an hour.

Frequency: Once or twice daily.

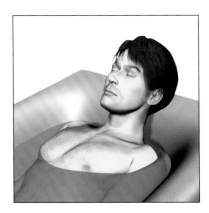

1. Submerge the entire body in the water, up to the neck.

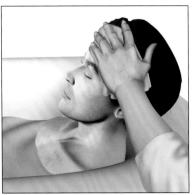

2. Refresh the forehead or the entire head with cool compresses if the patient feels congested or has a headache.

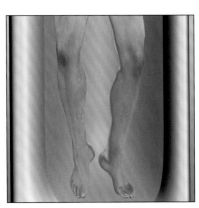

3. Make gentle movements in the water.

HOT PACKS ON THE BACK

Moist heat applied directly to the back has a sedating and relaxing effect that is very useful for a variety of central nervous system disorders.

Effects

• Sedation: Relieves anxiety.
• Promotes sleep.
• Relaxes tense muscles due to stress.

Indications

• Anxiety.
• Insomnia.
• Stress accompanied by muscle tension.

Caution: Be careful not to get burned when wetting the towel as well as when applying it.

Water temperature: As hot as possible; ideally, near-boiling.

Duration: 10-15 minutes. When the moist towel loses its heat (usually within two or three minutes), soak it in hot water again.

Afterward: Dry the skin on your back and cover up with wool blankets.

Frequency: Once or twice daily.

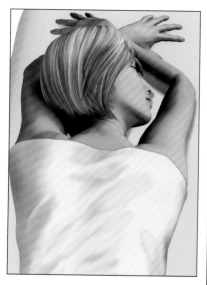

1. Protect the skin with a dry cotton cloth.

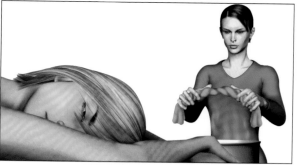

2. Soak and wring out a towel in very hot water.

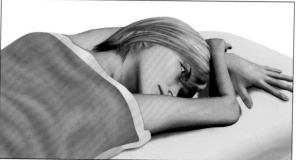

3. Apply the hot towel over the protective dry cloth

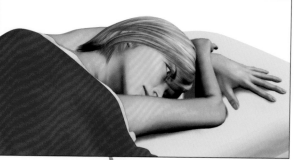

4. Cover these two cloths with a wool blanket. A few minutes later, soak the towel again in hot water and wring it out.

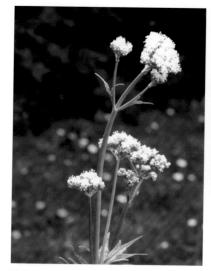

Valerian root

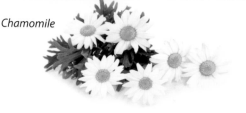

Chamomile

Lavender

NATURAL TREATMENTS FOR THE BRAIN - 2

*Water in the form of baths and rubdowns,
and the sun, have a healing influence on the brain*

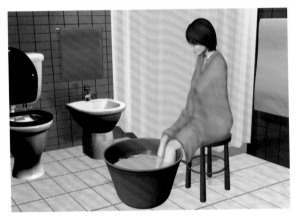

Submerge both legs at the same time to halfway up your calves. Add hot water when the temperature drops.

SOAKING FEET IN HOT WATER

Soaking the feet in hot water is a simple and effective remedy to decongest the brain, relieving heaviness and headaches.

Effects
- Decongestant.
- Sedates and relaxes the entire body, due to the reflex that is produced from the feet on up.

Indications
- Headache.
- Anxiety.
- Insomnia.

Water Temperature: 36-40 °C (97-104 °F).
Duration: 10-15 minutes.
Afterward: Rub your feet with a cloth soaked in cold water and put on wool socks.
Frequency: Up to three times daily.

ICE PACKS TO THE HEAD

Ice packs applied to the head reduce inflammation and congestion of the brain.

Effects
- Decongestant.

Indications
- Stroke: As an emergency treatment, it helps reduce brain temperature and therefore prolongs survival of the neurons that have lost their blood supply.
- Brain hemorrhage due to stroke or brain trauma, to reduce hemorrhage until medical care is provided.

Caution: Always place a towel or cloth over the skin, to protect it from extreme cold.

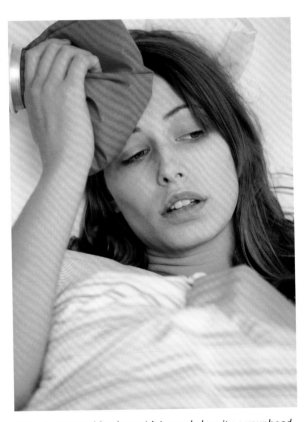

Fill a plastic or rubber bag with ice and place it on your head.

GLOVE RUBDOWN

This achieves an intense toning effect for the nervous system and circulation.

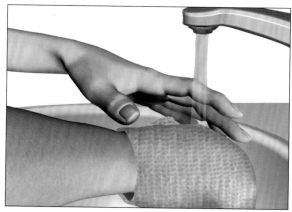

1. Soak a bath glove in cold water; do not wring out.

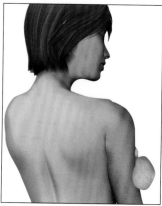

2. Rub vigorously over your skin until it becomes reddened.

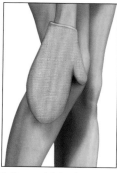

3. Start with both arms, then your thighs and legs, ending with your chest and abdomen.

Effects

- Toner.
- Immunostimulant.
- Increases blood pressure when it is low.

Indications

- Generalized weakness.
- Lack of resistance to infections or cold.
- Depression.
- Hypotension.

Caution: The room should be at a comfortable temperature, and the patient should not feel cold.

SUNBATH

Exposure to sunlight balances the nervous system and activates the metabolism as a whole. The sun causes vitamin D to be synthesized in the skin, which improves calcium absorption.

Effects

- Antidepressant.
- Immunostimulant.
- Mineralizer.
- Antianemic.

Indications

- Depression and asthenia.
- Neurovegetative imbalance.
- Weak defenses.
- Rickets and osteoporosis.
- Anemia.

Caution: Sun exposure should be progressive with regards to both time and the amount of skin surface exposed, with periods of rest in between. It is good to start exposing the feet and legs for 5-10 minutes, and increase the amount of skin exposed and the time each day, until the whole body is exposed (except the head) for two hours after 10 days.

- Always cover your head.
- Use sunscreens for more sensitive areas of your skin, applying them at least half an hour before going into the sun (their effect is not immediate).
- Wear sunglasses.

Contraindications

- Photosensitivity due to taking certain medications, or other causes.
- Skin cancer.

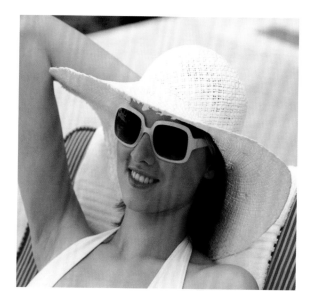

HOW TO IMPROVE YOUR MEMORY - 1

*It has been shown that certain foods
are able to stop age-related memory deterioration.*

Although many people complain about their bad memories, they should be comforted to know that losing a bit of memory can be beneficial. A little forgetting is necessary and healthy. Remembering everything is harmful to mental health, and even to happiness.

FOODS RICH IN VITAMIN E

Wheat germ and its oil, almonds and other nuts, sunflower seeds, and virgin olive oil are some of the foods highest in vitamin E. All of them are as much or more effective than supplements to increase the level of vitamin E in the blood and in the brain, which improves neuron function.

A study done by the University of Indiana (United States), with 4,809 people over the age of 60, showed that the nutrient that most influences the memory is vitamin E. The lower the level of vitamin E in the blood, the more problems there are with memory.[a] The role of vitamin E is explained by keeping in mind that it is a powerful antioxidant that neutralizes the free radicals that damage neurons. In addition, vitamin E promotes the stability of neuron cell membranes, allowing them to better preserve memories.

FOODS RICH IN BETA-CAROTENE

Carrots, mangos, oranges, apricots and squash or zucchini are good sources of beta-carotene. A study done of 5,182 people over 55 by the Erasmus University School of Medicine in Rotterdam (Holland) showed that those who consume less than 0.8 mg of beta-carotene per day have nearly double the risk of suffering memory deterioration, disorientation, and difficulty in problem solving, as compared to those who consume 2.1 mg or more.[b] Consuming

more than 2 mg of beta-carotene per day is not difficult at all, since just 100 grams of carrots (raw or cooked) is already 2.8 mg.

Carrots

FOODS RICH IN VITAMIN C

A study by the University of Bern (Switzerland) shows that people over 65 with high levels of antioxidants such as vitamin C and beta-carotene in the blood, have better memories.[c] Kiwis, citrus fruits, and fruits in general are good sources of vitamin C, and many of them also supply beta-carotene, such as oranges and mangos.

Kiwis and oranges

FRUITS RICH IN ANTHOCYANINS

Blueberries, blackberries, black olives, black currants, and strawberries are rich in anthocyanins, vegetable pigments with a bluish or reddish hue. Anthocyanins are polyphenolic flavonoids

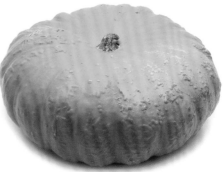

Squash or zucchini, rich in beta-carotene

a. Association of antioxidants with memory in a multiethnic elderly sample using the Third National Health and Nutrition Examination Survey. Perkins AJ, Hendrie HC, Callahan CM, Gao S, Unverzagt FW, Xu Y, Hall KS, Hui SL. Am J Epidemiol. 1999 Jul 1;150(1):37-44. PMID: 10400551

b. Jama JW, Launer LJ, Witteman JC, den Breeijen JH, Breteler MM, Grobbee DE, Hofman A. Dietary antioxidants and cognitive function in a population-based sample of older persons. The Rotterdam Study. Am J Epidemiol. 1996 Aug 1;144(3):275-80. PMID: 8686696

c. Perrig WJ, Perrig P, Stahelin HB. The relation between antioxidants and memory performance in the old and very old. J Am Geriatr Soc. 1997 Jun;45(6):718-24. PMID: 9180666

that have a strong antioxidant action. A study by the University of Barcelona (Spain) with research animals has shown that these vegetable pigments cross the hematoencephalic barrier and get into the neurons, specifically into the parts of the brain related to leaning and memory.[d] In neurons, the anthocyanins of blueberries and other bluish or reddish fruits regenerate the delicate biochemical mechanisms that serve to support memory, thanks to its antioxidant and neuroprotective action.

FOODS WITH LOW GLYCEMIC INDEX CARBOHYDRATES

This group includes muesli and other preparations from whole grains, bananas and tubers such as cassava. Over the period of 3 or 4 hours they take to digest, they provide quite a constant level of glucose in the blood, which improves brain performance.

It is especially beneficial to eat these types of foods for breakfast, in order to avoid the feeling

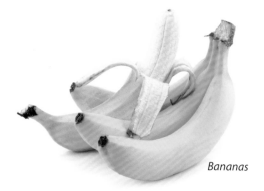

Bananas

of being run-down at midday due to a dip in glucose levels. Low glucose in the brain slows the synthesis of acetylcholine in the neurons, one of the primary neurotransmitters, needed for memory and other cognitive functions.

OMEGA-3 FATTY ACIDS

A study by the University of Siena (Italy) shows that omega-3 supplements taken over 35 days improve attention, memory and intellectual

function in healthy subjects.[e] This effect is due to the fact that these fatty acids promote neuron cell membrane stability and the transmission of nerve impulses over synapses.

The best food sources of omega-3 fatty acids are fish, flaxseed, walnuts and soy.

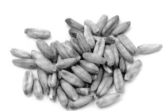

Whole grain wheat

e. Cognitive and physiological effects of Omega-3 polyunsaturated fatty acid supplementation in healthy subjects. Fontani G, Corradeschi F, Felici A, Alfatti F, Migliorini S, Lodi L. Eur J Clin Invest. 2005 Nov;35(11):691-9. PMID: 16269019

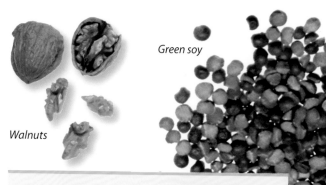

Green soy

Walnuts

Antioxidants Against Alzheimer's

Consuming antioxidants protects against degenerative brain diseases such as Alzheimer's and Parkinson's. But taking them for a short time is not enough –they should be taken over decades.

This is the reason that studies do not find benefits in occasionally taking antioxidant supplements. Rather, following a diet rich in antioxidants for the first five decades of life does indeed prove effective in preventing degenerative brain conditions.

Deep-colored fruits and vegetables, such as cherries, strawberries, pomegranates, blueberries and blackberries, have the most natural antioxidants.

d. Anthocyanins in aged blueberry-fed rats are found centrally and may enhance memory. Andres-Lacueva C, Shukitt-Hale B, Galli RL, Jauregui O, Lamuela-Raventos RM, Joseph JA. Nutr Neurosci. 2005 Apr;8(2):111-20. PMID: 16053243

HOW TO IMPROVE YOUR MEMORY - 2

Healthy habits, medicinal herbs and nutritional supplements,
along with the foods mentioned in the previous unit, improve memory
and the intellectual performance of adolescent students and the elderly.

OXYGEN

Good brain oxygenation is an absolute must for memory preservation. The brain consumes quite a bit of oxygen. Deep breaths of fresh air, aerobic exercise (such as a brisk walk) and a diet low in saturated fat and cholesterol, improve the supply of oxygen to the brain.

REST

Sleeping well for enough hours helps to preserve memory. During sleep periods, neurons are cleansed of the waste products they accumulate during active times, which improves their performance.

Physical or psychological stress and a lack of enough rest deteriorate memory. It is especially

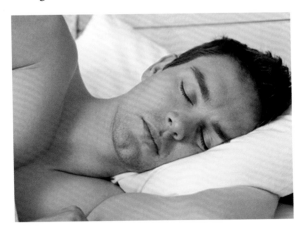

good to avoid the anxiety that comes from trying to do several things at once.

AN ACTIVE MIND

Reading, studying and solving exercises or problems exercise the mind (watching TV does not). It has been seen that intellectual exercise increases the number of interconnections between neurons (synapses), which improves memory capacity.

MEDICINAL HERBS

Ginkgo (Ginkgo biloba)

Improves short-term memory and reduces reaction time for bringing up a memory, thanks to an increase in blood flow to the brain and oxygen supply to neurons.

- How to Use: 120-360 mg of extract daily, divided into two or three doses, over several months.

Ginseng ("Panax ginseng")

Fights fatigue and improves mood, improving brain oxygenation.

- How to Use: 100-250 mg of extract, once or twice daily.

Ginkgo and Ginseng

The best results to fight against memory loss have been achieved through taking ginkgo and ginseng together. This was shown in a study by the University of Northumbria (United Kingdom) with young people who were volunteers to receive 360 mg of ginkgo extract and 400 mg of ginseng extract daily, over a period of 12 weeks.[a]

---

a. Modulation of cognition and mood following administration of single doses of Ginkgo biloba, ginseng, and a ginkgo/ginseng combination to healthy young adults. Kennedy DO, Scholey AB, Wesnes KA. Physiol Behav. 2002 Apr 15;75(5):739-51. PMID: 12020739

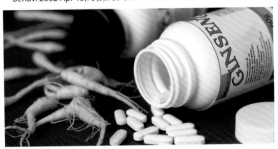

Ginkgo and ginseng extract.

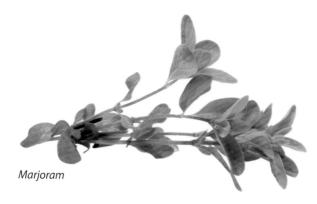

Marjoram

Aromatic Herbs

Many studies have shown that sage (*Salvia officinalis*), marjoram (*Origanum majorana*) and lemon balm (*Melissa officinalis*), improve cognitive function and promote memory. In the treatment of Alzheimer's, high doses of their essences are taken orally (up to 60 drops per day). Sage, marjoram or lemon balm can be taken several ways:

• Infusion: Two or three cups daily.
• Inhalation of the essential oil: Place several drops onto a cloth or the back of your hand several times per day, and inhale deeply.
• Consumption of essential oil: 10-20 drops daily, dissolved in half a glass of water or juice.

Foods Are Better than Supplements

Vitamin E and C supplements have been shown to be effective in improving memory and other cognitive functions (related to alertness). However, the food sources of these vitamins are even better than the supplements, according to a study done by Utah State University (United States).[a]

Regular consumption of foods rich in vitamin E (such as wheat germ, almonds and avocados) and in vitamin C (such as citrus fruits and kiwis) is more effective in memory preservation than supplements of these vitamins.

a. Association of antioxidants with memory in a multiethnic elderly sample using the Third National Health and Nutrition Examination Survey. Perkins AJ, Hendrie HC, Callahan CM, Gao S, Unverzagt FW, Xu Y, Hall KS, Hui SL. Am J Epidemiol. 1999 Jul 1;150(1):37-44. PMID: 10400551

NUTRITIONAL SUPPLEMENTS

Wheat Germ
A good source of B-group vitamins and of essential fatty acids needed for good brain function.

• How to Use: 1-3 tablespoons daily, preferably with breakfast.

Soy Lecithin
This is a good source of choline, a substance from which acetylcholine is produced in the brain. Acetylcholine is a neurotransmitter involved in the biochemical processes of memory.

• How to Use: One or two tablespoons daily.

Vitamin E
Vitamin E supplements have been shown to be effective for improving memory and other cognitive functions in several studies. The broadest study was carried out by Harvard University (United States) with nearly 15,000 women over 70.[b] The best results are obtained by taking 600 mg or more daily of vitamin E over a period of 10 years, along with vitamin C, which strengthens its effect.

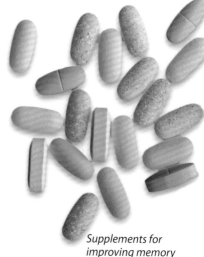

• How to Use: 600-1,000 mg of vitamin E, along with 1,000-1,500 mg of vitamin C daily, spread over two or three doses, preferably with meals.

Supplements for improving memory

Huperzine A
Alkaloid extracted from the Chinese herb *Huperzia serrata*. It improves the level of the neurotransmitter acetylcholine in the brain, and the memory along with it. It is also used in Alzheimer's.

• Dose: 60-200 µg daily, in capsules or tablets.

b. High-dose antioxidant supplements and cognitive function in community-dwelling elderly women. Grodstein F, Chen J, Willett WC. Am J Clin Nutr. 2003 Apr;77(4):975-84. PMID: 12663300

FOODS THAT FIGHT DEPRESSION - 1

Depression comes from a chemical imbalance among neurons.
Good nutrition can contribute to restoring balance.

FOODS RICH IN TRYPTOPHAN

Tryptophan is an essential amino acid that makes up part of the proteins we consume with our food, and which make up the human body.

Tryptophan influences mood because it is a precursor to an important neurotransmitter, serotonin. This is the chemical substance in the brain that is responsible for wellbeing and relaxation.

It is known that the amount of tryptophan in the foods we eat influence serotonin levels in the brain. And with higher levels of serotonin, there is an increased sensation of wellbeing and less risk of depression.

Sources of Tryptophan

Tryptophan is found in many proteins that make up foods. However, in order for tryptophan to be transformed into serotonin, in addition to proteins, you need to consume a large amount of carbohydrates, such as sugars or flours.

Good sources of tryptophan are beans and other legumes, as well as nuts, all eaten along with rice, pasta, bread or crackers, preferably whole grain.

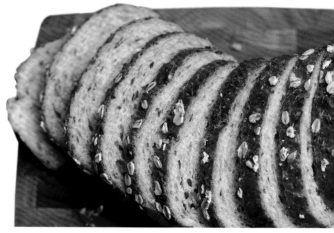

WHOLE GRAINS

Oats, wheat, rice, corn and other whole grains (with their bran and germ) promote good brain function and fight off depression, for the following reasons:

- During their digestion, which takes 3-5 hours, glucose is being released continually. In this way, by eating whole grains you keep a good blood glucose level, without causing surges. The same occurs with other foods that have a low glycemic index, such as legumes and nuts. Because glucose is the primary fuel for neurons, foods that provide a prolonged and relatively constant level of glucose:
  - Promote good brain function.
  - Prevent lightheadedness, such as can happen after a meal high in refined sugar (without fiber).
  - Prevent sudden mood swings.
- They provide B-group vitamins in the grain's germ and bran, which contributes to mental stability.
- They promote serotonin production in the brain, which is the chemical mediator of a good mood.
- They contain medicinal properties with a mild sedating and balancing action for the nervous system, such as the avenine in oats.

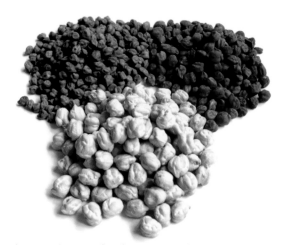

Legumes in general and nuts are good sources of tryptophan. This amino acid converts to serotonin, the chemical mediator in the brain responsible for a good mood.

OMEGA-3 FATTY ACIDS

It has been known for some time that a diet low in omega-3 fatty acids promotes depression. Now, a study by the University of Bristol (United Kingdom) shows a certain antidepressive effect in omega-3 fatty acids, which is even more intense in cases of extreme depression.[a]

The primary omega-3 fatty acid is alpha linolenic acid (ALA), found in plants. In the body, ALA partially converts into long-chain omega-3 fatty acids, called eicosapentaenoic acid, or EPA, and docosahexaenoic acid, or DHA, which are also necessary for brain development.

EPA and DHA omega-3 fatty acids are found in fish oil, but the body can synthesize them from plant alpha linolenic acid (ALA), which is found primarily in flaxseed, walnuts and soy.

The Disadvantages of Fish

Unfortunately, fish has some disadvantages that can counteract its benefits, such as:
- Growing levels of cardiotoxic methylmercury.
- Potential for contamination by parasites, bacteria and toxins.
- Ability to produce allergies.
- Uric acid formation.
- Depletion of marine resources due to overfishing.

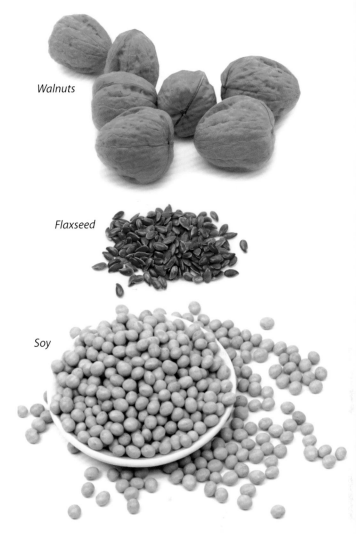

Walnuts

Flaxseed

Soy

Plant sources of omega-3 such as flax, walnuts and soy, are an interesting and healthy alternative to eating fish.

a. Effects of n-3 long-chain polyunsaturated fatty acids on depressed mood: systematic review of published trials. Appleton KM, Hayward RC, Gunnell D, Peters TJ, Rogers PJ, Kessler D, Ness AR. Am J Clin Nutr. 2006 Dec;84(6):1308-16. Review. PMID: 17158410

The Best Plant Sources of Omega-3 Fatty Acids

The daily allowances of the essential fatty acid, alpha linolenic acid 18:3 (known by the initials ALA), the most important omega-3 plant, have been set between 0.9 g for children and 1.6 for adult males. In cases of depression, this amount can be doubled or tripled.

Certain green-leafy vegetables such as corn salad or mâche ("Valerianella locusta") and common purslane ("Portulaca oleracea") also contain a significant, although small, amount of alpha linolenic acid.

Plant Food	Amount that Supplies the Recommended Daily Allowance of Omega-3
Flaxseed	10 g (about a tablespoon of seeds or their oil). The flour from germinated seeds has the advantage that it assimilates better than the seeds.
Walnuts	30 g of shelled walnuts (about 6 walnuts)
Soy	4 servings (one serving is a glass of soy milk, 60 g of tofu or a plate of cooked soy).

FOODS THAT FIGHT DEPRESSION - 2

*Depression is associated with a low level of folates in the bloodstream.
The Mediterranean diet, rich in vegetables, legumes and nuts,
provides large amounts of folates to fight depression.*

THE MEDITERRANEAN DIET

A study by the University of Las Palmas de Gran Canaria (Spain) shows that a Mediterranean diet rich in fruits, nuts, vegetables, legumes and, optionally, fish, prevents depression.[a]

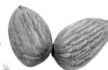

A raw vegetable salad, to which a handful of nuts and a tablespoon of wheat germ can be added, should be part of meals every day for people who want to beat depression.

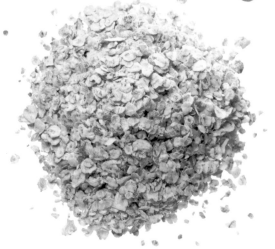

FOLIC ACID AND FOLATES

Folic acid and its salts, known as folates, are vitamins that are essential for the nervous system. Together, they are called folacin or vitamin B_9.

Historically, B-group vitamins have been considered important in the prevention and treatment of depression. However, recent studies have shown that the B vitamin that most influences depression is specifically B_9, or folacin, made up of folic acid and folates.

A meta-analysis (review of a group of studies) done at the University of York (United Kingdom) has confirmed that a low level of folates in the bloodstream is associated with depression.[b] A diet rich in folates, or folate supplements, contributes to the treatment of depression.

Currrently, the lack of folates or vitamin B_9 is one of the most common vitamin deficiencies in industrialized nations. It is not surprising that, therefore, depression is becoming more common. The lack of folates in women who are going to become pregnant causes spina bifida and other nervous system deformities in the fetus, which have permanent effects on children.

---

b. Is low folate a risk factor for depression? A meta-analysis and exploration of heterogeneity. Gilbody S, Lightfoot T, Sheldon T. J Epidemiol Community Health. 2007 Jul;61(7):631-7. PMID: 17568057

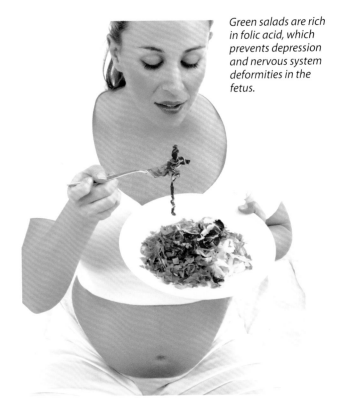

Green salads are rich in folic acid, which prevents depression and nervous system deformities in the fetus.

---

a. Mediterranean diet and depression. Sanchez-Villegas A, Henriquez P, Bes-Rastrollo M, Doreste J. Public Health Nutr. 2006 Dec;9(8A):1104-9. PMID: 17378948

Foods Rich in Folic Acid or Folates

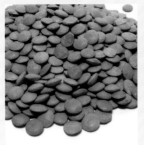

Lentils (433 µg/100 g)

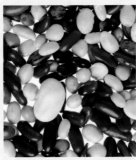

Beans (388 µg/100 g)

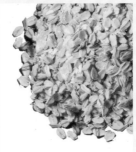

Wheat Germ (281 µg/100 g)

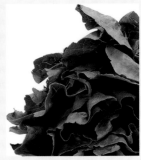

Spinach (194 µg/100 g)

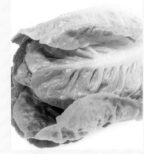

Lettuce (136 µg/100 g)

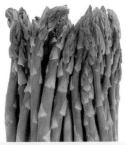

Asparagus (128 µg/100 g)

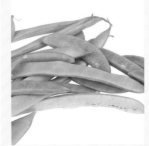

Lima Beans (96 µg/100 g)

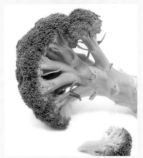

Broccoli (71 µg/100 g)

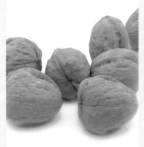

Walnuts (66 µg/100 g)

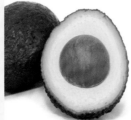

Avocados (62 µg/100 g)

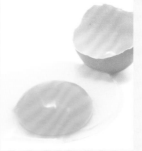

Eggs (47 µg/100 g)

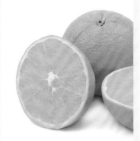

Oranges (30 µg/100 g)

Sources of Folic Acid and Folates

Legumes and vegetables (preferably raw) are the best source of folates, followed by nuts and fresh fruits.

There are also supplements, but it is not advisable to take more than 1 mg daily (= 1,000 µg), since high doses of folates can mask symptoms of possible vitamin B_{12} deficiency.

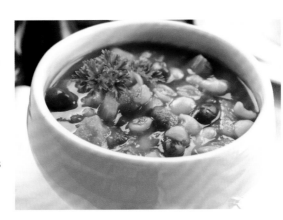

Losses with Cooking

Cooking destroys part of folates. In legumes, over 50% of folates can be lost with cooking. Even so, they are still a good source of folates.

MIND AND BEHAVIOR-ALTERING PRODUCTS

In addition to alcohol and other psychoactive drugs, certain foods eaten regularly can also have a negative effect on behavior, promoting sudden mood swings, anxiety and aggressiveness.

SUGARY PRODUCTS

Neurons need a constant supply of glucose, its primary fuel. If the blood glucose level that gets to the brain is under 80 mg/100 ml, the result is apathy, inability to concentrate, low intellectual performance and even lightheadedness.

Products that are high in refined sugar and low in plant fiber, such as cakes and sweets that have an elevated glycemic index, cause blood glucose levels to spike. This causes an increase in insulin secretion, which causes a sudden drop in blood glucose levels.

These fluctuations in blood glucose level interfere with the proper functioning of neurons, in addition to promoting type 2 diabetes.

Eating sugary products is associated with these mental conditions:
• Sudden mood swings.
• Irritability and anxiety, followed by apathy.
• Hyperactivity.
• Emotional imbalance.
• Aggressiveness and violent behavior.

CERTAIN ADDITIVES

It has been known for some time that food colorings, preservatives and artificial sweeteners can cause hyperactivity and anxiety.

A study done in the United Kingdom confirmed that certain additives that are usually in soft drinks, candies and other sweets, promote these behavioral disturbances, especially among children between the ages of 3 and 9:
• Hyperactivity, manifested by the inability to complete a task or play with a single toy, for example.
• Rowdy behavior.
• Loss of concentration.

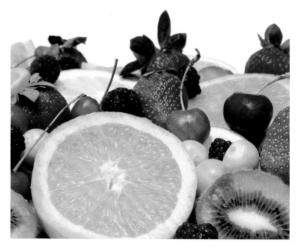

Fresh fruits increase the blood glucose very little (they have a low glycemic index) despite containing quite a bit of sugars. This is due to their fiber content, which regulates glucose absorption.
Although this makes fruits a sugary food, they promote a balanced mood and are well-tolerated by diabetics, unlike refined sugars.

The additives that can most affect the behavior of sensitive people are artificial colors, followed by preservatives, flavorings and some chemically-synthesized sweeteners. The following stand out among them:c
• Tartrazine (E102): A yellow coloring used widely in ice cream, candies, baked goods, cookies, luncheon meats, sausage and preserves. It is used as a substitute for saffron in pre-cooked rice meals.
• Quinoline Yellow (E104): A coloring used mainly in baked goods, cookies, ice cream, soft drinks, plant preserves and processed meats.
• Orange Yellow S (E110): A coloring used mainly in ice cream, candies, cookies, baked goods and orange soft drinks.
• Azorubine (E122): A red coloring used primarily in soft drinks, candies and ice cream.

- Cochineal Red A (E124): Used as a substitute for paprika and also in ice cream, candies, yogurts and processed meats.
- Aspartame (E951): A sweetener widely used in soft drinks, chewing gum and products made without sugar. It can cause anxiety and headache in patients with phenylketonuria and in people who are sensitive to this sweetener.
- Glutamate: A flavor enhancer.

Although the use of all of these additives may be legal, just as tobacco and alcohol are, that does not mean they are harmless. Avoiding them is a good way to protect the brain. These additives must surely cause some change in the subtle and delicate chemical balance of neurons when they cause such behavioral changes.

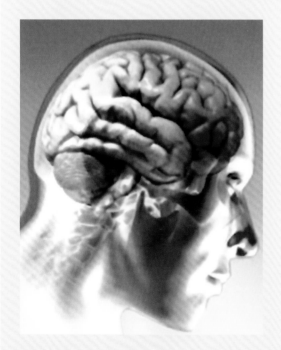

Meat Dulls the Mind

A health educator and writer of the 19th Century said, "Those who use flesh meats freely do not always have an unclouded brain and an active intellect, because the use of the flesh of animals tends to cause a grossness of body and to benumb the finer sensibilities of the mind."[a]

a. White G, Ellen. *Counsels on Health*, p 115.

Unfortunately, the food additives industry is very powerful, and it is not easy to end the use of superfluous and clearly harmful additives like chemical colorings.

PROCESSED AND REFINED PRODUCTS

Regular consumption of fast food, which is high in processed and refined products, and low in natural foods, can alter behavior and promote mental and emotional imbalance.

Nutrition based on meats, pre-packaged and canned goods, which are generally very high in chemical additives, salt, spices and preservatives, also promote nerve disorders.

The troubling effect of this type of nutrition is due to its lack of vitamins, minerals and polyunsaturated fatty acids such as omega-3, all of which are nutrients that are necessary for the nervous system to function well.

MEAT

Some evidence has shown that a diet including meat causes mental imbalance, favoring impulsive behaviors over rational thinking.[a] Meat contains hypoxantine, a stimulant similar to caffeine, and biogenic amines such as histamine and tyramine (especially in cured meats), which cause irritability.

In addition, it is known that fat from meat obstructs cerebral arteries and reduces blood flow to neurons, decreasing intellectual ability. It is also known that the arachidonic acid, a long-chain fatty acid found almost exclusively in meat, worsens the damage caused by ischemia (lack of blood flow) in the brain.[b]

a. Nedley, Neil. *Proof positive*. Neil Nedley, Oklahoma (USA), 1998, pág. 276.
b. Detrimental effects of post-treatment with fatty acids on brain injury in ischemic rats. Yang DY, Pan HC, Yen YJ, Wang CC, Chuang YH, Chen SY, Lin SY, Liao SL, Raung SL, Wu CW, Chou MC, Chiang AN, Chen CJ. Neurotoxicology. 2007 Aug 10; PMID: 17854901

DIET AND AGGRESSIVE BEHAVIOR

There are solid signs that certain food products in the Western diet, associated with a lack of vitamins, minerals and essential fatty acids, promote violent behavior.

The relationship between diet and temper or behavior has been a controversial topic among scientists for centuries, even though it is clearly true according to conventional wisdom. Only in the last few decades have there been studies published that show an objective relationship between what people are and what they eat.

One of the first steps in confirming that certain foods can promote violent behavior was taken at the Wales Swansea University (United Kingdom). There, it was shown that elimination diets, in which certain "suspect" products are omitted, reduce aggressiveness.[a]

As explained in the previous unit, among suspicious products that can promote hyperactivity and even violent behavior, the following stand out:
• Certain artificial additives (primarily food colorings).
• Industrially processed foods.
• Refined sugars.
• Meats.

If the elimination of a product from the diet is capable of reducing a person's aggressiveness, the relationship between diet and violence is confirmed. Although more research is still needed, what is already known would be enough to at least help stop the increase in violence and aggressiveness in the world.

HYPOGLYCEMIA

Studies by the University of Helsinki show that aggressive people are more tolerant to glucose, and suffer reactive hypoglycemia after eating sugars. In addition, they have lower serotonin levels in the brain.[b] Both conditions are favored by the consumption of alcoholic beverages.

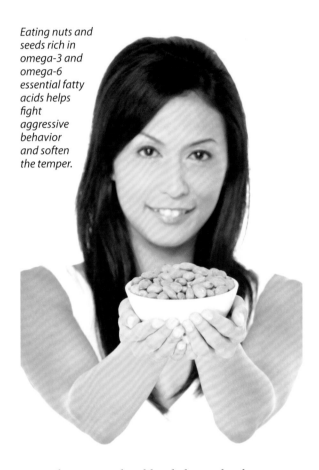

Eating nuts and seeds rich in omega-3 and omega-6 essential fatty acids helps fight aggressive behavior and soften the temper.

Hypoglycemia, or low blood glucose level, can present itself as a reaction after eating goods high in refined sugars and low in fiber, such as sweets, cakes and candies. It has been seen that certain people are more susceptible to the increase in glucose level caused by sweet products, and they react with a sharper decrease. These fluctuations in the blood glucose level promote aggressive behavior.

According to these studies, people who have a tendency toward aggressiveness or violent behavior should:
• Avoid especially the combination of refined sugars and alcohol.

• Increase foods rich in tryptophan in the diet, as it is a precursor to serotonin (see "Foods that Fight Depression").

a. The impact of diet on anti-social, violent and criminal behaviour. Benton D. Neurosci Biobehav Rev. 2007;31(5):752-74. Epub 2007 Mar 4. Review. PMID: 17433442
b. Low brain serotonin turnover rate (low CSF 5-HIAA) and impulsive violence. Virkkunen M, Goldman D, Nielsen DA, Linnoila M. J Psychiatry Neurosci. 1995 Jul;20(4):271-5. Review. PMID: 7544158

LACK OF VITAMINS AND MINERALS

One of the most revealing studies was done by Oxford University with jail inmates in the United Kingdom. They were given vitamin, mineral, and essential fatty acid supplements for at least two weeks, and committed 35% fewer infractions or crimes than the other prison inmates.[c]

Researchers of this study concluded that a diet that lacks vitamins, minerals and essential fatty acids, such as fast food, promotes antisocial and violent behavior.

Another study done by the California State University (United States) with young people from 13 to 26 years of age, who were in correctional facilities, confirms that a balanced diet in accordance with recommendations of the WHO, and rich in vitamins and minerals reduces the number of cases of antisocial behavior by half.[d]

LACK OF ESSENTIAL FATTY ACIDS

Essential fatty acids are fats that the body cannot produce from other fats, and because of that, they must be taken in with the diet. These essential fats are needed to form neuron membranes. Two types of essential fatty acids are known, both of which are polyunsaturated:

- Omega-3 Fatty Acids: The most important is alpha linolenic acid (18:3), known by initials ALA. Part of the ALA consumed turns into EPA omega-3 fatty acids (eicosapentaenoic acid) and DHA (docosahexaenoic acid) which are necessary for brain development and are present in fish oil. The primary dietary sources of alpha linolenic essential fatty acid (ALA) are:

  – Flaxseed.
  – Walnuts and other nuts.
  – Soy (seeds, oil and soymilk, but not soy protein extracts.
  – Certain leafy vegetables, such as corn salad or mâche *(Valerianella locusta)* and common purslane *(Portulaca oleracea)*.
  – Breastmilk.

- Omega-6 Fatty Acids: The most important is linolenic acid (18:2) which is found in all types of nuts and seeds (sunflower, corn, squash, etc.) and in a lesser amount, in chicken meat.

It is known that a lack of these essential fatty acids, present primarily in nuts, seeds and other plant foods, promotes aggressive and violent behavior. The lack of omega-3 fatty acid promotes depression (see the units "Foods that Fight Depression").

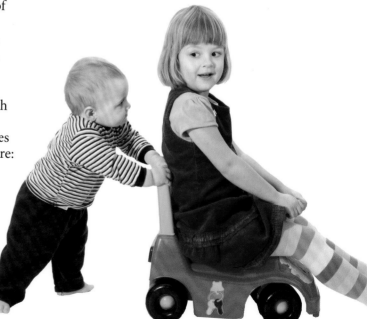

c. Influence of supplementary vitamins, minerals and essential fatty acids on the antisocial behaviour of young adult prisoners. Randomised, placebo-controlled trial. Gesch CB, Hammond SM, Hampson SE, Eves A, Crowder MJ. Br J Psychiatry. 2002 Jul;181:22-8. PMID: 12091259

d. The effect of vitamin-mineral supplementation on juvenile delinquency among American schoolchildren: a randomized, double-blind placebo-controlled trial. Schoenthaler SJ, Bier ID. J Altern Complement Med. 2000 Feb;6(1):7-17. PMID: 10706231

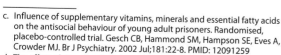

Antidepressants and other psychodrugs are being prescribed more and more, especially to hyperactive children. A proper diet could avoid many of these medications.

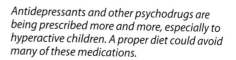

MEAT-EATING AND VIOLENCE

Meat-eating involves cruel violence against animals.
Could there be a link between increased meat consumption
and the increase in social violence?

Although there is evidence linking frequent meat consumption with behavior disturbances and, particularly, with aggressiveness, scientific research is needed in order to confirm it.

However, seeing the growing violence in so-called developed societies, which affects children, students, couples, adults and even animals, one must wonder if it could be associated with an increase in meat consumption, in addition to what is already known about alcohol consumption, and use of other drugs. Of course, violence has always existed. But what is interesting is that it increases precisely when it is unexpected, within well-educated societies with all needs seemingly met.

One of the principles of epidemiology says that coincidence does not necessarily indicate causation. That is, the fact that there is a parallel in the increase of meat consumption and violence rates does not necessarily indicate that one causes the other. But, in any case, this association proposes an interesting working hypothesis, still awaiting exploration by science.

Even without scientific data, there are events in the history of humanity that support a causative relationship between meat eating and increased violence.

It is said that the gladiators of ancient Rome ate raw meat before going into combat. In the Iliad, Homer tells how the warriors were offered meat-based feasts between one battle and the next. All throughout history, philosophers and moralists have pointed out that certain foods, such as meat and meat products, promote aggressiveness and violent behavior.

In the Book of Genesis, it is said that "the earth was filled with violence"[a]. Jesus himself referred to this fact when he said, "But as the days of Noah were, so also will the coming of the Son of Man be. For as in the days before the flood, they were eating and drinking…"[b] Could the violence of our times be related to abuses in eating and drinking, and the needless torture and murder of millions of creatures every day around the world to turn them into meat? Could we be living today a moral and social degradation such as what occurred in the days of Noah prior to the great flood? If so, according to what many believers understand by this and many other signs, this is the time to prepare for the greatest event in history: the coming of the redeemer Messiah. This preparation must include a change in the ways of living and eating, in order to get them aligned with the ideal as contemplated in the great law of love.

a. Genesis 6:11 (NKJV)
b. Matthew 24: 37-38 (NKJV)

Think of the cruelty to animals that meat eating involves, and its effect on those who inflict and those who behold it. How it destroys the tenderness with which we should regard these creatures of God!

Ellen G White. *Counsels on Diet and Foods*, p. 383

The Peace Diet

ELIMINATE OR DECREASE

- **Alcohol**: Alcoholic beverages, such as beer, wine and spirits, are the primary cause of violent behavior worldwide.
- **Refined sugars**: Eating refined sugars (unaccompanied by fiber) causes drastic fluctuations in blood glucose levels, with sudden increases that can be followed by decreases to below normal levels. Neurons are very sensitive to decreases in blood glucose levels.
- **Additives**: Eating certain additives, especially artificial colorings, can set off hyperactivity and even violent behavior, especially among children and sensitive persons (see "Mind and Behavior-Altering Products").
- **Fast food and processed foods**: These tend to be low in vitamins, minerals and polyunsaturated fatty acids, such as those found in walnuts, seeds and vegetable oils. The lack of these nutrients is associated with antisocial or violent behavior according to many studies. In addition, foods that are processed, canned and contain preservatives, tend to contain chemical additives related to behavior disorders, especially in children.
- **Stimulants**: Cocaine, and to a lesser degree, caffeine, are neuro-stimulants that alter the release of neurotransmitters between neurons and disturb the delicate chemical balance in the brain, which is responsible for mental and emotional stability.
  - In addition, because they are addictive drugs, cocaine as well as caffeine cause a real withdrawal effect when they are stopped.
  - For both reasons, nervous system stimulants promote violent behavior and aggressiveness.

INCREASE

- **Walnuts**: These are rich in tryptophan, a precursor to serotonin, the neurotransmitter for wellbeing. Plus, they are one of the best plant sources of omega-3 polyunsaturated essential fatty acids, such as alpha linolenic acid (ALA). Their phospholipid content also contributes to balance in the nervous system.
- **Other nuts and seeds**: They are all rich in polyunsaturated essential fatty acids, which when lacking promote antisocial and violent behavior.
- **Whole grains**: Thanks to being rich in fiber, the digestion of the starch in grains releases glucose slowly, which prevents drastic fluctuations in blood levels. In addition, their germ is a good source of B vitamins, which are necessary for neuron stability.
- **Fruits and vegetables**: Good sources of vitamins and minerals, which when lacking promote violent behavior.

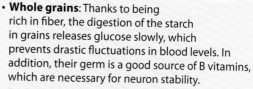
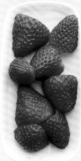
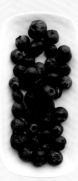
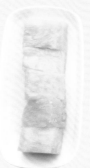

The greatness of a nation and its moral progress can be judged by the way it treats its animals.

Mahatma Gandhi (1869-1948)

WILLPOWER

*Taking care of the brain promotes willpower,
a powerful tool to improve health.*

A VERY HUMAN ABILITY

Of all of the mind's abilities, the ability to make rational decisions and follow through with them is possibly the most specific to humans. Animals can feel, and to some level even think; but their ability to decide what behavior to follow is quite limited or simply does not exist, and it is always conditioned by hereditary behaviors (instincts) and hormones.

On the other hand, the human being has been given the ability to decide freely, above all hereditary, instinctive or hormonal conditioning; and thanks to willpower, decide to follow the most healthful behavior, despite what sounds good or what one likes.

WHAT IS GOOD AND WHAT SOUNDS GOOD

Willpower is the ability to do what is good, which does not always go along with what is desired. Putting this ability in practice, which is necessary to achieve health and true wellbeing, requires primarily a brain that is well oxygenated, nourished, rested and protected, such as what is shown in this chapter.

Thanks to willpower, man regains control over himself, and exercises complete control over body and mind. In this way, and not through the complacency of unhealthy habits, true freedom and happiness are achieved.

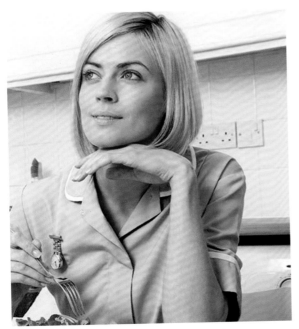

The mind can be defined as the element of a human person that allows him to be conscious of reality, think, feel and choose. The mind is seated in the brain.

Uses for Willpower

Application of Willpower	Example of the Need to Exercise It
To resist hereditary tendencies and desires which are harmful to health.	"My body asks for red meat, but my cardiologist has recommended that I stop it because of my high risk of a heart attack."
To free oneself from being so-called "ruled by hormones".	"The days before my period I feel like I need to eat something sweet, but I'm gaining weight."
To break addictions, whether physical or psychological.	"I can't go without coffee, even though it causes me heartburn."
To break bad habits that are not good for health.	"I feel like plopping onto the couch, but I need to exercise every day."

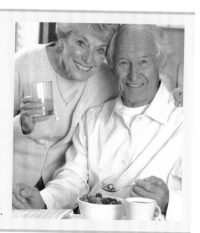

Choose What is Best

In order to make healthy decisions and choose what it is good to drink, eat or do, you often have to exercise willpower against what sounds good.

But as you practice healthy behavior, willpower develops like a muscle that has been exercised. Then, choosing what is healthy does not require so much effort, but instead happens spontaneously.

So, for example, many smokers need willpower to stop smoking. But once they are successful at it, and their appetite has been educated to not smoke, the enjoyable and easy thing to do becomes breathing fresh air.

"Choose what is best. The habit will soon make it enjoyable and easy."
Pythagoras, 5th Century B.C.

Health Depends on Good Choices

Living is making decisions. Whether actively or passively, we are always deciding something, choosing among available options. Even if they seem insignificant, the decisions of daily life widely affect health.

Health depends more on the decisions we make every day regarding lifestyle, than heredity or environment.

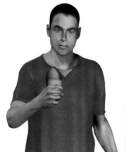 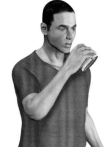

Should I have some ice cream or some fruit juice?

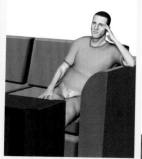 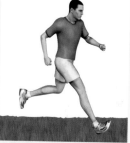

Should I sit watching TV. or do I go out and exercise?

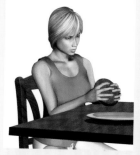 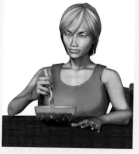

Should I eat a hamburger or a salad with seeds?

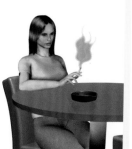 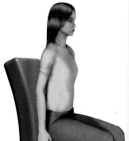

Should I smoke a cigarette or do some deep breathing?

Watch your decisions, for they turn into actions.
Watch your actions, for they become habits.
Watch your habits, for they determine your health and shape your character.
Oriental Proverb

How to Increase Your Willpower

Willpower is like a muscle: The more it is exercised, the more powerful it becomes. However, in order to achieve success, you must keep the brain's physiological needs and certain psychological principles in mind.

Meet the Needs of the Brain

When the brain has everything it needs for good functioning, the mind is in the best condition to make decisions, and follow through with them. This includes the following:

- Basic physiological needs: Constant supply of oxygen and glucose (see how to improve the oxygen and glucose supply in the units "Basic Needs of the Brain").
- Physical, chemical and microbiological protection for the brain (see the corresponding units).
- Sufficient rest.
- Keep the blood free from alcohol and other psychoactive drugs and practice "Healthy Habits for the Brain" (see the corresponding unit).

Avoid an Excess of Calories

In addition to food quality, its quantity also affects mood, intellectual performance, and willpower. It is known that overeating can cause deterioration in brain performance and mental slowness.

Large meals, in which one thousand or more calories are consumed, especially if they come from animal origin with saturated fats, cause a decrease in blood flow to the brain. After a big meal, blood is directed to the stomach, and other digestive organs, taking it away from cerebral blood flow.

Additionally, those large meals tend to be high in fat, which slows the absorption of foods and forces an increased blood flow to remain in the digestive organs.

These are some examples of the effects that a large meal can have on the mind:

- Decreased intellectual performance.
- Decrease in the ability to pay attention and concentrate, even extending to drowsiness.
- Decrease in the ability to make healthy decisions.

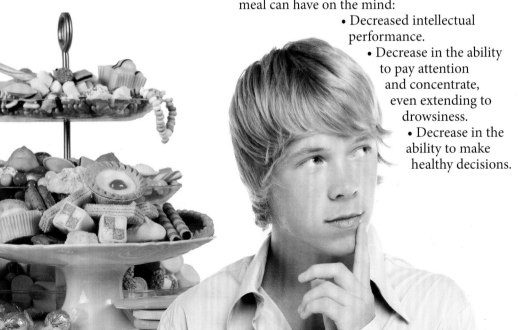

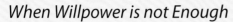

When Willpower is not Enough

People who suffer from chemical substance addiction or deeply rooted unhealthy habits often lack the willpower needed to become free from them. Sometimes, they feel completely incapable of overcoming the habit that enslaves them, and not even medical or psychological help is enough.

In this situation of personal helplessness, many believers successfully turn to a Supreme Power, outside of themselves: *"Lord, I cannot stop using this drug (or kick this habit) that dominates me. I have tried everything. I now submit to your power and your promises, trusting that you will make me victorious".*

When willpower isn't enough, besides putting the recommendations of this unit into practice, there is still a supernatural resource, which is always available to whomsoever shall turn to it: "Ask, and it will be given to you" (Luke 11:9, NKJV).

Prayer is one of the most powerful forms of energy man can generate.
Alexis Carrel (1873-1944),
French physician, Nobel Prize Laureate in Physiology and Medicine, 1912.

INCREASE KNOWLEDGE

Knowledge is necessary, although not enough, to be able to decide freely. Studying the effects of a certain habit or product helps strengthen the decisions made about it.

However, information alone does not necessarily modify behavior. The best example of this (and the saddest) is that of the physician or healthcare professional who smokes. In order to attain healthy habits, in addition to knowledge and information, good motivation is needed.

SET YOUR MOTIVATIONS

Motivations are powerful leverage tools to move the mind and change behavior. Every person should look for and set their own; the more, the better. Some of the motivations that most contribute to willpower are health, family, spirituality, and environmental ones.

EDUCATE YOUR APPETITE

An educated and controlled appetite bolsters the will and facilitates healthy decision-making. Those decisions that promote health strengthen the mind and increase willpower.

The units that follow show strategies to educate and control the appetite.

The Frontal Lobes: Willpower Central

(3) Thalamus
Nerve center of feelings

(1) Frontal Lobes
Anatomic center of the ability to decide, expressed through willpower.

(4) Hypothalamus
Nerve center of the appetite

(2) Cerebellum

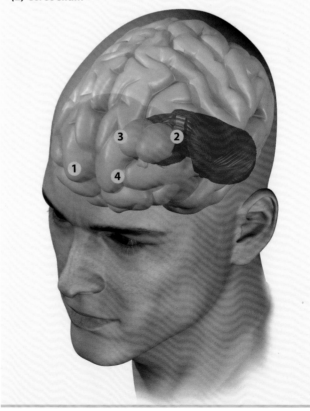

APPETITE AND HEALTH

The appetite, the command center of which is found in the brain, influences everyday habits. These habits eventually influence the state of one's health –more than heredity or environment.

Appetite is an instinctive impulse that drives us to satisfy desires or needs. Although appetite is associated primarily with the desire to ingest food for the purpose of preserving an individual's life, it is also used to refer to the reproductive impulse.

Appetite drives behavior. When you feel hunger, appetite moves you to prepare or search for food to satisfy this need. When you feel a sexual desire, appetite moves you to look for a partner.

Animals satisfy their appetite automatically, guided only by instinct and without having in mind the suitability or timing of such action.

However, as humans we have been given a brain structure that is capable of filtering and rationalizing the calls of the appetite: The cerebral cortex, especially the part located in the frontal lobes.

Just like any motor, the appetite needs to be controlled.

GIVE THE BODY WHAT IT ASKS FOR?

There is a theory that the appetite should always be satisfied, giving it everything it demands: "The body is wise, give it what it asks for".

But this theory presumes a serious mistake, especially applied to the education of children. Giving in to an appetite that is uneducated and uncontrolled is one of the primary causes of illness and unhappiness in the world.

Responses to the Call of the Appetite

Animals only have one option when they feel the call of the appetite: Satisfy it. Humans, on the other hand, can decide whether to respond, how to respond and when to respond to the call of the appetite. Willpower is the ability of humans to control the response to the call of the appetite (see "How to Increase Your Willpower").

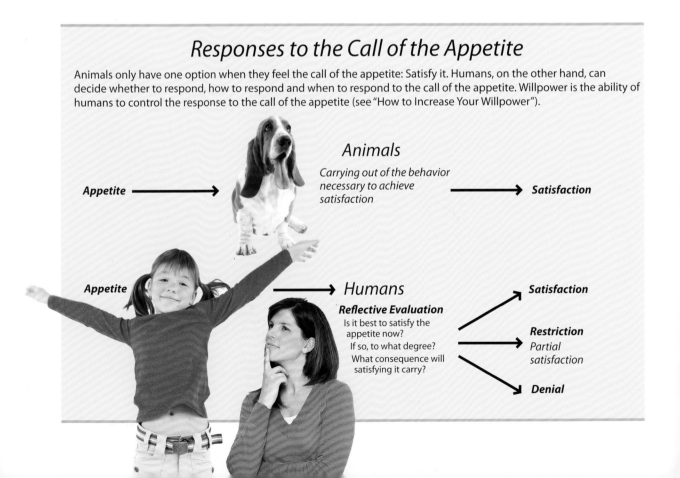

Animals

Appetite → *Carrying out of the behavior necessary to achieve satisfaction* → **Satisfaction**

Humans

Appetite → **Reflective Evaluation**
Is it best to satisfy the appetite now?
If so, to what degree?
What consequence will satisfying it carry?

→ **Satisfaction**

→ **Restriction** *Partial satisfaction*

→ **Denial**

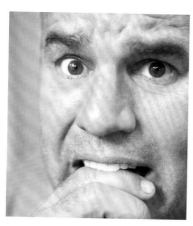

Slaves to the Appetite?

"I know that I shouldn't eat candies, because they throw off my diabetes; but I feel like I can't stop having them. I don't have any willpower."

Is this person condemned to be a slave to his appetite?

Is it possible to change what we like to find satisfaction in healthy behavior? Absolutely; the appetite is teachable, and the recommendations on these pages help achieve this.

Here are some practical ideas to stop a voracious appetite:

1. Eat more slowly, chewing food well.

2. Drink water with lemon juice between meals.

3. Drink a fucus extract (**seaweed**) or **soluble fiber** in a glass of water ten minutes before meals.

Appetite Command Center

The appetite has its organic command center in the hypothalamus, a nerve structure that measure a little more than a centimeter across, located at the base of the brain, on top of the pituitary gland.

The hypothalamus is the center of autonomic nervous system. From this small but very important nerve center come the impulses to eat, drink and have sexual activity, impulses which need to be evaluated and controlled in the cortex of the brain's frontal lobes.

In addition, the hypothalamus controls the sensation of fullness, body temperature, reaction to stress and the secretion of hormones in the pituitary gland.

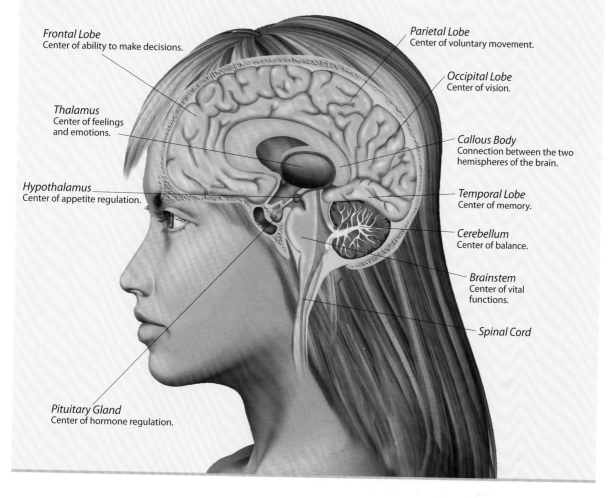

Frontal Lobe
Center of ability to make decisions.

Parietal Lobe
Center of voluntary movement.

Occipital Lobe
Center of vision.

Thalamus
Center of feelings and emotions.

Callous Body
Connection between the two hemispheres of the brain.

Hypothalamus
Center of appetite regulation.

Temporal Lobe
Center of memory.

Cerebellum
Center of balance.

Brainstem
Center of vital functions.

Spinal Cord

Pituitary Gland
Center of hormone regulation.

EDUCATING THE APPETITE - 1

The education of the appetite is, along with exercising willpower, the way to achieve the behavioral change needed to improve health and prevent disease.

DO NOT GET RID OF THE APPETITE, JUST EDUCATE AND CONTROL IT

The function of the frontal lobes of the brain is not to suppress the appetite, because it is vital for life, but rather to educate and control it, so that it can contribute to the health and well-being of ourselves and others. Just like a car's horsepower must be controlled by the driver, the horsepower of the appetite must be directed by the upper layers of the brain. This is achieved by:

- **First: Educate the appetite**, so I will like healthy things and find satisfaction in healthy behaviors.

- **Second: Control the appetite**, so I will feel satisfied with a sensible amount of what is healthy and good.

Although it requires a certain discipline, replacing hereditary or acquired tastes with others

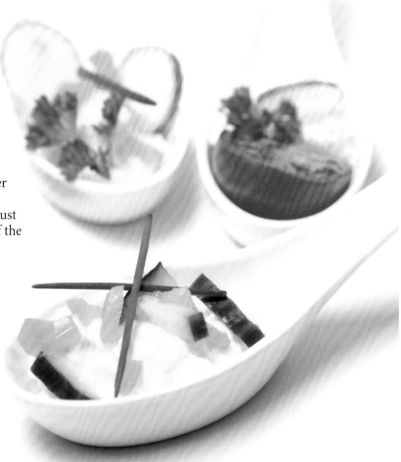

First Educate, Then Control the Appetite

The appetite should first be educated in quality, so that it will like to eat, drink or do what is healthy; and then, control amounts, so that it will be done in appropriate amounts.

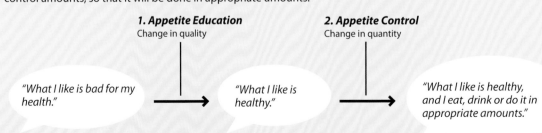

1. Appetite Education
Change in quality

2. Appetite Control
Change in quantity

"What I like is bad for my health."

"What I like is healthy."

"What I like is healthy, and I eat, drink or do it in appropriate amounts."

that are healthier is possible. The outcome for health and the true quality of life more than compensate the effort.

BENEFITS OF EDUCATING THE APPETITE

- It prevents obesity, and all that goes with it. Appetite education is the most effective tool to fight childhood obesity, which is more and more common.

- It prevents many cases of cancer that are related to diet.

- It prevents much of the damage promoted by drinking alcoholic beverages:
  - Physical, such as accidents and violent behavior.
  - Mental, such as decreased intellectual output and deterioration in personality.
  - Social, such as domestic violence and social isolation.

- It prevents addiction to psychoactive drugs, with all their physical, mental and social consequences.

THE TASTE FOR MEAT IS HEREDITARY

In order to evaluate the influence of heredity and of the environment in food preferences in children, researchers at University College of London (United Kingdom) looked at 103 sets of monozygotic twins (who are genetically identical) and another 111 sets of dizygotic twins (fraternal).[a]

The results showed that meat and fish preference is highly hereditary, while the preference for fruits and vegetables is a result of life experiences. When they see their parents showing enthusiasm or displeasure for fruit and vegetables, children learn to do the same.

That is, according to this research, children inherit the taste for meat, while they learn to have a taste for or reject the taste for plant foods according to the behavior they see in their parents.

a. Heritability of food preferences in young children. Breen FM, Plomin R, Wardle J. Physiol Behav. 2006 Jul 30;88(4-5):443-7. Epub 2006 Jun 5. PMID: 16750228

The Path to Health

Health education is able to change behavior through an increase in willpower and appetite education.

This behavioral change results in health benefits and disease prevention.

The brain is the organic support of this personal development process toward health and well-being; by taking care of it, and paying attention to its needs, as this chapter shows, a person's whole health benefits.

Health Education
Activities that motivate and show how to maintain and improve health.

Increase in willpower

Appetite education

Change in Behavior
Stop unhealthy habits and start healthy habits

Better Health
Increased ability to achieve personally and respond to the challenges of the environment.

Disease Prevention
Reduced risk of suffering a disease, eliminating or modifying the factors that promote it.

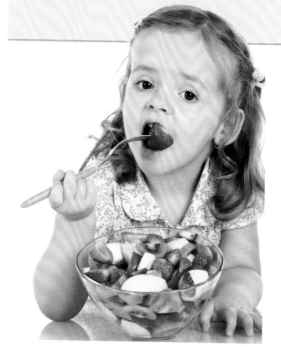

EDUCATING THE APPETITE - 2

Many people already know what is good for health; but they have a hard time putting it into practice, and they ask themselves, "What can I do so that I will like what is good and healthy, and enjoy doing it?"

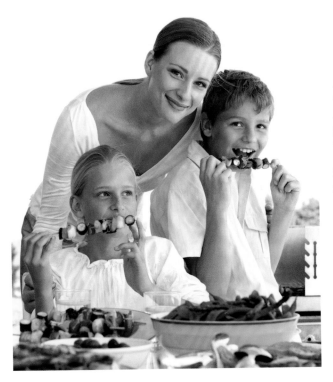

PHASES IN APPETITE EDUCATION

Appetite education is a gradual process, something that each individual must live for themselves as a personal growth experience.

Appetite education begins with increasing knowledge about the advantages of healthy behavior that can be incorporated (cognitive phase). Reading is the best way to increase knowledge. Audiovisual materials may be more attractive, but they are potentially less able to set information to memory.

After this, there is the emotional phase ("falling in love" with what is healthy) and the pragmatic phase (putting it into practice and repetition). Finally, healthy behavior can be integrated such that it starts to come "from inside".

Phases in Appetite Education

Phase	Description	Example
1. Cognitive	Acquiring knowledge about healthy foods or behavior. - Reading is the primary method to acquire and retain knowledge.	"I'm learning about the composition of apples, their properties and their health benefits."
2. Affective	Praising what is healthy and good, verbalizing expressions about the enthusiasm about the healthy product or behavior.	"I love apples! What a beautiful color and shape they have! "The soft, crispy taste is delightful to chew!" "And what a delicious taste they have!"
3. Pragmatic	Repetition of the good and healthy behavior.	"I'm going to have an apple every day after coming home from playing sports."
4. Integration	Spontaneity of the good and healthy behavior. This comes spontaneously without the need to tell yourself to do it.	"What I feel most like eating is an apple."

Following the four phases of appetite education is the only sure and lasting way to practice healthy habits. If they are forced to be practiced, without the person starting to enjoy them, it will be hard for them to last, and in the end, they will be given up.

REINFORCEMENT TECHNIQUES

During the process of educating the appetite, the following mental reinforcement techniques can be used to help solidify healthy behaviors.

- **Mental Preparation**: "I'm convinced by everything that I've read that having a salad every day is good, so I'm going to end up liking it".

- **Imitation**: "My friend has 5 pieces of fruit per day, and he's doing great. Maybe it would do the same for me".

- **Constant Repetition**: "I'm going to get out and walk every day, and eventually I will end up liking it".

- **Autosuggestion**: "What a beautiful apple! And it smells so good! Plus, it's so healthy! I have to like it!"

- **Asking for Help from a Friend**: "I'd like to call you every time I am tempted to smoke. Will you help me stop tobacco?"

THE BRAIN'S REWARD CIRCUIT

All humans need to feel rewarded and satisfied, especially after going through stressful adverse circumstances.

- The student, after passing the test.
- The athlete, once his efforts are finished.
- The worker, after a day of giving his best.

Research in neurophysics has identified what is known as the "reward circuit". After going through an adverse or stressful experience, there is a need to compensate for it through a gratifying or pleasurable experience. When you live it, certain neurotransmitters are released between neurons, such as serotonin, which produce satisfaction.

Everybody chooses the pleasurable experience they want for gratification. Educating the appetite makes them choose healthy behaviors that, when repeated, become set in the reward circuit.

Some people erroneously search for satisfaction in alcohol or drugs, or in risky behavior. These experiences can achieve temporary satisfaction, but their repetition eventually leads to frustration and personal decline: First, it is taken to feel good (the drug), but then it has to be taken in order to not feel bad.

Incorporating healthy habits into the brain's reward circuit is the big challenge in educating the appetite..

The Reward Circuit

Educating the appetite achieves a feeling of satisfaction and reward with experiences derived from healthy behaviors.

Adverse or stressful circumstance

↓

Search for a gratifying experience
You can search for a healthy behavior or a habit that is harmful to your health

↓

Releasing of serotonin between the neurons

↓

Feeling of satisfaction

↓

Feeling of reward

Repetition

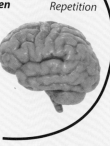

EDUCATING THE APPETITE - 3

Fasting and other ways of limiting foods have therapeutic and educational value. Incorporating a restriction on sweets and fast food is beneficial for the health of children and adults.

THE VALUE OF FASTING

It is interesting that Judaism, Christianity, Islam and other religions, recommend periods of fasting or limitations on foods as a way to promote mental clarity and spirituality.

It might seem that when no food is consumed, the glucose supply to the brain would be reduced and, therefore, so would mental abilities. However, the body has physiological mechanisms to maintain the energy supply to the brain, whether in the form of glucose or other energy sources.

- On the first day of fasting, glucose is obtained from the glucogen reserves in the liver and the muscles (about 500 g).

- From the second day of fasting on, the glucose needed for neurons is obtained first from dispensable proteins, the body's reserves, fat, and later, from structural proteins. In this way, the supply of glucose to the brain is ensured.

- When fasting is prolonged (more than three weeks), the blood glucose level decreases, and it is unable to completely satisfy the needs of the brain. In this extreme situation, the neurons of an adult are able to use energy sources other than glucose, which is also what happens in the brains of newborns and infants. This alternative energy sources are called ketone bodies, made from body fats and lactic acid. In this way, although not without metabolic efforts, the brain can continue functioning in situations of extremely low glucose levels.

The Advantages of Short-Term Fasting (1-2 days)

- It improves brain performance, especially in people who are weighed down by overeating or unbalanced nutrition.

- It alleviates the metabolic overload when it temporarily replaces the diet that is high in calories, refined sugars and saturated fats

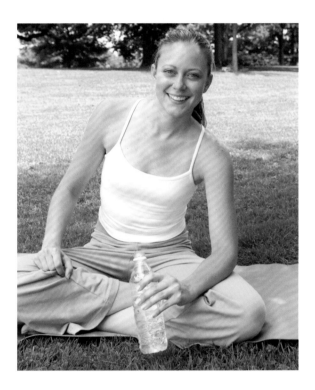

of animal origin, common to industrialized nations. As it is indicated in "Mind and Behavior-Altering Products", this type of diet redirects the blood flow to the digestive organs, decreasing oxygen supply to the brain and mental clarity.

- Helps educate the appetite: Fasting, or short-term food restrictions are valuable as educational tools to increase will-power and dominion over one's appetite.

However, even better than sporadic fasting is following a healthy diet day by day, which for adults would be hypocaloric (frugal) and low in saturated fats.

It has been shown in research animals that calorie restriction in the adult diet prolongs life.

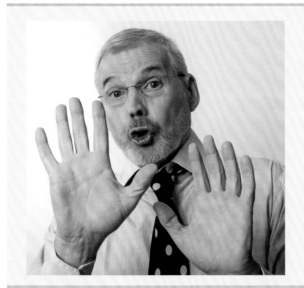

Eat Less to Feel Better

The voluntary limitation of food consumption on certain days of the year, or certain foods over the whole year, is part of humanity's religious culture.

In addition to the physical benefits, such as reducing the tendency toward obesity, occasional food restrictions also have an educational effect on the appetite.

The inhabitants of modern opulent societies, in which an excess of food causes disease, would gain many benefits by going back to the traditional practice of temporary restriction of food intake.

David Did Not Control His Appetite

According to a famous legend, Michelangelo's "David" one of the sculptures that best reflects the beauty of human anatomy, was taken to the United States to be exhibited on a tour of several cities.

After spending time in that great country, a paradigm of food abundance, David returned to Italy with quite a few extra pounds. David did not control his appetite, and the impulses of his hypothalamus won out over the reasoning of his cerebral cortex.

The historical record shows that the true David, king of Israel from the year 1011 to 971 B.C., did not control his appetite either. In Chapter 11 of the second book of Samuel, it tells how David did not control his sexual appetite when he saw an unclothed woman from his terrace, which led him to commit several crimes for which he had to bitterly repent.

However, a descendent of King David, Jesus of Nazareth, about a thousand years later, gave an awe-inspiring example of appetite control. After fasting for 40 days, he resisted the temptation to use supernatural powers to convert stones into bread.

Where Eve, Adam, David and many others failed due to not controlling their appetites, Jesus prevailed, demonstrating how humans can also prevail. This triumph has given courage and inspiration to many people throughout history to control themselves in favor of their physical and spiritual health.

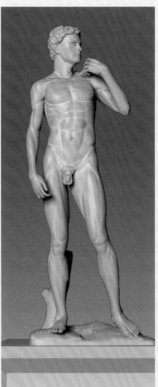 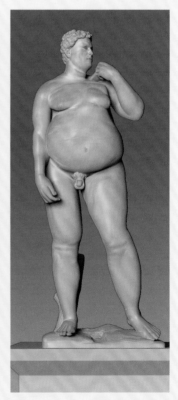

Before the tour　　　　After the tour

Eyes

They supply up to 80% of all the information that enters the brain.

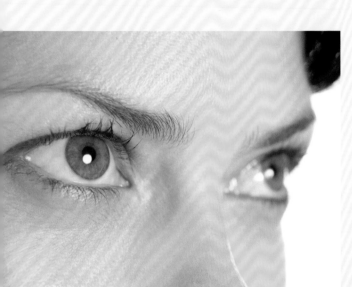

A simple look can express more than a thousand words.

The shape of the human eye is approximately that of a sphere with a 24 mm diameter. Concentrated within it is the greatest anatomic complexity of our entire body, due to the smallness and precision of its structures.

Although it could be compared to a photography device because of the functions it carries out, the eye is much more than that. It is the location of one of the great miracles of life: sight.

The extraordinary complexity of the eye is one of the greatest arguments against the theory of evolution. This was already true in Darwin's times, when the eye was not as well known as it is today; despite this, in his famous work "The Origin of the Species" Darwin states: *"To assume that the eye, with all of its mechanisms that cannot be duplicated… could have been formed by natural selection, seems, I freely admit, totally absurd."*[a]

More excellent in their own right than other sensory organs, which are nothing more than a differentiation of the epidermis, our eyes are an extension of the brain.

a.　DARWIN, Charles. *The Origin of Species*. Oxford University Press, p. 152.

Facts and Figures About the Eyes

0.07 mm (= 70 μ)	Resolution power of the human eye. It is the minimum distance that must exist between two points situated 25 cm from the eye that can still be seen as distinct points.
1 mm	Diameter of the macula, the most sensitive area of the retina.
14-20 mm Hg	Normal intraocular pressure.
70-80 mV (millivolts)	Electrical charge in the retinal cell membranes upon receiving bright light.
100 000	Number of eye movements in one day.
1 600 000	Number of nerve fibers in each optic nerve.
120 000 000	Total number of light-sensitive cells in the retina.

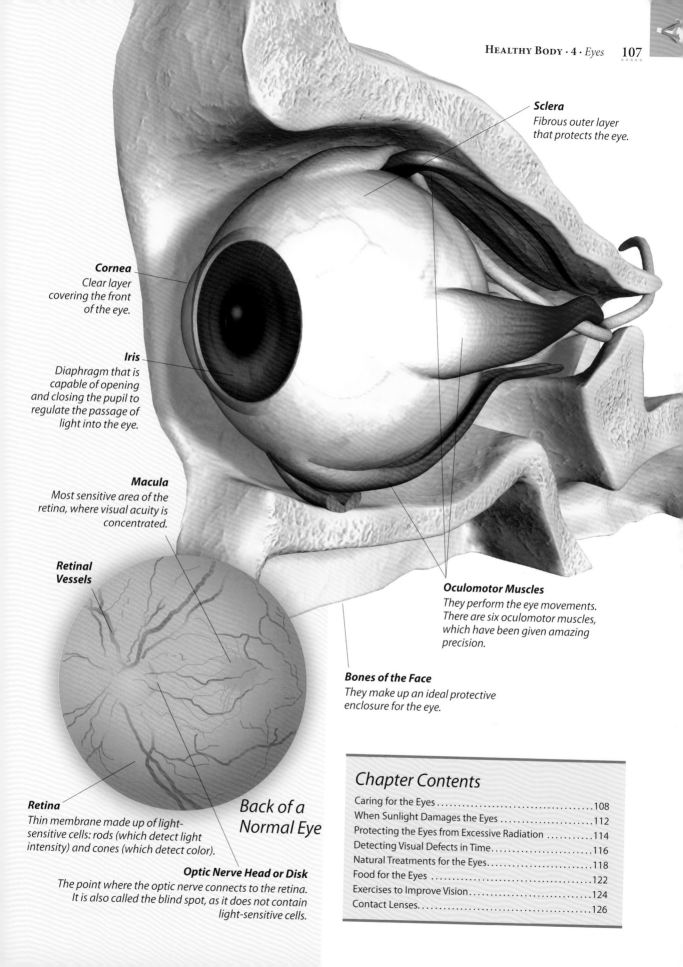

Sclera
*Fibrous outer layer
that protects the eye.*

Cornea
*Clear layer
covering the front
of the eye.*

Iris
*Diaphragm that is
capable of opening
and closing the pupil to
regulate the passage of
light into the eye.*

Macula
*Most sensitive area of the
retina, where visual acuity is
concentrated.*

**Retinal
Vessels**

Oculomotor Muscles
*They perform the eye movements.
There are six oculomotor muscles,
which have been given amazing
precision.*

Bones of the Face
*They make up an ideal protective
enclosure for the eye.*

*Back of a
Normal Eye*

Retina
*Thin membrane made up of light-
sensitive cells: rods (which detect light
intensity) and cones (which detect color).*

Optic Nerve Head or Disk
*The point where the optic nerve connects to the retina.
It is also called the blind spot, as it does not contain
light-sensitive cells.*

Chapter Contents

CARING FOR THE EYES - 1

Wearing glasses, not only sunglasses but also protective glasses for certain jobs, is the simplest and most effective way to care for the eyes

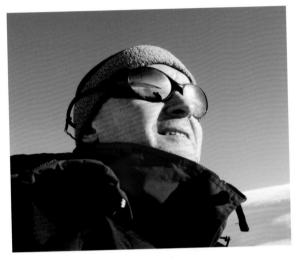

WEAR SUNGLASSES OUTDOORS

Due to the current deterioration of the ozone layer of the stratosphere, more and more invisible ultraviolet light is reaching us along with solar radiation. These rays promote the development of cataracts and retinal damage, among others.

Sunglasses protect the eyes against excessive solar radiation and the wind. Good sunglasses should filter:

- Part of the visible solar radiation.
- All or most invisible ultraviolet radiation (UV-A and UV-B rays) that is potentially dangerous to the eyes.

When Sunglasses are a Must

- Retinal diseases: Macular degeneration and retinitis pigmentosa.
- Conjunctivitis or other eye infections.
- Cataracts.
- Use of photosensitizing medications, such as certain antibiotics, oral contraceptives, sedatives, cholesterol medications and others (listed in warning information). These medications worsen the damage that ultraviolet rays cause to the eyes.
- After an accident or surgical procedure involving the eyes.

When Sunglasses are Recommended

- With light-colored eyes (a light-colored iris is more sensitive to light).
- When visiting places where ultraviolet radiation is intense, especially near the snow or the ocean, and in high mountains.
- When it is cloudy or foggy: Even though the sun is not shining, clouds and fog allow the passage of ultraviolet rays that are potentially dangerous to the eyes.

WEAR PROTECTIVE GLASSES

When doing any task in which liquids or solid fragments could splash into the eyes, protective glasses must be worn.

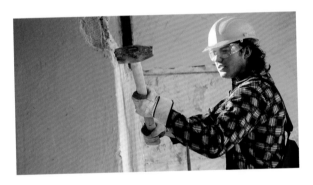

PRECAUTIONS WITH MONITORS

- Use flat-screen monitors whenever possible: Screens made from cathodic tubes, in both computers and televisions, fatigue the eyes more than modern flat screens.
- Avoid screen glare.
- Get as far away from the monitor as possible.
- Adjust the monitor to below eye-level for a more comfortable visual angle.

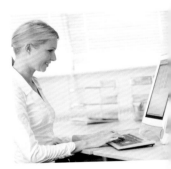

AVOID EYE IRRITANTS

Several physical or chemical agents are aggressive to the eyes, especially:

- Wind.
- Smoke (including tobacco smoke).
- Dust.
- Volatile chemical substances (gasoline, solvents, etc.).
- Pollen from certain trees and plants in springtime.

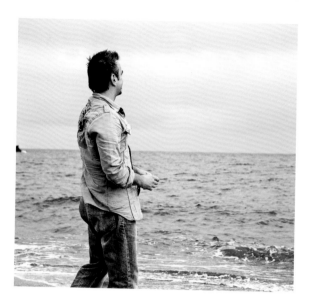

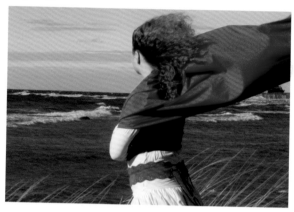

NO EYE-RUBBING

Hands tend to carry a number of bacteria and other germs that, when they come into contact with the eyes, can cause conjunctivitis and other serious infections, such as trachoma.

TAKE CARE OF THE EYES' SILENT ENEMIES

The silent enemies of eye health are:

- High cholesterol.
- High blood glucose.
- Hypertension.

Periodic medical checkups are recommended to control these silent enemies in particular, before they cause irreversible damage to the vision.

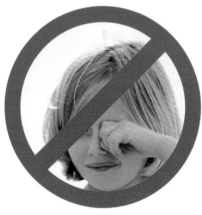

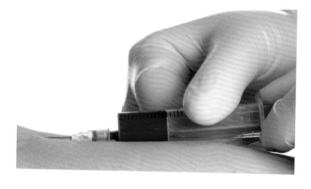

REST THE EYES

Look off into the distance once in a while. They say that sailors have beautiful eyes because they spend so many hours looking off into the distance.

Reading or looking close-up for too long should be avoided, especially in low lighting conditions.

Reasons You Must See a Doctor

- Any eye injury.
- Generalized or localized loss of vision in part of the visual field.
- Eye pain.
- Loss of strength in the eye muscles.

CARING FOR THE EYES - 2

Just like any high-tech precision machine, the eyes require a regular maintenance plan over the entire lifetime.

BLINK OFTEN

With each blink, the eyes are cleansed and refreshed, thanks to the secretion of tears that continually bathe their surface.

CAREFUL WITH LIGHTING

The light from non-electronic fluorescent tubes also oscillates, turning on and off continually –50 or 60 times per second. That is the reason they cause more eye fatigue than incandescent or halogen lamps, which give off a constant light.

A DIET RICH IN ANTIOXIDANTS

The eyes are very sensitive to the oxidation produced by free radicals. Cataracts, macular degeneration of the retina and other significant causes of vision loss are a result of an excess of free radicals.

A diet rich in antioxidant fruits and vegetables neutralizes free radicals and protects the delicate structures of the eye that allow vision (see "Food for the Eyes").

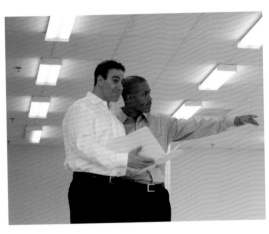
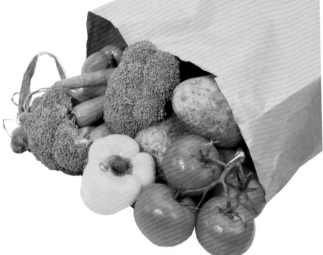

GET ENOUGH SLEEP

During sleep, the retinal pigments necessary for vision regenerate, thereby recovering from the day's wear-and-tear. A lack of sleep exhausts the retina's visual capacity and causes redness and irritation of the conjunctive membrane that covers the anterior pole of the eye.

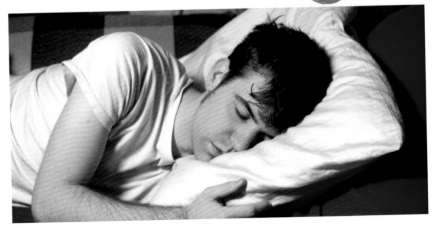

AVOID TOBACCO AND ALCOHOL

Tobacco smoke irritates the eyes. But a smoking habit damages the eyes much more, as it reduces blood flow to the retina, increases the level of free radicals that damage the lens and the retina, and finally decrease or loss of vision.

It has been well proven that **smokers** are at greater risk of suffering two of the primary causes of vision loss:

• Macular degeneration of the retina.
• Cataracts (the risk increases greatly in smokers who also drink).

Smokers also suffer more cases of glaucoma and Graves' ophthalmopathy (bulging eyes).

Alcohol consumption is also harmful to the vision:

• It increases intraocular pressure and promotes glaucoma.
• It promotes the formation of cataracts.
• It reduces the visual field and causes diplopia (double vision).

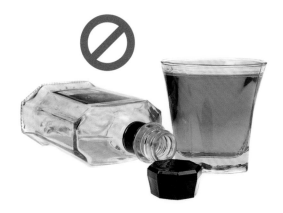

HAVE REGULAR EYE EXAMS

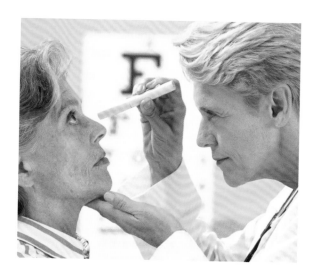

It is recommended to follow a schedule of eye exams suggested for the general population, such as the one shown in the adjacent table. However, should there be any of the following risk factors, more frequent exams are recommended.

• Premature children.
• Children of mothers who had German measles, sexually transmitted diseases, drug use, or other medical problems during their pregnancy.
• A family history of diabetes, hypertension or glaucoma.
• Severe nearsightedness (myopia), farsightedness (hyperopia) or astigmatism.
• Belonging to the Black or American Indian racial groups, due to their higher risk of glaucoma.

Plan for Eye Exams

Age	Examiner	Objective
Birth	Pediatrician or family physician	Evaluation of the overall condition of the eyes.
Age 3	Pediatrician or family physician or ophthalmologist	Determination of visual acuity.
Age 5	Ophthalmologist	Preschool exam, ocular motility test.
Between ages 6 and 39	Ophthalmologist	Complete exam any time there are eye symptoms or injuries that involve the eyes.
Age 40	Ophthalmologist	Complete exam.
Up to age 65	Ophthalmologist	Exam every 2 or 4 years.
After age 65	Ophthalmologist	Exam every year or every 2 years.

WHEN SUNLIGHT DAMAGES THE EYES

What we do not see can blind us: Ultraviolet radiation is not visible to the eyes, but in excess it causes eye damage and decreased vision.

The eyes are designed to receive light, and in a specific way: from the Sun. In addition, they need light to continue to function and not become atrophied. Not only the eyes, but also our entire body and all of nature require light from the Sun.

However, although it may seem contradictory, that same sunlight needed by the eyes can damage them. This is primarily due to the fact that, for the last several decades, the light from the Sun that reaches the Earth carries too much ultraviolet radiation. A little is necessary, but a lot will damage the eyes.

HAS THE SUN BECOME AN ENEMY?

The planet Earth has the optimal conditions for the development of life as we know it. Therefore, any small variation in the physical conditions that surround us, including the intensity and type of radiation received, can make life impossible. The human mind infers naturally that this planet has been designed intelligently to sustain life and, specifically, humankind. That is what is stated in the anthropic principle, which has been studied extensively by science.

Humankind, however, with its often-destructive activities, is changing these ideal conditions for life on our planet. Therefore, for example, because of the thinning of the ozone layer of the stratosphere caused by pollution, a little more radiation reaches us than normal. This change, which seems to be of very little importance, has been enough for a dramatic increase in many eye disorders, such as shown in this unit, as well as skin disorders.

Humankind has broken the anthropic principle, and in addition to that, physical pollution as well as moral pollution could make this planet uninhabitable, contrary to what was initially formed. Human science and wisdom do not seem to be achieving improvement in the situation – at least not globally.

For believers, there is a hope that is far beyond all that science has to offer: a supernatural intervention that, like the Apostle Peter says, will give way to "a new heaven and a new earth, the home of righteousness".

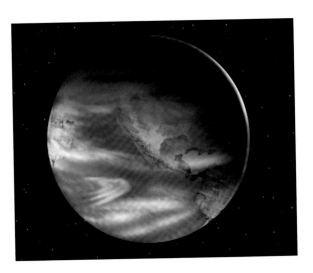

DAMAGE CAUSED BY EXCESSIVE SOLAR RADIATION TO THE EYES

Of all of the radiation that makes up sunlight, ultraviolet rays are the most harmful to the eyes.

On the Eyelids
• **Basal cell carcinoma**, a type of skin cancer.

On the Cornea
The cornea absorbs a good part of the ultraviolet radiation that reaches the eye. It has been shown that high intensities of UV-C and UV-B rays trigger the production of interleukin in the cornea, a substance that causes inflammation, promoting these disorders:

- **Photokeratitis**: Superficial burn on the cornea, accompanied by severe inflammation. Also known as "snow blindness".

- **Pterygium**: Also known as a "growth on the eye". It is an abnormal growth on the conjunctiva, similar to a scar, that eventually covers the cornea. By covering the cornea, it causes vision loss, and even blindness. It is common to warm regions, where there is intense sunlight, dryness, wind and dust. Its surgical removal restores the vision that had been lost. Sunglasses prevent it from developing.

On the Choroid

The choroid is the layer of blood vessels and connective fibers that surround the retina.

- **Melanoma of the choroid**: This is the most common type of malignant eye tumor in adults.

On the Lens

- **Cataracts**: Cloudiness of the lens, more common with age. It is currently the most significant cause of blindness in the world. Each decade that goes by, the number of cases in the world doubles, which is without a doubt influenced by the destruction of the ozone layer of the stratosphere.

Retina

The retina is the innermost layer of the eye, where light-sensitive cells are located.

- **Solar retinitis**: Caused by the intense action of visible and infrared light on the retina. It is caused by staring at the sun, for example, when trying to see a solar eclipse without eye protection.

- **Macular degeneration of the retina**: This is the most significant cause of vision loss in people over age 65, in developed countries. An excess of ultraviolet radiation is one of the contributing factors.

- **Retinitis pigmentosa**: Hereditary degeneration of the retina, worsened by excessive ultraviolet radiation.

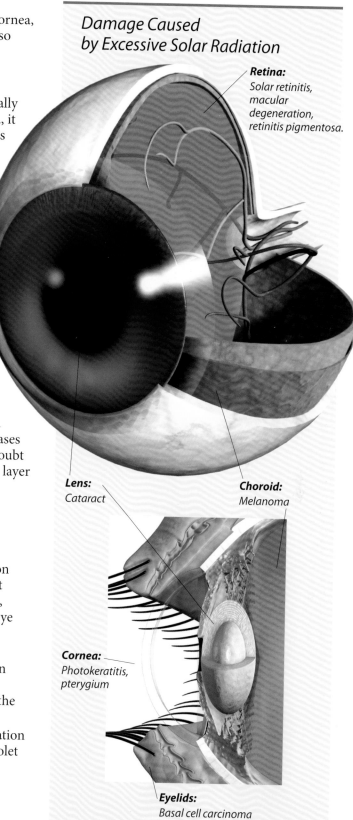

Damage Caused by Excessive Solar Radiation

Retina: *Solar retinitis, macular degeneration, retinitis pigmentosa.*

Lens: *Cataract*

Choroid: *Melanoma*

Cornea: *Photokeratitis, pterygium*

Eyelids: *Basal cell carcinoma*

PROTECTING THE EYES FROM EXCESSIVE RADIATION

Knowing how to protect against overexposure to ultraviolet "invisible light" is essential to caring for the eyes and preventing vision loss.

SUNLIGHT AND THE EYES

Light is a special type of electromagnetic radiation that is capable of causing an impression on the retina of our eyes.

Our eyes are constantly receiving electromagnetic radiation with different wavelengths. However, not all of it causes an impression on the retina, but rather only when its wavelength is between 390 and 750 nanometers (1 nm or nanometer is a millionth of a millimeter). This is the radiation that makes up visible light.

However, there is radiation that our retina does not see, that is to say, that it does not transform into electrical signals, but that can damage the eyes. This is specifically the most dangerous kind, and the kind that needs to be carefully protected against.

Of all the radiation that we do not see, the most damaging to the eye is ultraviolet (UV-A, UV-B, and UV-C). Its primary source is the sun.

WHEN ULTRAVIOLET RADIATION IS THE MOST INTENSE

Ultraviolet radiation is most intense in the following places and circumstances. Avoiding them as much as possible protects against eye-damaging overexposure.

Near Reflective Surfaces

Snow reflects 80% of the ultraviolet radiation received from the sun; sand: 17%; and water: 5%. Grass reflects less than 1% and dirt, hardly any.

Summertime and Near the Equator

In both cases, the sun's rays are directed more vertically toward the earth, and therefore have to pass through a lesser thickness of the atmosphere. All of this results in receiving more intense radiation.

Near the South Pole

The protective ozone layer of the stratosphere has thinned all around the planet, but especially around the South Pole.

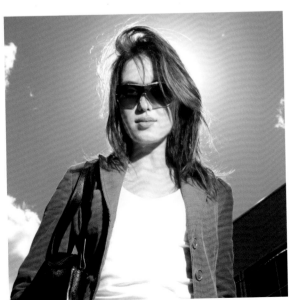

What Causes the Most Eye Damage

A combination of these three factors greatly increases the risk of suffering eye damage and reduced or loss of vision:

1. Exposure to intense ultraviolet radiation.

2. Absence of protective barriers against ultraviolet rays (for example, not wearing sunglasses).

3. Diet low in plant antioxidants.

Protecting Yourself Against Ultraviolet Rays Is More Necessary than Ever

When we are exposed to sunlight, we are also exposed to invisible ultraviolet radiation, which, when excessive, can damage the eyes.

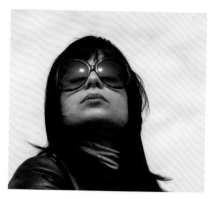

Because clouds allow ultraviolet rays to pass through them, the eyes must also be protected on cloudy days.

Cloudy Days

Although clouds retain part of the visible solar radiation, they allow invisible ultraviolet rays to go through them. Therefore, on cloudy days, we are exposed to a greater intensity of ultraviolet rays than we would expect when there is less light.

Middle of the Day

Between 10 am and 3 pm, 75% of the day's ultraviolet radiation is received.

Altitude

The sun's ultraviolet rays pass through a smaller layer of protective atmosphere as elevations rise farther above sea level, thereby reaching us with greater intensity. With every 1,000 m increase in altitude, ultraviolet radiation increases by 12%.

Barriers Against Ultraviolet Rays

OZONE LAYER

The ozone layer of the stratosphere filters most of the UV-C rays and a good portion of the UV-B rays.

The thickness of the ozone layer has been reduced each year in recent decades, especially in the southern hemisphere. This causes more potentially dangerous ultraviolet radiation to reach the earth and our eyes, such as UV-B rays.

The blue blotch on the image shows the hole in the ozone layer over Antarctica in 2005, according to NASA.

GLASS

Although transparent, glass filters most of the invisible ultraviolet rays. This fact has its positive side, as far as eye protection is concerned. However, keep in mind that sunbathing with the sun on the other side of a window nullifies part of the sun's therapeutic effects, such as vitamin D synthesis in the skin.

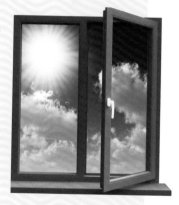

THE AIR IN THE ATMOSPHERE

The air (not the clouds) filters part of the ultraviolet rays that come from the sun. The lower the sun is, the thicker the atmosphere is that its rays must pass through, and the less ultraviolet radiation that reaches us.

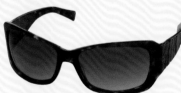

SUNGLASSES

Be sure that the ones you get have lenses that provide maximum protection against ultraviolet rays.

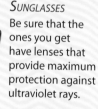

HAT WITH A BRIM

This reduces the ultraviolet radiation that reaches the eyes. It is also helpful to wear it in addition to sunglasses, since these always allow some radiation to get in from the sides.

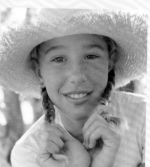

DETECTING VISUAL DEFECTS IN TIME

This is how the eyes see when they are affected by the most common visual defects. Detecting visual defects in time is essential to preventing the underlying disease from progressing and seriously affecting the ability to see.

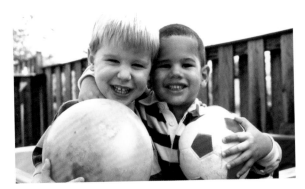

Normal Vision

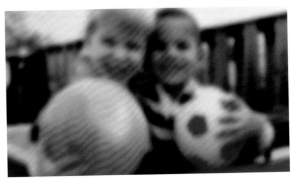

Cataracts
Blurry and dimmed vision in the entire visual field, due to the lens losing its transparency.

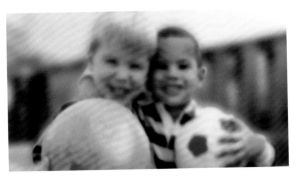

Myopia
Blurry vision caused by deformity of the eye.

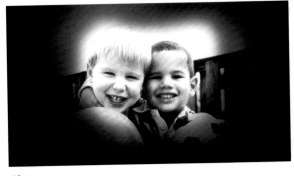

Glaucoma
Loss of peripheral vision, due to increased pressure in the eye, which compresses and weakens the optic nerve.

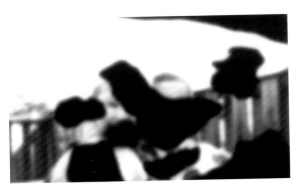

Exudative Diabetic Retinopathy
Blurry vision with areas of visual loss (scotomas) due to capillaries and exudates that form on the retina.

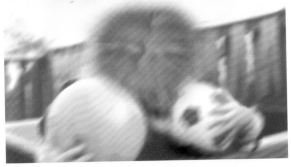

Age-Related Macular Degeneration of the Retina
Loss of vision in the middle area, and blurry peripheral vision.

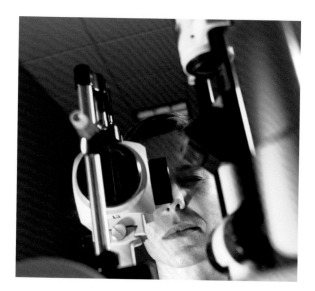

Measurement of intraocular pressure using a tonometer. This test is vital to the diagnosis of glaucoma.
- Normal range: 14-20 mm Hg.
- Suspected glaucoma: 21-35 mm Hg.
- Confirmed diagnosis: over 35 mm Hg.
Note: There have been cases of glaucoma with normal intraocular pressure.

A Snellen eye chart, a simple but very effective tool to detect visual disturbances.

Figures on these two pages: United States National Eye Institute. http://www.nei.nih.gov/health/examples/

Amsler Grid

The Amsler Grid is a graphic used for early detection of macular diseases, especially age-related macular degeneration.

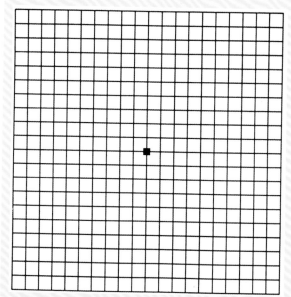

Cover one eye, and stare at the dot in the middle with the other eye. If the boxes look blurry, or distorted, there could be an injury to the macula (the most sensitive area of the retina).

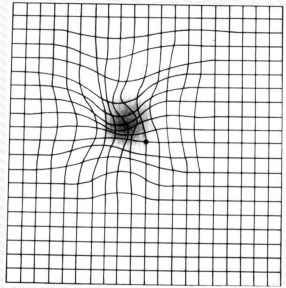

This is how the Amsler grid appears to someone who has macular degeneration of the retina.

NATURAL TREATMENTS FOR THE EYES - 1

Water is very beneficial for the eyes, whether used for rinses or baths. Vegetable foods such as cucumbers, applied directly over the eyelids, are also beneficial.

EYE RINSE

The eye rinse is basic hygiene. It is very recommendable for conjunctivitis and other infections. It is one of the easiest treatments to administer to children.

Uses

- To cleanse the eyes of dirt or foreign matter.
- In the morning, to clear nighttime secretions.
- At nighttime, to eliminate dust or smoke residues accumulated during the day.

Water temperature: Lukewarm.

Duration: 3-5 minutes.

Afterward: Dry the face with a clean cotton cloth or towel.

Frequency: Two or three times per day.

Caution

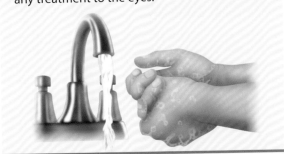

Wash your hands thoroughly before applying any treatment to the eyes.

CUCUMBER SLICES OVER THE EYELIDS

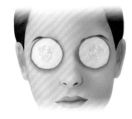

Cucumber is a great friend of the eyelids. It is applied directly over the eyes as raw, intact slices

Uses

- To refresh and decongest fatigued eyelids.
- To relieve eye fatigue.
- To reduce sagging eyelids.
- To strengthen skin tissues and contribute to the eyes' beauty, thanks to their sulfur content.

Cucumber Temperature: Cold (from the refrigerator).

Duration: Two half-hour sessions per day, or one one-hour session.

Afterward: Wash your face with water, then dry.

How to Do: The slices must remain in place at least an hour a day, preferably after your afternoon or evening meal, while resting. If they dry out, they must be replaced

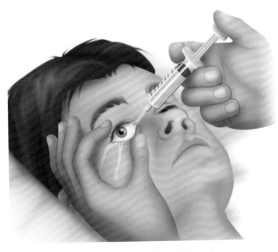

Apply the water with a sterile, if possible, syringe, allowing it to flow over the eye without any pressure, toward the temple, to avoid contaminating the other eye.

Open and close eyes during the rinse.

Use special liquid for eye rinses, normal saline or water boiled with salt at 14 g (a tablespoon) per liter of water.

EYE BATH

The eye bath allows a more prolonged contact between the liquid and the eye than an eye rinse.

Caution: If using medicinal plant infusions as liquid for the eye bath, such as chamomile (*Matricaria chamomila*) or common thyme (*Thymus vulgaris*), be careful, because they can cause allergic reactions in people who are sensitive to them or who are allergic to pollen.

Uses

- To relieve irritation and itching in the eyes.
- To stimulate blood circulation in the front of the eye, thereby strengthening defenses against infection and ability to regenerate.

Liquid Temperature: Lukewarm.

Duration: 2-3 minutes per eye.

Afterward: Dry your face with a clean cotton cloth or towel.

Frequency: Up to three times per day.

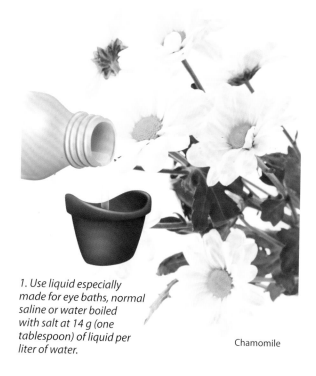

1. Use liquid especially made for eye baths, normal saline or water boiled with salt at 14 g (one tablespoon) of liquid per liter of water.

Chamomile

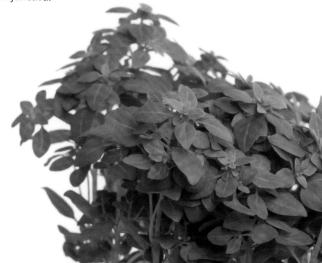

2. Fill the eyecup with the liquid and apply it over your eye, while looking up.

3. Open and close your eyes, and move your eye all around so that the liquid is able to get into good contact with the whole conjunctiva.

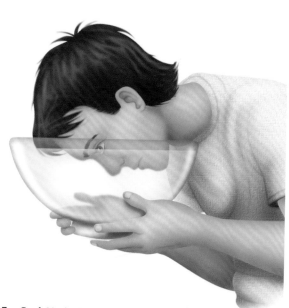

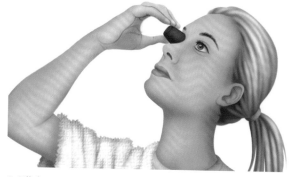

Eye Bath Variation

Instead of using a cup, submerge your eyes and part of your face in a clean container with the liquid you are going to use. Open your eyes and move them around in the water.

NATURAL TREATMENTS FOR THE EYES - 2

Medicinal plants and charcoal cleanse and reduce inflammation of eyes that are loaded with impurities.

COMPRESS WITH PLANT BAGS OVER THE EYE

Herbal tea bags are a very practical way to apply herbs to the eyes. The most common of them, for their medicinal effects and availability, are:

- Chamomile (*Matricaria chamomilla*).
- Dog rose (*Rosa canina*).
- Green tea (*Thea sinensis*).

Uses

- To reduce inflammation and tone the eyes in eye infections (blepharitis, keratitis and others).
- To reduce sagging eyelids.

Bag Temperature: Warm.

Duration: 5-10 minutes.

Afterward: Wash your face with water, then dry.

Frequency: Two or three times per day.

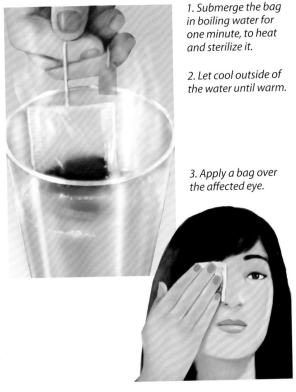

1. Submerge the bag in boiling water for one minute, to heat and sterilize it.

2. Let cool outside of the water until warm.

3. Apply a bag over the affected eye.

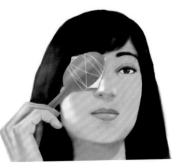

EYE COMPRESS

An eye compress consists of placing a water-soaked piece of gauze over the eye. Depending on the water temperature, there are different effects and uses.

- **Warm Water**: This is the most common and easy to tolerate. It reduces inflammation and relaxes the eye.
- **Hot Water**: This increases blood flow to the eye, which promotes curative processes. It is helpful in all eye disorders, including inflammations such as iridocyclitis, conjunctivitis, and glaucoma. When there is infection, it is recommended to soak the compress in a preparation of an antiseptic plant, such as:
  – Eyebright (*Euphrasia officinalis*).
  – Common thyme (*Thymus vulgaris*).
- **Cold Water**: This uses ice-cold water. An ice cube wrapped in gauze can also be applied. It relieves eye inflammation and itching in viral conjunctivitis. It is also used when there is inflammation and pain in the eye.

Water temperature: Warm, hot or cold (ice-cold).

Duration: 3-5 minutes.

Afterward: Dry your face with a clean cotton cloth or towel.

Frequency: Two or three times per day.

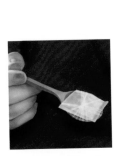

Variation of Eye Compress
Secure the gauze onto a long-handled spoon. Submerge the spoon with the gauze in water and apply it to the affected eye.

VEGETABLE CARBON POULTICE OVER THE EYE

Powdered vegetable carbon has an amazing ability to retain toxins and foreign substances. When applied over the eyes in infections, edema or congestion of the eyelids, the conjunctiva or lachrymal ducts, a carbon poultice is an excellent alternative treatment that attains surprising results.

Uses

• To cleanse and reduce inflammation in the eyes in cases of conjunctivitis, blepharitis (infection of the eyelids), dacryocystitis (infection of the tear sac), sties or other external eye infections.

Poultice Temperature: Warm (room temperature).

Duration: 20-30 minutes, or more. It may be left on overnight while you sleep.

Afterward: Wash your face with water, then dry.

Frequency: Two or three times per day.

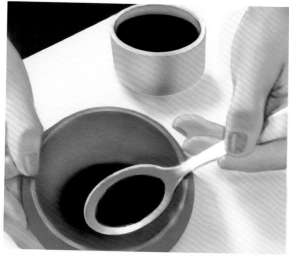

1. Place a tablespoon of activated vegetable carbon in a glass or other container, add a few drops of cool water until the mix acquires a pasty consistency.

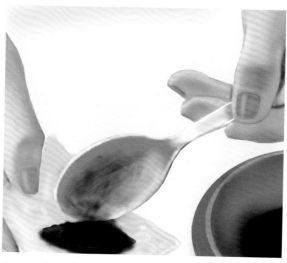

2. Place the carbon paste onto a piece of gauze.

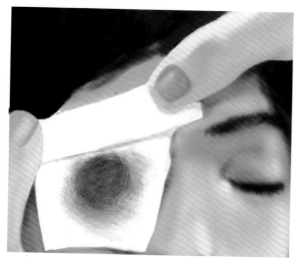

3. Apply the gauze with carbon directly over the affected eye.

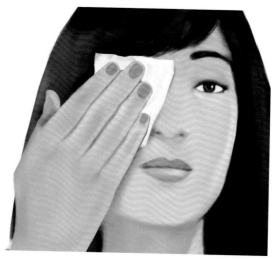

4. Cover the gauze with a cloth to prevent the carbon from dripping onto your face. The poultice can be secured in place with a loose bandage.

FOOD FOR THE EYES

*Food should provide antioxidants to fight off free radicals,
and the vitamins needed for vision.*

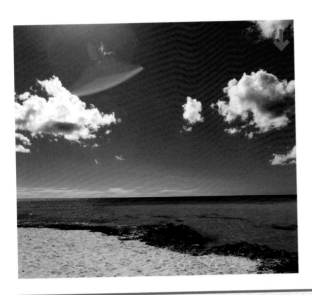

Food provides the eyes multiple nutrients that they need in order to transform the light that reaches them into electrical signals. These are then analyzed and interpreted by the brain, giving way to the complex phenomenon we call vision.

FREE RADICALS HARM THE VISION

Free radicals are oxydated molecules, which are chemically unstable due to their lack of electrons, that behave aggressively against our bodies. Free radicals damage cells and tissues in general, causing early aging, degenerative diseases and even cancer.

Antioxidants that Protect the Retina

All of these antioxidants protect the eyes in general, and specifically the retina, improving vision.

Antioxidant	Effect on the Retina	Food Sources
Vitamin C	Present in retinal cells, which protect from the damage caused by free radicals generated by ultraviolet light, tobacco and chemical contamination.	Fruit (especially kiwi and citrus) and fresh vegetables.
Vitamin E	Very abundant in photoreceptor cells (cones) of the retina. It prevents perioxidation (degradation) of fats, and protects against free radicals.	Wheat germ, dried oleaginous fruits and avocado.
Beta-carotene	Transforms into vitamin A. Thanks to this vitamin, rhodopsin is regenerated, which is a light-sensitive pigment found in retinal cells, and that is used up when transforming light waves into electrical signals.	Carrots, mangos, oranges, sweet potatoes, zucchini or squash, and all orange-colored vegetables.
Carotenoides	Especially lutein and zeathanthin, greenish-yellow in color. These vegetable pigments act as powerful antioxidants that neutralize free radicals and protect retinal cells against the harmful effects of ultraviolet radiation.	Spinach, chard, corn, lettuce, green cabbage, turnip greens, lamb's lettuce or mâche.
Flavonoids	Vegetable pigments that are widespread in the vegetable world. The most active on the retina are the dark blue or red ones, called antocyanines or antocyanidines. These are powerful antioxidants capable of stopping the progression of macular degeneration in addition to improving the sensitivity of the retina to light and night vision.	Blueberries, strawberries, black grapes, pomegranates, blackberries, and black olives.
Minerals	Zinc, copper, magnesium and selenium are necessary for the action of antioxidant enzymes.	Dried fruits and legumes are excellent sources of these minerals.

Sources of Free Radicals

- Ultraviolet rays from the sun are the primary source of free radicals for the eye.
- Tobacco.
- Drugs.
- Chemical contamination.
- Inflammation and infection in the eyes and the body in general.
- Ionizing radiation.

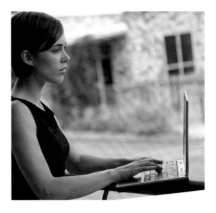

People who spend many hours in front of computer screens or reading need more antioxidants and vitamins for their retinas.

EYE DAMAGE CAUSED BY VITAMIN DEFICIENCY

The eyes need several vitamins for good vision, and so its delicate tissues will stay in good condition. A lack of certain vitamins, such as A, can cause serious eye damage, and even vision loss.

- **Vitamin A Deficiency**:
  - Blepharitis (inflammation of the eyelids), sties, conjunctivitis and other eye infections.
  - Xerophthalmia (dryness and inflammation of the conjunctiva) that can lead to blindness, especially in children.
  - Night blindness (lack of adjusting to darkness).

- **Vitamin B Deficiency**:
  - Atrophy of the optic nerve, inflammation of the conjunctiva and the cornea.
- **Vitamin C Deficiency**:
  - Glaucoma.
  - Cataracts.
  - Eye infections.
  - Retinal bleeding.
- **Vitamin K Deficiency**:
  - Retinal bleeding.

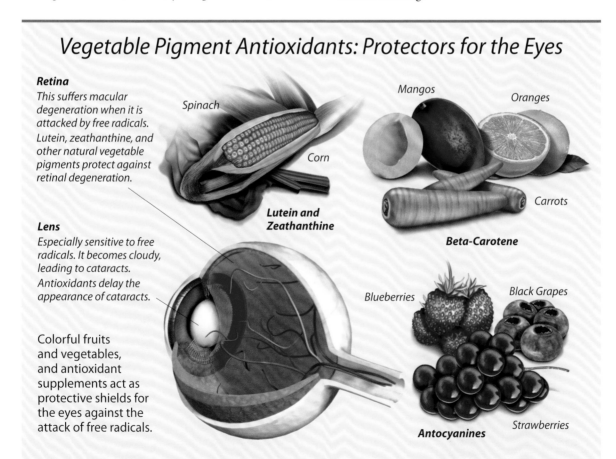

Vegetable Pigment Antioxidants: Protectors for the Eyes

Retina
This suffers macular degeneration when it is attacked by free radicals. Lutein, zeathanthine, and other natural vegetable pigments protect against retinal degeneration.

Lens
Especially sensitive to free radicals. It becomes cloudy, leading to cataracts. Antioxidants delay the appearance of cataracts.

Colorful fruits and vegetables, and antioxidant supplements act as protective shields for the eyes against the attack of free radicals.

Spinach

Corn

Lutein and Zeathanthine

Mangos

Oranges

Carrots

Beta-Carotene

Blueberries

Black Grapes

Strawberries

Antocyanines

EXERCISES TO IMPROVE VISION

The muscles both inside and outside the eye need to be exercised in order to enjoy good vision.

The job that is least demanding on the eyes is looking into the distance (more than 50 meters) without concentrating on any single fixed point. However, modern lifestyles require a fixed gaze for many hours every day on objects that are very close, such as books or computers. This tires and weakens the eyes, which promotes the progression of visual defects.

The eye exercises presented here can compensate for eye fatigue and, according to some, stop the progression of visual defects such as myopia, presbyopia (farsightedness) and astigmatism.

In each exercise session for improving vision, you can do one, some or all of the exercises shown in this unit.

It is recommended to always start with an eye rinse, and finish by resting the eyes.

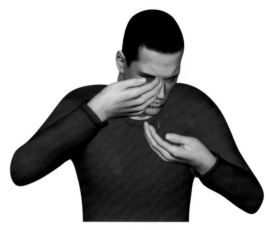

1. Eye Rinse
Wash your eyelids with warm water for about 10 seconds, then with cold water for another 10 seconds. Repeat several times.
This is the ideal exercise to begin the session.

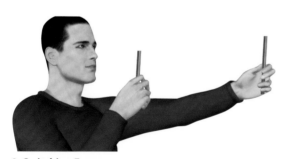

2. Switching Focus
Hold two objects at different distances, one in each hand. Fix your vision on one of them, then after blinking for a few seconds, fix it on the other.
Repeat at least ten times in a row.

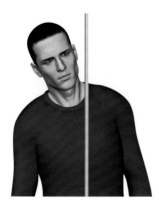

3. Dowel Exercise
Move your head from one side of a dowel to the other, keeping your eyes fixed on it. Keep doing this for 2 or 3 minutes.

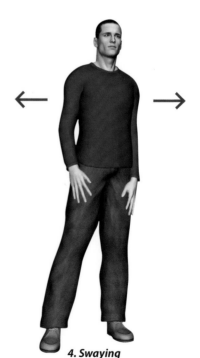

4. Swaying
In a standing position, fix your vision on an immobile object. Sway your body side to side without taking your eyes off the selected object, blinking continuously.
Repeat at least ten times.

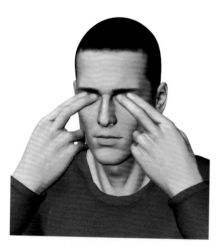

5. Eye Massage

Done gently, on yourself as well as by a massage therapist, an eye massage is a complement to the rest of the exercises.

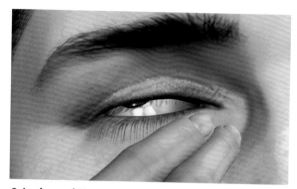

8. Lachrymal Massage

Use your fingertips to glide over your lower eyelid, from the temple toward the nose.

This exercise facilitates the drainage of tears through the tear duct, which is located at the internal or nasal aspect of the eye. This is recommended for dacriocystitis (inflammation of the lachrymal sac) and watery eyes.

For bags under the eyes, this exercise helps them to be reabsorbed.

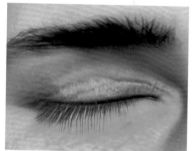

9. Rapid Blinking

While keeping the vision fixed on a far away object, blink rapidly for one or two minutes.

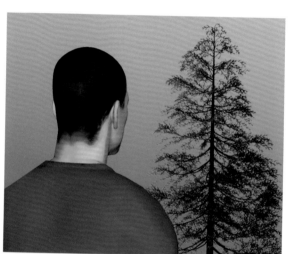

6. Paint with Your Eyes

Look at an object that is a moderate distance away, such as a tree or a car, and trace its outline with your eyes, without moving your head.

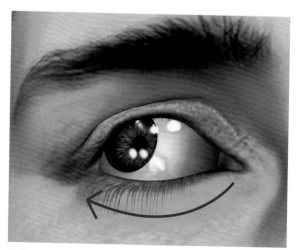

7. Eye Gymnastics

Move your eye in every direction, making a circle. Repeat three or four times in a row.

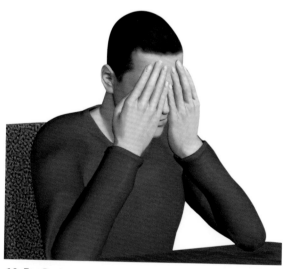

10. Eye Rest

Close your eyes and cover them with the palms of your hands, but without touching the eyes themselves. Stay in this position resting your eyes for a few minutes.

Eye rest an ideal ending to exercise session for vision improvement.

CONTACT LENSES

*The user should know that without the right attention and care,
contact lenses could cause serious damage the cornea and the conjunctiva.*

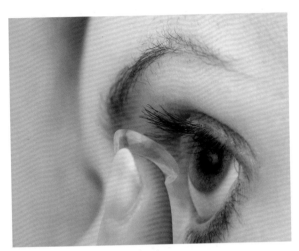

*Contact lenses are an alternative to glasses, with many
advantages and some inconveniences.*

PRECAUTIONS FOR CONTACT LENSES

- Do not wear them for more than the recommended number of hours, and do not sleep with them in place.
- Do not share them with anyone, as they can damage others' eyes, even if they have been disinfected.
- If your eyes become red or irritated, remove the contact lenses and consult a specialist.
- Abide by the expiration date on the contact lenses and on the maintenance solutions.
- Wash, rinse and disinfect them with appropriate solutions each time you change them. Wash your hands first.
- Never use non-distilled water or non-sterilized saline solution.

COMPLICATIONS WITH CONTACT LENSES

Giant Papillary Conjunctivitis

Inflammation of the conjunctiva that covers the inner aspect of the upper eyelid, caused by contact lenses.

- **Causes**: Intolerance to maintenance solutions; deposition of proteins on the lens. More frequent with soft lenses.

- **Symptoms**: Itching, sticky secretion.
- **Prevention**: Change maintenance solutions for something less allergenic. Wear rigid or semi-rigid gas permeable contact lenses.

Corneal Abrasion from Contact Lenses

Irritation of the cornea due to the presence of one or more particles between the backside of the lens and the cornea.

- **Causes**: Tends to be more common with rigid lenses. A speck of invisible dust on the backside of the contact lens can be enough to cause it, especially if the eyes are rubbed with the lens in place.
- **Symptoms**: Sensation of a foreign object.
- **Prevention**: Clean the contact lens well.

Corneal Neovascularization Due to Contact Lenses

Appearance of small capillaries over the cornea.

- **Causes**: Corneal oxygenation deficiency due to lenses that are too tight.
- **Prevention**: Change the type of contact lens.

Corneal Edema Due to Contact Lenses

Swelling of the cornea due to fluid retention. Its sensitivity decreases, due to which it becomes weak and more prone to infection. It is the most common serious complication from wearing contact lenses.

- **Causes**: Insufficient oxygenation (asphyxia) of the cornea due to:
  - Lenses that are too tight or too small, which impede the circulation of tears between the cornea and the contact lens.
  - Insufficient blinking, due to a an inhibition reflex: when it bumps the edge of the contact lens, the eyelid does not close completely. This reduces the circulation of the tear fluid between the contact lens and the cornea, which is necessary for oxygenation of the cornea.
- **Symptoms**: Pain and blurry vision after removal of the contact lens.
- **Complications**: If it continues, a corneal ulcer may develop.
- **Prevention**: Avoid contact lenses that are too tight. Do not leave them on overnight.

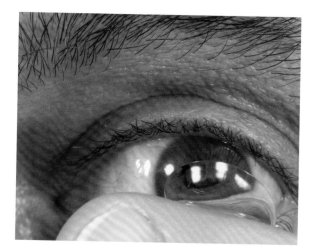

Corneal Ulcer due to Contact Lenses

Loss of corneal substance with added bacterial infection. It is the most serious complication from wearing contact lenses.

- **Causes**:
  - Insufficient cleansing of the contact lenses.
  - Excessive continuous use.
- **Symptoms**: Pain, sensation of a foreign object, secretion, redness of the eye

What to Do if You Have Complications

- Remove the contact lenses immediately: this is usually enough to alleviate the discomfort.
- Do not strain your vision for 24 hours.
- Apply an eye compress.
- Do an eye massage.
- A corneal ulcer requires specialized attention by an ophthalmologist.

Contact Lenses and the Cornea

The cornea does not receive any blood flow, therefore its cells are oxygenated from the oxygen dissolved in the lachrymal fluid that continuously bathes it.

For this reason, contact lenses should not be too tight over the cornea, so they will allow the lachrymal fluid to freely circulate behind them.

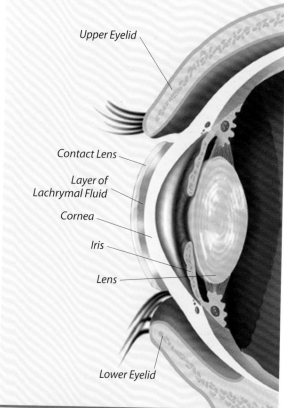

Upper Eyelid

Contact Lens

Layer of Lachrymal Fluid

Cornea

Iris

Lens

Lower Eyelid

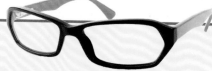

Contact Lenses and Glasses

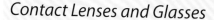

Advantages of Contact Lenses over Glasses

- More effective in correction of visual defects (myopia, hyperopia and astigmatism), especially when these are not severe.
- They can stop the progression of visual defects, especially myopia.
- They increase the visual field.
- They help to see distances better.
- Recommended for driving and sports

Inconveniences of Contact Lenses as Compared to Glasses

- They require a certain adjustment period and strict hygiene.
- Risk of corneal edema, which can become complicated by a corneal ulcer.
- Risk of eye infection, caused more often by Pseudomonas bacteria and fungus.
- Risk of intolerance to cleansing and maintenance products.
- Poorly tolerated in cases of dry eyes with insufficient tear production.
- Unsatisfactory results in cases of presbyopia (farsightedness).

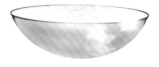

Nose

Filters infectious agents and senses aromas that are capable of stirring emotions.

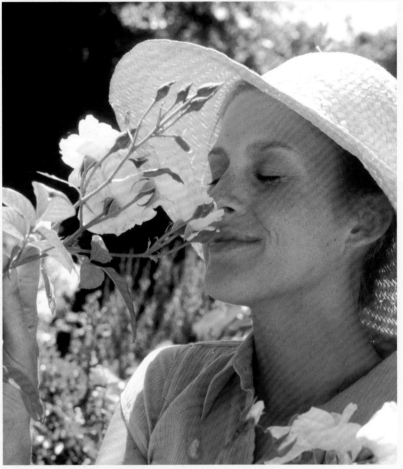

Love Enters Through the Nose
Olfactory sensations influence the nerve centers related to feelings and sexuality.

When a virus gets into the body, the first line of defense that tends to confront it is contained in the mucosa inside the nasal passages. That is where antibodies and secretions capable of eliminating infectious agents are produced. This is why it is so important to keep the nasal mucosa in good condition.

The nose and paranasal sinuses make up a single anatomical and functional unit. The sinuses are cavities inside the facial bones. They are called paranasal because they are found alongside the nasal passages.

Both the inside of the nasal passages and the inside of the paranasal sinuses are lined with a mucous membrane that is capable of secreting and moving mucus.

Facts and Figures About the Nose

3 cm² (0.46 sq in)	Surface area of the pituitary membrane or sensitive area of the nose (in dogs, 30 cm²)
1 000	Number of chemical receptors in each olfactory neuron.
4 000	Number of different scents that can be perceived.
10 000 000	Number of olfactory neurons.

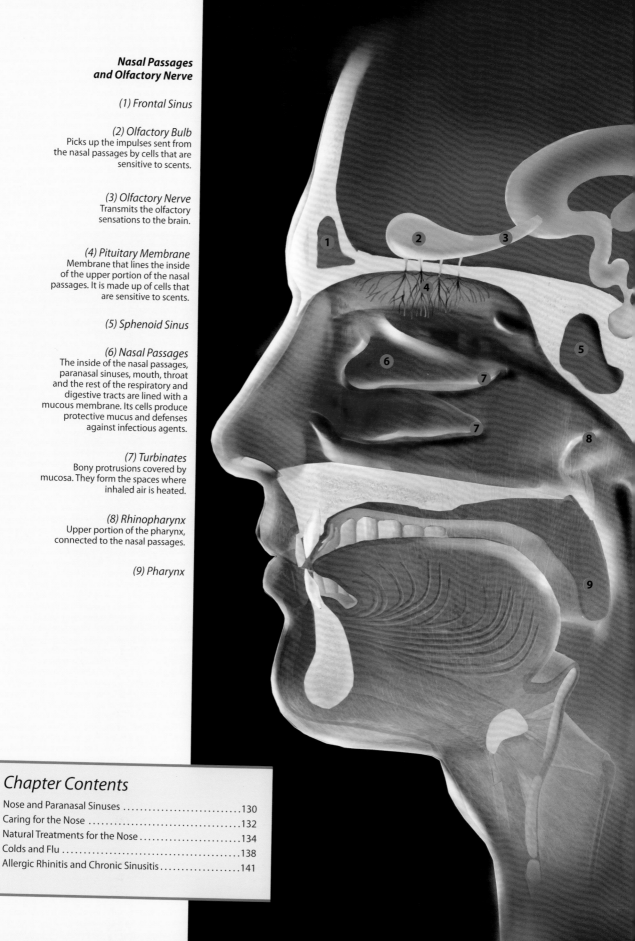

Nasal Passages and Olfactory Nerve

(1) Frontal Sinus

(2) Olfactory Bulb
Picks up the impulses sent from the nasal passages by cells that are sensitive to scents.

(3) Olfactory Nerve
Transmits the olfactory sensations to the brain.

(4) Pituitary Membrane
Membrane that lines the inside of the upper portion of the nasal passages. It is made up of cells that are sensitive to scents.

(5) Sphenoid Sinus

(6) Nasal Passages
The inside of the nasal passages, paranasal sinuses, mouth, throat and the rest of the respiratory and digestive tracts are lined with a mucous membrane. Its cells produce protective mucus and defenses against infectious agents.

(7) Turbinates
Bony protrusions covered by mucosa. They form the spaces where inhaled air is heated.

(8) Rhinopharynx
Upper portion of the pharynx, connected to the nasal passages.

(9) Pharynx

Chapter Contents

NOSE AND PARANASAL SINUSES

The nasal passages are connected to the paranasal sinuses, forming a single anatomical unit, whose primary function is to warm inhaled air and allow the sense of smell. Taking care of the nose also promotes the health of the paranasal sinuses.

FUNCTIONS OF THE NOSE

1. To Warm Inhaled Air

The nasal passages, with their cavities and the spongy mucosa that lines them, constitute a veritable air-warming unit. When it passes through the nose, air acquires the temperature and humidity level required for entering the lungs.

2. To Cleanse Inhaled Air

The layer of mucus that adheres to the mucous membrane is like a treadmill that cleans. Dust particles, bacteria and other particles transported by air adhere to this layer of mucus.

3. To Smell

Inside the upper portion of the nasal passages there are nerve endings that are capable of perceiving smells.

FUNCTIONS OF THE PARANASAL SINUSES

1. Reduce the Weight of the Cranium

By forming cavities in the bones of the cranium, the sinuses allow it to weigh less.

2. Mucus Production

Mucus produced in the paranasal sinuses goes to the nasal passages and contributes to humidifying and warming the air that enters the lungs.

3. Resonance Chamber

Sinuses serve as a resonance chamber for the voice. When the sinus cavities are obstructed or full of mucus due to sinusitis, voice tone changes.

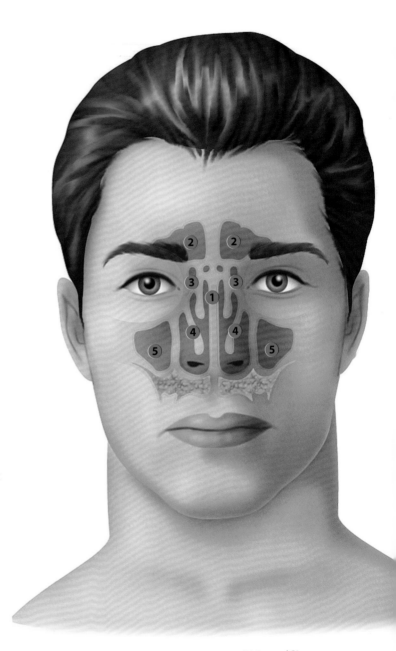

(1) *Nasal Septum*
Deviation due to a congenital defect or trauma causes breathing difficulty and promotes infection of the paranasal sinuses.

(2) *Frontal Sinuses*
(3) *Ethmoid Sinuses*
(4) *Nasal Passages*
(5) *Maxillary Sinuses*

Smell and Taste

The sense of smell goes with the sense of taste. Therefore, when we say that we like a certain food, what we really like most is how it smells. Smelling foods before eating them is a good way to promote digestive function.

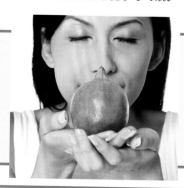

How to Blow the Nose Correctly

Blowing the nose is necessary to eliminate excess mucus that clogs the nasal passages. This improves breathing and speaking.

However, in order to avoid ear damage and contaminating others with infectious germs, certain precautions must be taken when blowing the nose.

Avoid Blowing Hard

The high pressure that comes from blowing the nose hard, especially when one of the nasal passages is stuffy, can cause damage to the nose and to the ear.

In addition, in the case of sinusitis, it is strongly recommended against, as the increased pressure pushes mucus into of the paranasal sinuses.

Good Hygiene

Nasal mucus can contain a number of infectious agents, primarily the viruses responsible for colds and flu. In order to avoid the spread of infection, very strict hygiene should be followed when blowing the nose, such as that shown on this page.

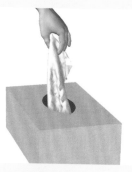

1. Use a clean tissue.

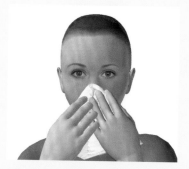

2. Hold the tissue with both hands.

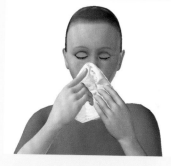

3. Blow gently, blocking only one nostril at a time. Do not start blowing by blocking both nostrils, as this causes a big increase in the pressure inside the nose that can cause ear damage.

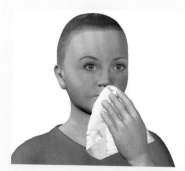

4. Clean the nose with the clean part of the tissue, or with another tissue.

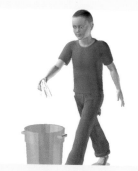

5. Discard the tissue in the trash (do not store in a pocket)).

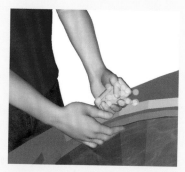

6. Wash hands with soap and water, then dry well.

CARING FOR THE NOSE

*The nose is the entry point to the respiratory system.
By taking care of the nose, good respiratory function is promoted
and infection of the bronchial tubes and lungs are prevented.*

BREATHE FRESH AIR

Smoke and irritant gases inflame the inside of the nasal passages and paranasal sinuses, promoting infection.

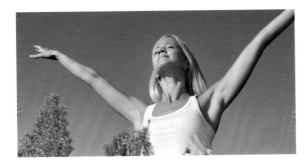

FOLLOW STRICT NASAL HYGIENE

Do not put fingers inside the nose. It is much better to irrigate the nasal passages in order to eliminate mucus, dust and infectious agents that accumulate in the nose (see "Natural Treatments for the Nose").

DO NOT PLACE FOREIGN OBJECTS INTO NASAL PASSAGES

Teach children not to place any object into their nasal passages. Food pieces, seeds, pieces of wood, paper bags or any object that enters the nose can cause infection and bleeding in the nose, along with difficulty breathing.

In Case of a Foreign Object in the Nose

- Do not try to remove it with tweezers or other devices, since this usually pushes it in deeper.
- Block the other nasal passage and have the person blow their nose gently to try to expel the foreign body.
- Seek medical care if the foreign body is not easily removed.

AVOID DRASTIC TEMPERATURE CHANGES

The mucous membrane lining the inside of the nose and paranasal sinuses is very sensitive to temperature changes, such as when entering a very cold room on a hot day.

When suddenly entering a cold place, the vessels of the mucosa must dilate in order to heat the air that enters the lungs. Similarly, when entering a hot place, the vessels of the mucosa must contract. These drastic changes weaken the mucous membrane's resistance to infectious agents.

The best air-warming unit is the one we have in our nasal passages. If the external air-warmer is abused, the nose suffers.

USE A VAPORIZER OR HUMIDIFIER

The spongy mucous membrane lining the inside of the nasal passages and paranasal sinuses secretes about 200 ml of water every day to warm the air that enters the lungs. This must reach a humidity of 70-80%, and a temperature of about 32 °C (= 90 °F).

Steam cleanses the nasal and sinus cavities, loosening secretions and making them easier to expel.

When environmental air is too dry (less than 50% relative humidity), usually due to the use of a heater inside homes, the nasal mucosa does not produce enough steam, drying and damaging it. Nasal and sinus secretions become thicker and the air that enters the lungs is not clean and warm enough.

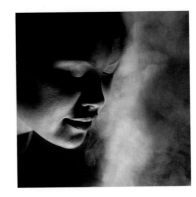

In this situation, it is necessary to use a vaporizer or humidifier. The kinds that turn cold water into steam without the need to heat it up use less electricity. They should be filled with distilled water in order to avoid the spread of germs and other impurities that non-distilled water may contain.

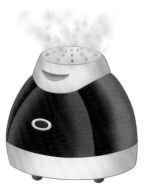

Caution

Humidity promotes the development of mites and mold on drapery and carpet. These microscopic creatures can cause allergic rhinitis. Therefore, if using a humidifier, carpets, drapery and other home fabrics clean must be kept extremely clean, or be removed from the home.

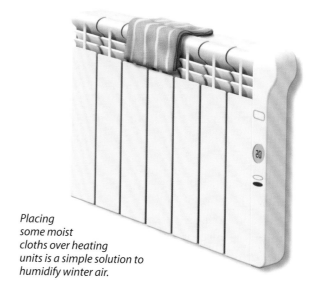

Placing some moist cloths over heating units is a simple solution to humidify winter air.

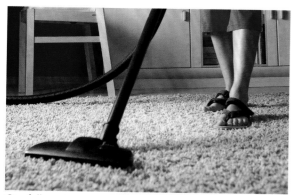

Carefully vacuum rugs and carpets, especially if using a humidifier.

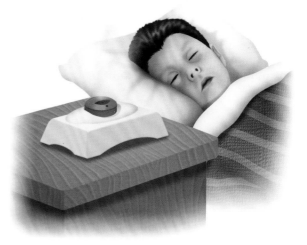

A vaporizer used at night maintains the humidity needed to protect the mucous membranes of the nose and the paranasal sinuses.

DO NOT USE COCAINE

In addition to its many damaging effects on the brain, sniffing powder cocaine through the nose produces vasoconstriction (narrowing of blood vessels) inside the nose. With less blood flow, the nasal mucosa loses sensitivity and becomes more susceptible to infection.

Because of all of this, sniffing powder cocaine causes perforation of the nasal septum and ulcers inside the nose.

Reasons You Must See a Doctor

- Obstruction of one or both nasal passages for more than two weeks, unrelated to a cold.
- Loss of the sense of smell or taste in the absence of a cold.
- Headache that worsens with lowering or moving the head, with yellowish or greenish mucus discharge.
- Nasal discharge of mucus with blood.

NATURAL TREATMENTS FOR THE NOSE - 1

There are natural treatments able to clear the nose and contribute to relieving the underlying infection or allergy. Nasal decongestants are also effective, but only temporarily, and with a potential for side effects.

IRRIGATION OF NASAL PASSAGES

This clears the inside of nasal passages of mucus, dust and infectious agents.

Irrigation of the nasal passages is the most useful technique to clear and reduce inflammation of the nasal passages. At first, it can be a bit bothersome, but it is easy to get used to doing it.

Liquids for Nasal Irrigation

Any of these liquids works for nasal irrigation:

- **Nasal saline solution** already made (sold over-the-counter).
- **Water** (preferably bottled or distilled) with table salt in the amount of 1 teaspoon (about 5 g) per half liter of water, or half a teaspoonful per cup. An excess of salt dries out the nasal mucosa. Baking soda is an alternative to salt.
- **Saline solution** (9 g of salt per liter).
- **Infusion** of one or several of these medicinal herbs (to which a teaspoon of table salt can be added per liter of water):
  – Chamomile (*Matricaria chamomilla*): Anti-inflammatory.
  – Common thyme (*Thymus vulgaris*): Antiviral.
  – Hamamelis (*Hamamelis virginiana*): Anti-inflammatory and softener.
  – Malva (*Malva silvestris*): Softener.

Caution: If are allergic to pollen, it is preferable to avoid the use of herbal infusions.

How to Introduce Liquid into the Nasal Passages

- **Irrigation with a Syringe or a Bulb Syringe**: Introduce the liquid into a nostril until it gets to the throat and is swallowed or spit out.

- **Continuous Rinse**: Tip head to one side and use a syringe or suitable container to introduce the liquid into the higher nostril. The water comes out the other nostril.nasal.

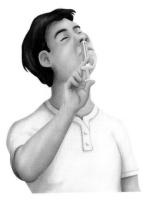

Nasal irrigation with syringe. It is best to do the irrigation in the morning and in the evening over one to two weeks.

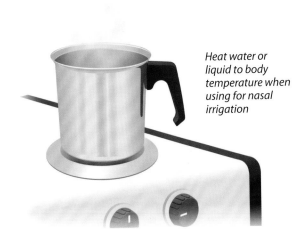

Heat water or liquid to body temperature when using for nasal irrigation

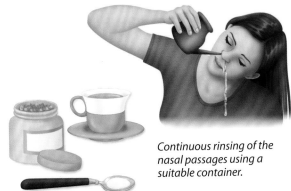

Continuous rinsing of the nasal passages using a suitable container.

For nasal rinsing and irrigation, it is best to add half a teaspoon of salt per cup of infusion.

- **Nasal inhaler** or atomizer.
- **Dropper**: Ideal for small children with nasal mucus. In children, it is best to place several drops of sterile saline solution in each nasal passage, with the head tipped back.
- **Palm of the Hand**: Place a few drops of the nasal rinse liquid into the palm of the hand. Inhale it through the nose, blocking one of the nasal passages. The water should go in through the nose and come out the mouth. Repeat with the other nasal passage.

INHALATION OF AROMATIC ESSENCES

All aromatic herbal essences are antiseptic and antiviral. Inhaling them clears the nose and relieves congestion. This can be done several times throughout the day.

Most Recommended Essences

- Common Thyme (*Thymus vulgaris*).
- Lavender (*Lavandula angustifolia*).
- Rosemary (*Rosmarinus officinalis*).
- Eucalyptus (*Eucalyptus globulus*).

Tomillo

Ways to Use the Essence

- In the palm of the hand.
- On a cloth.
- Adding a few drops of essence to a container of hot water.

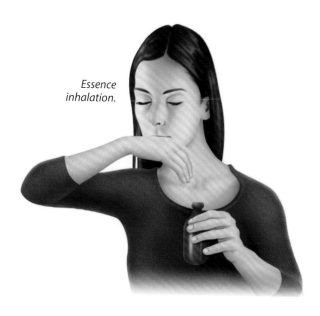

Essence inhalation.

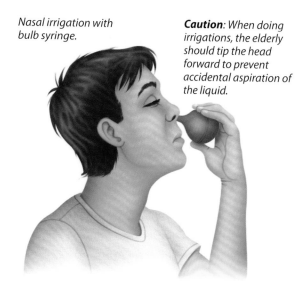

Nasal irrigation with bulb syringe.

Caution: When doing irrigations, the elderly should tip the head forward to prevent accidental aspiration of the liquid.

NASAL DECONGESTANTS

These are vasoconstrictor medications (they narrow the blood vessels) used in spray, drops, pills or syrups.

By narrowing the blood vessels inside the nose, blood flow is reduced and the mucous membranes shrink. This produces an almost immediate sensation of a clear nose.

Caution

If using nasal decongestants, keep the following precautions in mind:

- Nasal decongestants only relieve certain symptoms such as nasal obstruction, but they do not cure the cold.
- By reducing blood flow in the mucous membrane lining the inside of the nasal passages, defenses are also reduced. As a result, the viral infection that causes the cold can worsen or take longer to resolve.
- They can cause a rebound effect, increasing congestion after the initial favorable effect wears off.
- Never use them more than three times per day nor more than three days in a row.
- It is not recommended to use them in cases of heart disease, hypertension, hyperthyroidism or glaucoma, due to their potential side effects.

NATURAL TREATMENTS FOR THE NOSE - 2

Clogged nasal passages due to cold viruses or allergies force mouth-breathing, which alters the physiology of respiration. These natural treatments help unclog the nose.

SOAKING FEET IN HOT WATER

Soaking the feet in hot water decongests the nose and head in general, contributing to unclogging the nose.

Water Temperature: 36-40 °C (97-104 °F).

Duration: 10-15 minutes.

Afterward: Rub feet with a cloth soaked in cold water and put on some wool socks.

Frequency: Up to three times per day.

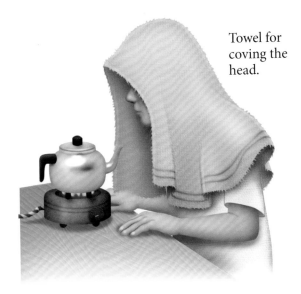

Towel for coving the head.

Container of boiling water.

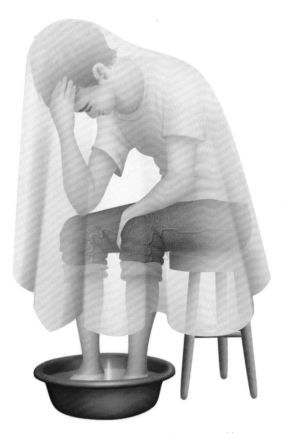

Submerge both legs at once up to above the ankles. Add hot water when the temperature decreases.

FACIAL STEAM BATH

Humidity is essential to keeping the mucosa of the nasal passages and paranasal sinuses in good condition. A facial steam bath allows a good amount of humidity to enter the nasal passages and the paranasal sinuses. In this way, impurities are cleansed and resistance to infectious agents is improved.

Taking a hot shower and inhaling the steam is also a simple way to decongest the nose.

Water Temperature: As hot as possible, to help steam production. Ideally, it should be near-boiling.

Duration: 5-10 minutes.

Afterward: Rub face and neck with cold water in order to close the skin's pores.

Frequency: One to three times per day.

COLD FACIAL COMPRESS

Cold produces vasoconstriction of the nasal passages, which relieves congestion. It also relieves the pain in cases of frontal or maxillary sinusitis. The compress can be placed on the forehead or over the cheekbones.

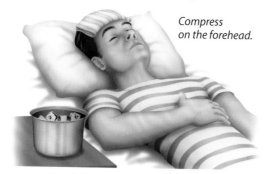

Compress on the forehead.

Moisten the cloth in cold water once every minute.

Water Temperature: 0-4 °C (32-39 °F).
Duration: 3-5 minutes.
Afterward: Cover head with a blanket or scarf.
Frequency: Up to three times per day.

SMELL AN ONION

The essence given off by onions alleviates nasal congestion, loosens mucus and fights disease-causing germs.

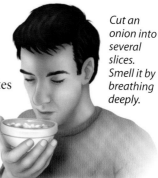

Cut an onion into several slices. Smell it by breathing deeply.

Nosebleeds

Nosebleeds, or epistaxis, is easily stopped in the majority of cases. The most important thing is to take preventive measures so that it does not happen again.

PREVENTION

With repeated nosebleeds, in addition to seeking specialized medical care, keep these preventive measures in mind:

- Do not put a finger in the nostrils.
- Do not blow nose frequently.
- Humidify air in the bedroom and the room where most of the day is spent by using a humidifier or a vaporizer.
- Apply a little bit of petroleum jelly inside the nostrils, two or three times per day.
- Do not take aspirin or other anticoagulant medications.
- Control blood pressure.
- Include sources of the following two vitamins in the diet:
  - Vitamin K, needed for blood coagulation. It is found in all green vegetables, and especially in alfalfa sprouts, Brussels sprouts and spinach.
  - Vitamin C, needed so capillaries will be tear-resistant. The bioflavonoids present naturally in bright-colored fruits and vegetables increase its effect. Citrus fruits, berries such as gooseberries, strawberries and blackberries, and kiwi, are good sources of vitamin C and bioflavonoids.

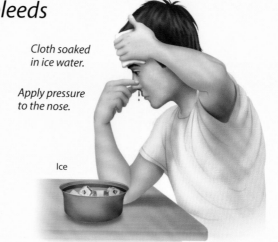

Cloth soaked in ice water.

Apply pressure to the nose.

Ice

FIRST AID FOR A NOSEBLEED

- Sit or stand (do not lie down) to reduce the flow of blood to the head.
- Tip head forward to avoid swallowing the blood.
- Place a cotton cloth that has been soaked in ice water on the forehead, face and/or back of the neck.
- Apply pressure to the sides of the nose with the thumb and forefinger. Ninety-nine percent of nosebleeds stop after 10 minutes of pressure on the soft parts of the nose.
- Soak a cotton ball in hydrogen peroxide and place it into the bleeding nostril.
- If the bleeding does not stop within 10 or 15 minutes, go to a hospital.

COLDS AND FLU - 1

PREVENTION

Cold temperatures make the cells of the mucous layer lining the inside of the nose and throat more sensitive, causing colds. Preventing a cold is easier than treating it.

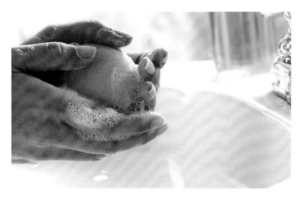

WASH HANDS

Hands are the primary transmitter of cold-causing viruses. Frequent hand washing, especially after shaking hands or being with other people, prevents the spread of viruses.

DO NOT TOUCH THE FACE WITH HANDS

When the nose, eyes or mouth are touched by hands, these can introduce infectious agents into the body.

AVOID CROWDS

Cold-causing viruses travel by way of saliva droplets projected when speaking, coughing or sneezing. The more people we have around us, and the closer they are to us, the greater the risk of their transmitting the cold virus or other infectious agents to us.

VENTILATE ROOMS WELL

Poorly ventilated rooms can harbor viruses and other infectious agents. Windows need to be opened in order to circulate the air, for at least a little while each day.

CAREFUL WITH AIR CONDITIONING

- Avoid the drastic changes in temperature when coming into a chilled environment due to very cold air conditioning, or when leaving.
- Be sure that there is adequate maintenance of the air conditioning unit, including regular changing of filters, where viruses can nest.

BREATHE FRESH AIR

Although it is cold, the fresh air in forests and mountains is preferable for cold prevention, as compared to the air in confined environments and where there is tobacco smoke. Whenever possible, get out to the countryside to breathe in the fresh air of the forest.

GET ENOUGH REST

Keeping regular rest periods, not staying up all night and avoiding stress help keep the immune system in good condition and prevent colds.

WARM CLOTHING

When it is cold, the neck, ears, hands, and feet, as well as the abdomen, should be especially protected. These body parts are sensitive areas, and when they get cold, there is a vasoconstriction reflex (narrowing of the blood vessels) in the mucosa of the nose.

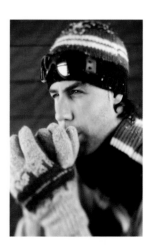

DRINK ENOUGH WATER

Staying well-hydrated by drinking at least 6-8 glasses of pure water per day contributes to protecting the respiratory mucosa against viruses.

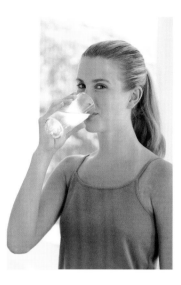

HUMIDIFY THE ENVIRONMENT

Indoors where it is dry due to heating, it is good to use humidifiers. Dry air due to a combination of heating and insufficient ventilation irritates the respiratory mucosa and promotes colds.

WEAR A PROTECTIVE MASK

In case of an epidemic, a facial mask is a very effective way to stop the spread of the viruses responsible for colds and flu.

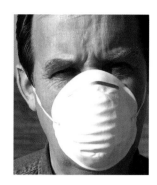

AVOID ABUSE OF ANTIBIOTICS

Do not take antibiotics unnecessarily, since they weaken defenses. Viral infections such as colds, flu, and many cases of bronchitis and of sinusitis are not cured or improved with antibiotics.

Having nasal mucus does not necessarily require the use of antibiotics. Actually, mucus is a defense mechanism to eliminate viruses from the nasal mucosa.

When mucus stops being fluid and transparent, and becomes yellowish or greenish, it could be due to a bacterial superinfection of the nasal passages or paranasal sinuses (sinusitis). Antibiotics should only be taken if prescribed by a doctor.

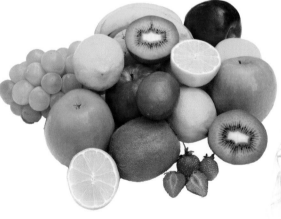

WATCH THE DIET

- Eat lots of fruits and vegetables that are rich in vitamin C and other antioxidants, such as fruits in general and particularly oranges and other citrus fruits, kiwi and dog rose (*Rosa canina*).
- Eliminate or reduce consumption of cow's milk and dairy products, as they promote mucus production in the nose and airways.

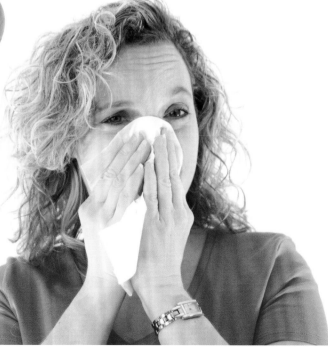

COLODS AND FLU - 2

NATURAL TREATMENT

*The immune system's defenses against infection are what
eventually overcome the viruses responsible for nose colds and the flu.
These natural treatments strengthen the defenses.*

When prevention has not worked and a cold has finally begun, the infection has to run its course. It is the body's defenses –not antibiotics– that truly eliminate the viruses that cause colds, as well as restore the nasal and respiratory mucosa.

If the cold is not complicated by sinusitis, otitis, pneumonia or asthmatic bronchitis, these simple natural remedies are generally enough to fight the infection, strengthen the nasal mucosa and promote a speedy recovery.

HYDRATION AND REST

Drink plenty of fluids and rest at home, for at least three days.

NATURAL TREATMENTS

These are the most effective in relieving nose colds and flu (see "Natural Treatments for the Nose"):
- Irrigation of the nasal passages.
- Facial steam bath.
- Soaking feet in hot water.
- Inhaling antiviral aromatic essences such as lavender and common thyme.

VITAMIN C

Vitamin C is necessary for immune system health. It can be taken as supplements, in addition to increasing fruit consumption in general, especially oranges, lemons and other citrus fruits, kiwi and dog rose.

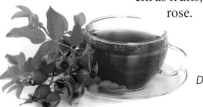

Dog rose infusion

BETA-CAROTENE

Vegetable beta-carotene or pro-vitamin A is a natural colorant in many fruits and vegetables, which has an intense antioxidant effect. In the body, beta-carotene is converted into vitamin A, which needed for the good health of the cells of the mucosa.

A glass of carrot juice a day during a cold guarantees the supply of vitamin A. Mangos, squash, oranges and spinach are also good sources of the antioxidant carotenoids that are converted into vitamin A.

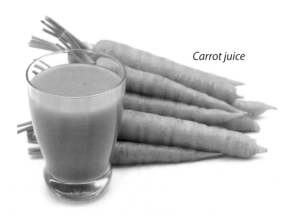

Carrot juice

GARLIC AND ONION

It has been shown that garlic and onion essences eliminate viruses; in addition, they are antioxidants and immunostimulants (they boost the defenses).

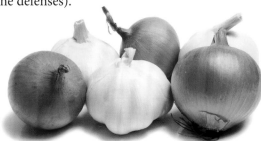

Garlic and onions

ALLERGIC RHINITIS AND CHRONIC SINUSITIS

PREVENTION

It is easier to prevent these conditions than to treat them.

Allergic rhinitis is the inflammation of the nasal mucosa triggered by an allergic reaction, generally to the pollen of certain plants or house dust. It manifests as nasal drainage, itching and congestion, usually in springtime.

Chronic sinusitis is the persistent infection of the paranasal sinuses, often after an acute sinusitis. It can also be allergy-based.

The following recommendations are useful in the prevention of both allergic rhinitis and chronic sinusitis.

WATCH INDOOR AIR QUALITY

- Keep bedrooms and other rooms well-ventilated.
- Remove or frequently vacuum and clean carpets, drapery, rugs, wool blankets, down comforters and other objects that retain dust.
- Do not allow dogs and cats indoors.

CAREFUL WITH CERTAIN MEDICATIONS

- Avoid continuous use of nasal decongestants, which can have a "rebound effect" and promote inflammation of the nasal mucosa.

LOCAL HYGIENE

- Irrigate the nasal passages to wash away allergens that may have entered the nose (see "Irrigation of Nasal Passages" under "Natural Treatments for the Nose").

WATCH THE DIET

- Check to see of the allergic rhinitis could be due to some food allergy. Cow's milk and dairy products are the foods that most often cause allergies. By simply eliminating milk and all types of dairy products, allergic rhinitis improves in many cases.
- Follow an antialleric diet, based on raw fruits, vegetables, and seeds. This diet can be followed for a day or two every week, or for a whole week during periods of greater allergy activity.
- Supplements: Vitamin C (500 mg per day) and zinc (30-50 mg per day) contribute to the good condition of the nasal mucosa.

ALLERGY VACCINATION

Allergy vaccinations prescribed by an allergy doctor have good results in preventing repeated attacks of rhinitis and sinusitis.

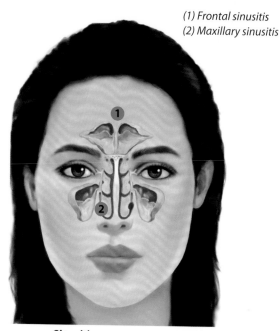

(1) Frontal sinusitis
(2) Maxillary sinusitis

Sinusitis
Buildup of mucus and inflammation of the mucosa in the paranasal sinuses.

Ears

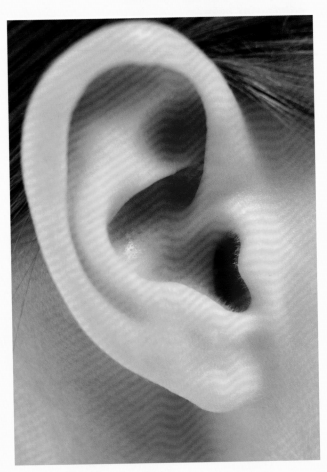

The ear's high degree of sensitivity can be lost if it is subjected to noise, or in other words, unpleasant sounds.

The organs of hearing and balance

The ears stand out for their sensitivity, not only to the pressure of sound waves transmitted through the air, but also to minor head movements. The ear's range of sensitivity to pressure is extremely broad, varying from 20 μp (micropascals, a unit of pressure) which is equivalent to a sound at 0 dB (decibels), up to 20 000 000 μp, which is the pressure of a sound at 120 dB. In other words, the ear is capable of detecting not only a very soft sound, but also one that is 2 million times louder.

The balance organ located in the inner ear is able to make a geometrically precise determination of the head's exact position.

Such sensitive organs should not be subjected to the rough sound stimuli of modern technology, such as amplifiers with hundreds or thousands of watts, or to headphones set at a loud volume. Just as ear hygiene is important to its care, so much more is preventing the wear caused by loud sounds and the continuous noise of modern life.

Facts and Figures About the Ear

1 x 0.5 x 0.5 cm (0.39 x 0.2 x 0.2 in)	Measurement of the middle ear (height x length x depth)
16 to 30 000	Number of vibrations per second (Hertz) that a child can detect with his ear. In an adult, it is up to 4 000.
55 mg (0.002 oz)	Weight of the 3 tiny bones in the middle ear that transmit sound vibrations.
4 000	Number of wax-producing glands in the auditory canal.
30 000	Number of nerve fibers that make up the auditory nerve.

(1) Outer Ear
Outer auditory canal.

(2) Middle Ear
Picks up, transmits and amplifies sound vibrations from the eardrum to the inner ear, by way of three tiny interconnected bones.

(3) Inner Ear
Inside of it, sound vibrations convert to electrical impulses thanks to the auditory receptor cells located inside the cochlea.

(4) Eardrum
Taut membrane that vibrates when sound waves reach it.
The vibration of the eardrum is amplified and transmitted to the auditory nerve by way of three tiny interconnected bones

Otoscopy

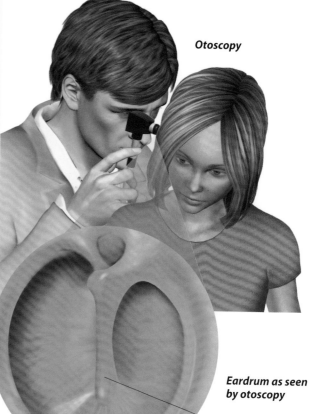

Eardrum as seen by otoscopy

Protrusion caused by the hammer bone.

Stirrup

Anvil

Hammer

(5) Cochlea
Contains the Organ of Corti, made up of hearing receptor cells.

(6) Auditory or Vestibulocochlear Nerve
Transmits information to the brain about sound and about changes in head position.

(7) Semicircular Canals
These are the balance organ. They are located in the three directions of space. They contain a gelatinous fluid called endolymph that stimulates balance receptors.

Chapter Contents

Caring for the Ears - 1

The obsession with completely eliminating wax from the ear should be avoided.
Having a little wax is not bad hygiene, but rather normal and necessary.

Protect the Ears from the Cold and the Wind

On cold days, especially when it is windy, the ears should be protected. Children's ears are especially sensitive to cold, which can trigger otitis.

- Wear a scarf.
- Place a cotton ball in each ear, but not too tightly.

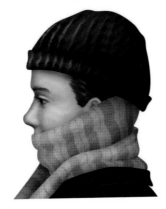

Wear a Helmet for Head Protection

When riding a bicycle, skating or skateboarding, wear a helmet that protects the head. Blows to the ears can permanently damage the eardrum.

In addition, an accidental fall can cause a temporal bone fracture with an associated permanent hearing loss.

Do Not Blow the Nose Hard

With hard nose blowing, especially if both nostrils are blocked at the same time, air pressure greatly increases within the nasal passages. This increase in pressure is transmitted to the middle ear by way of the Eustachian tubes, which connect the nasal passages to the middle ear on either side.

The middle ear is affected by increased pressure in the nasal passages. In addition, with hard nose-blowing, germ-filled mucus in the nose is pushed through the Eustachian tubes toward the middle ear, which can cause otitis media.

See the correct technique for nose blowing in Chapter 5, which is dedicated to the nose.

Avoid Exposure to Smoke

Exposure to tobacco smoke, whether actively or passively, weakens the immune system and promotes ear infections, which can later lead to hearing loss.

A study by the University of Oslo (Norway) with 2 549 children who were followed until the age of 10 has shown that those who have parents who are smokers are more likely to get respiratory infections, including otitis media.[a]

Exposure to smoke caused by a wood fire for cooking indoors is an important risk factor for otitis media in children. At the University of Awolowo of Ile-Ife (Nigeria), it has been shown that children who live in an environment where there is smoke indoors are much more likely to suffer middle ear infections.[b]

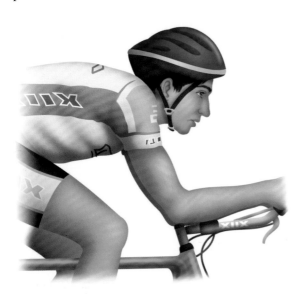

a. Early acute otitis media: predictor for AOM and respiratory infections in schoolchildren? Bentdal YE, Karevold G, Nafstad P, Kvaerner KJ. Int J Pediatr Otorhinolaryngol. 2007 Aug;71(8):1251-9. Epub 2007 Jun 7. PMID: 17559950

b. Epidemiology of otitis media in a local tropical African population. Amusa YB, Ijadunola IK, Onayade OO. West Afr J Med. 2005 Jul-Sep;24(3):227-30. PMID: 16276700

Do not smoke during pregnancy

Tobacco smoke harms the fetus in many ways, one of which is weakening of the ear. A study done at the maternity hospital in South Brisbane (Australia) with 8,556 women showed that children of those who smoked during pregnancy had up to 3.3 times more risk of acute ear infections than children of those who did not smoke.[a]

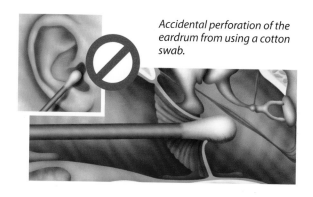

Accidental perforation of the eardrum from using a cotton swab.

PROPER WAX CLEANING

The presence of ear wax is normal and necessary to protect the eardrum. Wax is produced by glands located in the auditory canal.

Purpose of Ear Wax

- Waterproofing (repels water).
- Traps dust and even insects.
- Antiseptic (barrier against infectious agents).
- Skin protection and softening.

Cleaning Techniques

- Clean the wax only when it is visible at the opening of the auditory canal. Bathing and chewing tend to move wax and make it visible from the outside. Use a cloth or gauze that has been moistened, never dry.
- Use pharmaceutical saltwater diffusers, which soften and eliminate the wax plug.

Avoid Cotton Swabs

- Children should be taught never to place any object into the auditory canal, such as swabs, pencils or other objects.

- Swabs and other objects placed in the ear tend to push wax inward, completely closing the canal and potentially injuring the delicate eardrum.
- Use of cotton swabs can injure the skin within the canal, and even the eardrum, especially in children, whose auditory canal is shorter than it seems.
- Rubbing stimulates wax production in the ear. Therefore, rubbing the auditory canal with the dry cotton on the swabs, or with the tip of a cloth, causes skin irritation and increases wax production.

PRECAUTIONS FOR SWIMMERS

- Wear silicon or wax earplugs if there is a tendency toward external otitis, or when swimming in public pools.
- Upon getting out of the water, the head should be shaken to get rid of the water that could still be in the ears.
- Dry the external ear gently, without scrubbing it with the towel. Do not rub inside the ear with dry cloths or cotton. The skin of the external auditory canal is very delicate, and scrubbing it eliminates the natural protective wax.
- Do not use shampoo or soap directly on the external auditory canal.
- Gently rub the auditory canal with the tip of a cloth that has been soaked in lemon juice or vinegar, as the skin on the ears needs a certain level of acidity.
- Do not remove earwax unless it is visible from the outside.

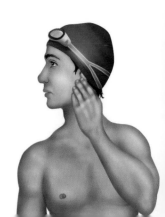

---

a. Maternal cigarette smoking during pregnancy is an independent predictor for symptoms of middle ear disease at five years' postdelivery. Pediatrics. Stathis SL, O'Callaghan DM, Williams GM, Najman JM, Andersen MJ, Bor W. 1999 Aug;104(2):e16. PMID: 10429134

Reasons you Must See a Doctor

- Pus or blood in the ear, with or without associated pain.
- Sudden loss of hearing in one or both ears.
- Sudden onset dizziness or vertigo.

CARING FOR THE EARS - 2

*Wax plugs should be eliminated by taking certain precautions,
more than anything, by not introducing any object into the auditory canal.*

EAR HYGIENE

- Wash your ears gently with a cloth soaked in soap and water.
- Tip your head toward the side where you are washing your ears, to avoid water getting into the auditory canal.
- Apply petroleum jelly or a hydrating cream onto the external auditory canal when it is dry or irritated.

DO NOT ATTEMPT TO REMOVE FOREIGN OBJECTS FROM THE EAR

Removal of a foreign object from the ear should be done by specialized healthcare providers.

Never put tweezers or pointed objects into the ear, as they tend to push the foreign object in farther.

BALANCE THE PRESSURE IN THE INNER EAR

When there are sudden changes in the atmospheric pressure (trips by airplane, going up or down mountain passes), the pressure in the middle ear must become balanced with that on the outside by way of the Eustachian tube. This canal connects the middle ear to the throat.

Methods to balance the pressure in the middle ear.
- Open and close your jaw.
- Swallow often or chew gum.

ELIMINATE WAX PLUGS

Sometimes, earwax becomes hard and dry, forming a plug in the auditory canal. This can cause:
- Bothersome noises in the ear, especially with chewing.
- Hearing loss: This occurs only rarely, when the wax plug completely obstructs the canal. A small crack between the plug and the skin is enough to allow the passage of sound.

Ear Irrigation

Removal of wax plugs in the ear merits the help of healthcare providers. It can also be done carefully at home if the following precautions are taken:

- Never place tweezers or other objects into the auditory canal, as this only impacts the wax even more. In addition, it can damage the eardrum.
- For two or three days before irrigating the ear, apply two or three drops of an oleosome solution or olive oil each day in order to soften the wax. After applying the drops, lay down on the side of the opposite ear for 5-10 minutes. When you get back up, clean the oil with a cloth, if it comes out of the ear. A little cotton can be gently placed in the opening of the auditory canal.
- Irrigate the auditory canal with lukewarm water (body temperature).
- Direct the stream up and back, so that it hits the wax plug laterally. If the stream impacts the plug directly, it compacts it even more.

Avoid Saturated Fats

Hard fats, such as those in meat, luncheon meats, bacon and other meat products, contribute to increased earwax production, and makes the earwax harder.

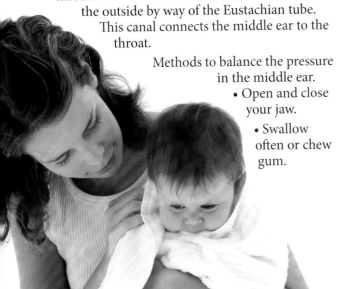

Hot Cone for the Ear

This is a method used traditionally in South America for ear hygiene. In the past, the cone was made out of plant leaves, but today there are paper cones with a protective disk available in stores in many countries.

The beneficial effect of burning the cone is due to a combination of two factors:

- The heat, which softens the wax.
- The air suction inside the cone, due to the chimney effect.

Caution: Do not do this on yourself, in order to avoid fire accidents.

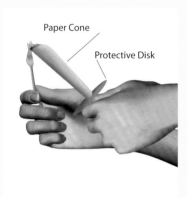

Paper Cone

Protective Disk

1. Light the paper on fire.

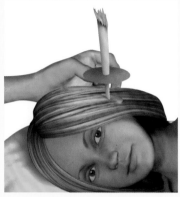

2. Place the paper cone and its protective disk over the ear, in the auditory canal.

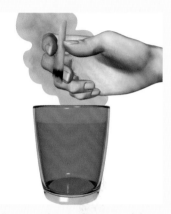

3. Leave in place in the ear until the paper burns all the way down.
4. Remove from the ear and extinguish in a glass of water.

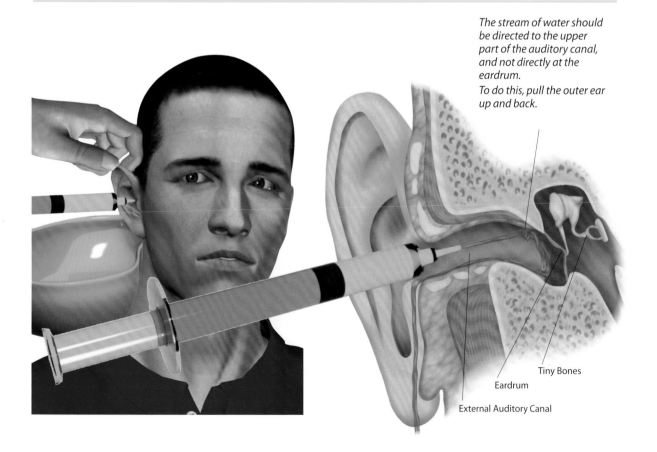

The stream of water should be directed to the upper part of the auditory canal, and not directly at the eardrum.
To do this, pull the outer ear up and back.

Tiny Bones

Eardrum

External Auditory Canal

CARING FOR THE EARS - 3

HEARING PROTECTION

*Loud sounds, such as those that may come from headphones
for listening to music, are an attack on the ear.*

SEE A SPECIALIST REGULARLY

It is recommended to see an otorhinolaryngologist for an ear exam at least once a year for both children and adults. This way, infection can be prevented and possible hearing loss can be detected.

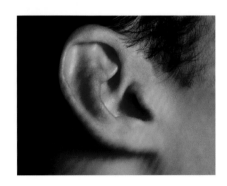

USE PROTECTIVE HEADGEAR IN LOUD ENVIRONMENTS

When they are well placed, headgear can reduce sound intensity between 15 and 30 decibels. Keep in mind that exposure to a sound over 90 decibels, such as that produced by a heavy truck 6 meters away, can temporarily damage hearing.

DECIBELS: THE INTENSITY OF SOUND

Exposure to a sound over 90 decibels can cause a temporary hearing disorder.

If exposure to loud sounds is continuous, it will cause permanent hearing loss. The first symptom of hearing damage is a permanent ringing after the loud sound or noise stops.

Common Causes of Hearing Damage

- Dance clubs.
- Headphones on electronic music devices, such as MP3 players.
- Explosives.
- Nearby jet engines.
- Jackhammers or other machinery.
- Motorcycles or cars without a muffler.

PAY ATTENTION TO MEDICATIONS

There are around 200 medications classified as ototoxic, which means that they can damage the ear (see "Improving Hearing").

Carefully read the information about the medication to be taken, especially if there are already hearing problems.

LOWER HEADPHONE VOLUME

Some electronic devices can provide the ear with up to 120 decibels, a sound intensity that is equivalent to an airplane taking off.

The general rule for ear protection is to lower headphone volume enough to be able to hear the voice of someone nearby.

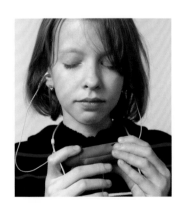

If a person speaking two or three meters away cannot be understood, headphone volume is too high.

Decibels: The Intensity of Sound

The decibel is the unit of measure for sound intensity.

Decibels follow a logarithmic scale. That is, a 10 dB (decibel) increase represents a sound that is 10 times louder. If the increase is 20 dB, the sound intensity increases 100 times.

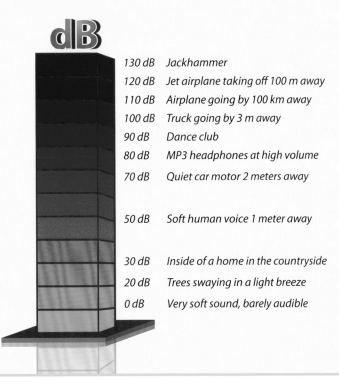

130 dB	Jackhammer
120 dB	Jet airplane taking off 100 m away
110 dB	Airplane going by 100 km away
100 dB	Truck going by 3 m away
90 dB	Dance club
80 dB	MP3 headphones at high volume
70 dB	Quiet car motor 2 meters away
50 dB	Soft human voice 1 meter away
30 dB	Inside of a home in the countryside
20 dB	Trees swaying in a light breeze
0 dB	Very soft sound, barely audible

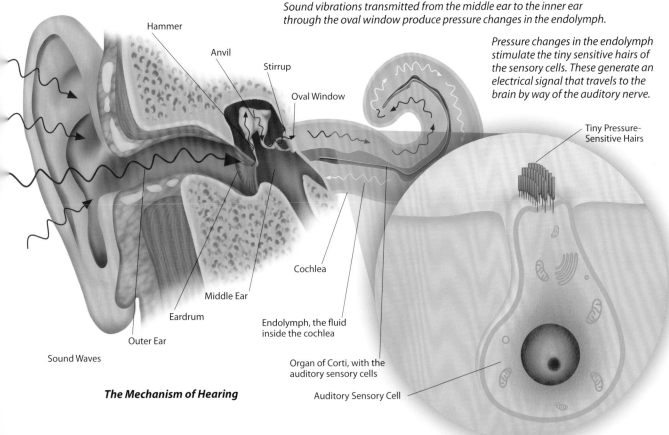

Sound vibrations transmitted from the middle ear to the inner ear through the oval window produce pressure changes in the endolymph.

Pressure changes in the endolymph stimulate the tiny sensitive hairs of the sensory cells. These generate an electrical signal that travels to the brain by way of the auditory nerve.

Hammer · Anvil · Stirrup · Oval Window · Tiny Pressure-Sensitive Hairs · Cochlea · Middle Ear · Eardrum · Endolymph, the fluid inside the cochlea · Outer Ear · Sound Waves · Organ of Corti, with the auditory sensory cells · Auditory Sensory Cell

The Mechanism of Hearing

NATURAL TREATMENTS FOR THE EARS

Heat and oil are two great remedies for the ears.

HOT BAG ON THE EAR

Heat, especially moist heat, is the most effective remedy to relieve ear pain from otitis media, especially in children.

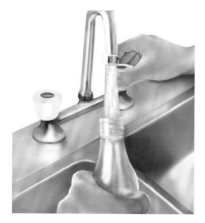

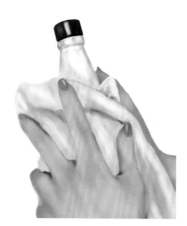

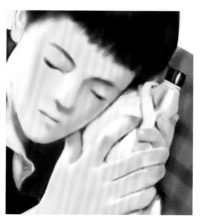

1. Fill a bag or bottle with hot water. The water should be at a comfortable temperature (around 32 °C, about 90 °F), so it will produce a pleasant sensation.

2. Wrap the bag or bottle with a soft towel or cloth.

3. Support the aching ear with the hot bag or bottle.

HOT COMPRESS ON THE EAR

This is a pleasant and effective way to apply heat to the ear.

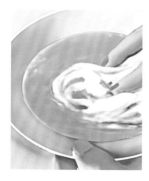

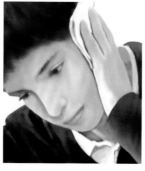

1. Soak a small towel or cloth in hot water.

2. Wring out, then apply onto the affected ear.
If the water is very hot, a thin cloth can be placed in order to protect facial skin. Soak the towel again when it cools down.

AUDITORY CANAL IRRIGATION

Wet the tip of a cloth with lemon juice or vinegar and gently rub the irritated auditory canal.

The skin on the auditory canal is quite sensitive, and needs a certain level of acidity. When the skin becomes irritated, acids such as lemon or vinegar help regain balance.

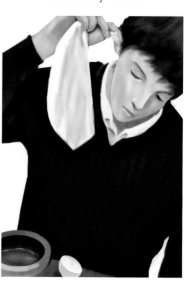

OIL EARDROPS

Two or three drops of oil in the ear relieve the pain of inflammation in otitis media. Heat the oil slightly before placing it into the ear, up to a temperature of 32 °C (about 90 °F).

Caution: Do not use oil when the ear is draining, as the eardrum could be perforated. In this case, the oil could get into the middle ear, where it would act like a foreign object.

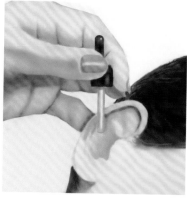

1. Heat a little oil to body temperature. Place two or three drops into the affected ear with the help of a dropper.

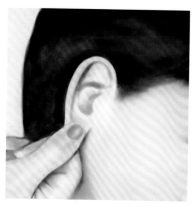

2. Pull on the ear to help the oil penetrate.

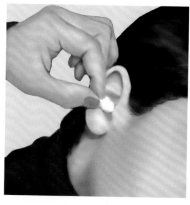

3. Gently cover the ear opening with a cotton ball.

Garlic Oil

For a better effect against infection, garlic oil can be placed in the ear, in either pearls or capsules, or homemade.

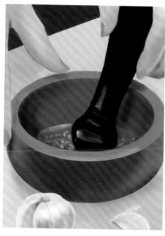

1a. To make homemade garlic oil, crush garlic and place it to marinate in olive oil for three or four hours.

1b. To use a garlic oil pearl or capsule, heat it up first then poke a pinhole in it.

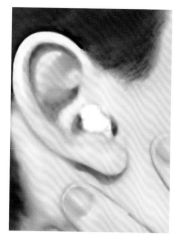

2. Place some drops into the ear and gently cover the opening with a cotton ball.

Medicinal Flowers for the Ears

With the flowers of common mullein (*Verbascum thapsus*) and pot marigold (*Calendula officinalis*), pharmacies make medicinal oils that are anti-infective and anti-inflammatory, recommended for use in ear infections. These oils are applied as eardrops to relieve pain and fight infection.

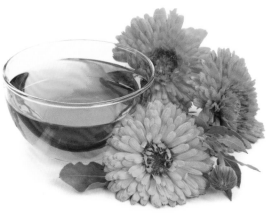

Pot Marigold Oil

IMPROVING HEARING

Hearing loss is usually a slow and unnoticeable process.
When it is noticed, the hearing loss already tends to be significant.
Protecting against excessive environmental noise is the most effective
measure to prevent hearing loss.

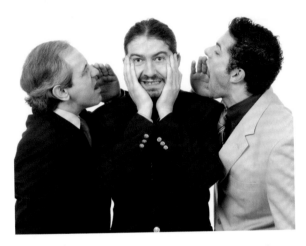

Having to strain the voice to keep up a conversation indicates that there is too much background noise that is potentially dangerous to the ears.

PROTECT AGAINST NOISE AND LOUD SOUNDS

Before starting a noisy activity, protect against noise with headgear or earplugs. Noise over 90 decibels irreversibly damages hearing.

If using headphones to listen to music, the volume should be low enough to be able to hear the voice of someone nearby.

PREVENTION OF CONGENITAL HEARING DEFECTS

Get vaccinated against rubella, if you have not been already. It is ideal to vaccinate girls before puberty. A blood test can be done to determine immunity to this virus.

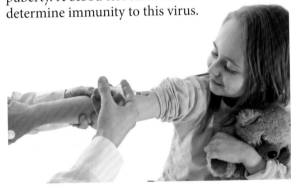

Hearing Loss Due to Noise

Noise causes permanent degeneration in the auditory nerve cells in the cochlea, within the inner ear. Once the sensory cells of the inner ear become damaged, there is no possibility for recovery.

Hearing loss due to noise is not generally noticed in early phases, unless a hearing test is done.

Noise exposure starts affecting the perception of high frequencies, over 4,000 cycles (that is, the first to go is the ability to hear very shrill sounds).

EFFECTS OF NOISE ON THE BODY
- Deteriorates the sense of hearing
- Triggers physiological reactions to stress
- Causes anxiety
- Speeds up the pulse and increases blood pressure
- Speeds up breathing
- Dilates the pupils
- Affects the ability to pay attention and concentrate
- Reduces intellectual performance
- Slows reflexes

Before Pregnancy
Get vaccinated against rubella, if you have not been already. It is ideal to vaccinate girls before puberty. A blood test can be done to determine immunity to this virus.

During Pregnancy
Avoid contact with children who are ill with fever and skin rash, as they could have rubella and spread the virus to the pregnant woman.

Infection with cytomegalovirus and the herpes virus, toxoplasmosis, and syphilis during pregnancy can also cause congenital deafness.

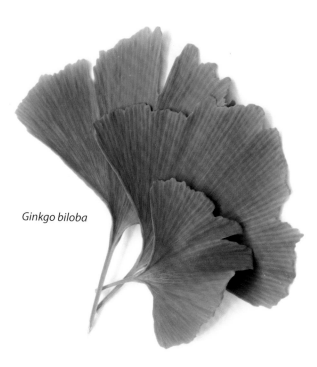

Ginkgo biloba

USE GINKGO BILOBA

Leaves from the ginkgo tree, whether as an infusion or extract, are good for the ears. Due to its vasodilation effect, blood flow is increased in the inner ear and the brain, strengthening the sense of hearing. In addition, they are antioxidants, so they neutralize free radicals, which are toxic molecules that deteriorate the delicate auditory receptors.

The effectiveness of ginkgo leaves has been shown specifically in the following cases:

• Sudden deafness: A study done by the University of Heidelberg (Germany) showed that ginkgo extract offers better results than pentoxifylline (a vasodilator) for the treatment of sudden deafness.[a]

• Tinnitus (ringing in the ears): Ginkgo extract (80 mg twice a day) taken over 12 weeks has been shown to be effective and safe for the treatment of tinnitus, according to a study by St Georg de Hamburgo hospital (Germany).[b]

AVOID TOBACCO AND COFFEE

Both nicotine and caffeine tighten arteries and reduce blood flow in the delicate inner ear.

WATCH OUT FOR OTOTOXIC MEDICATIONS

• Aminoglycosidic antibiotics such as streptomycin and gentamicin: They damage the ears' sensory cells. When a pregnant woman takes these antibiotics, the fetus' hearing is also affected.

• Diuretics, such as furosemide (Seguril).

• Interferon and antiviral medications used for the treatment of hepatitis C and AIDS: They can cause temporary hearing loss, which generally resolves after stopping the treatment.

• Chemotherapy: Cisplatin and other drugs used in chemotherapy can cause a mild to moderate hearing loss, accompanied by tinnitus (ringing in the ears).

• Quinine, used for malaria (tonic water has a certain amount) and chloroquine, used in the treatment of rheumatoid arthritis.

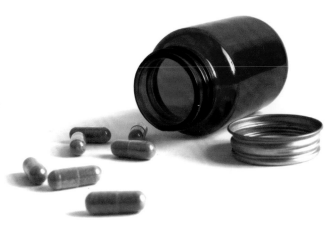

a. Ginkgo biloba extract EGb 761 or pentoxifylline for the treatment of sudden deafness: a randomized, reference-controlled, double-blind study. Reisser CH, Weidauer H. Acta Otolaryngol. 2001 Jul;121(5):579-84. PMID: 11583389

b. The efficacy of Ginkgo special extract EGb 761 in patients with tinnitus. Morgenstern C, Biermann E. Int J Clin Pharmacol Ther. 2002 May;40(5):188-97. PMID: 12051570

PREVENTION OF OTITIS MEDIA

The middle ear forms a closed chamber that is susceptible to inflammation and infection. Although at first it is benign, recurring otitis can end up damaging hearing.

Serous otitis media is the most common inflammation of the ear. It consists of the formation of serous fluid (not infected) in the middle ear, behind the eardrum.

At some point in their lives, most children suffer from serous otitis media, which manifests as pain and discomfort in the ear. In 85% of cases, the fluid disappears spontaneously after 10 or 15 days. In some cases, it may take months to disappear, with a risk of the following complications:

- Permanent hearing deficiency due to after-effects suffered by the eardrum and the chain of tiny bones.
- Bacterial infection in the middle ear (septic otitis media) which can spread to the inner ear.

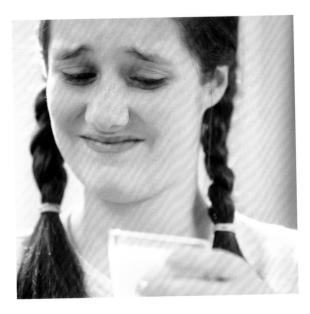

GUIDELINES FOR PREVENTION

- Avoid cold hitting the ear. Protect the ears, especially on cold, windy days.
- Adequately treat respiratory infections of the nose or throat, in order to avoid them spreading to the ears.
- Keep the nose as clear of mucus as possible. Saltwater irrigation of the nose is very effective in protecting the ears.
- Blow the nose correctly, avoiding the excess pressure that occurs when both nostrils are blocked at the same time (see how to blow the nose correctly in the chapter on the nose).

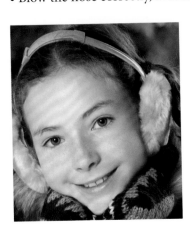

WATCH OUT FOR MILK AND DAIRY PRODUCTS

Clinical experience shows that children with otitis, rhinitis, bronchitis and other recurring respiratory infections get better when they stop drinking cow's milk. These children with recurring respiratory infections and excess mucus may suffer from some type of allergy to the proteins in cow's milk.

The worst manifestation of an allergy to cow's milk is known as Heiner syndrome, which manifests as otitis and persistent respiratory infections. It usually affects children between the ages of 6 months and 2 years.[a]

Even if there is not a clear allergy to cow's milk, many children with recurring otitis, rhinitis and upper respiratory infections, accompanied by an excess of mucus, improve by reducing or eliminating milk and dairy products. Soy drinks and yogurts are good alternatives to dairy products.

a. Milk-induced pulmonary disease in infants (Heiner syndrome). Moissidis I, Chaidaroon D, Vichyanond P, Bahna SL. Pediatr Allergy Immunol. 2005 Sep;16(6):545-52. PMID: 16176405

FINDING HEARING PROBLEMS IN TIME

*The sooner a potential hearing deficiency is detected,
the greater the possibility is to correct it.
Therefore, babies must be observed to confirm that they are
progressing in their hearing ability as they grow.*

These are some signs of hearing deficiency in babies and children. If any deficiency is noted, it must be brought to the attention of a pediatrician or otorhinolaryngologist.

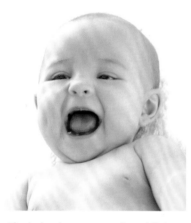
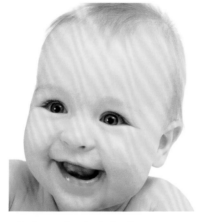
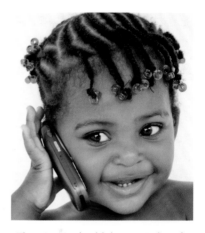

- The baby does not startle or blink with unexpected sounds.
- The baby does not turn to look when spoken to from one side.
- The baby does not calm down or smile upon hearing his mother's voice.

- At 6 months, the baby does not start making sounds.
- The one-year-old does not understand a verbal "no" without some guiding gesture.

- The 18-month-old does not identify his own name clearly.

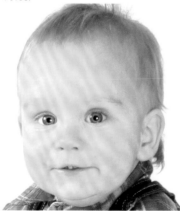
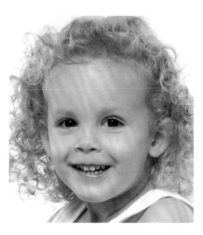
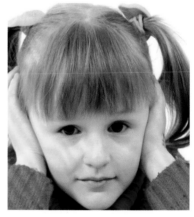

- The 2-year-old does not pay attention when he is told a story.

- The 3-year-old does not know how to respond to simple questions.

- The older child does not pay attention to a conversation, speaks very loudly or needs to increase TV volume.

Face

Capable of expressing as much or more with gestures than the mouth can with words.

The human face evokes a special interest in oneself and in others. A newborn, despite his visual limitations, already shows a special interest for his mother's face. It is known that there is a specific area of the brain charged with analyzing and recognizing faces. When that part of the brain is altered, familiar faces are not recognized. This disorder is known as prosopagnosia.

Without a doubt, what stands out the most about the human face is its ability to express emotions and mood: Happiness and sadness; serenity and fear; peace and strife; pleasure and pain, and so many other emotions are expressed better through facial muscles than with speech. In addition, these facial expressions are universal, and it has been shown they can be picked up by people from any culture, tongue or age.

Facial expression is truly a universally valid language, a system of non-verbal communication that brings all humans together; and one more piece of evidence of the singular origin of the human species.

However, in addition to emotions, the face is the most obvious expression of the condition of a person's physical and mental health. Many diseases and conditions are reflected in the face.

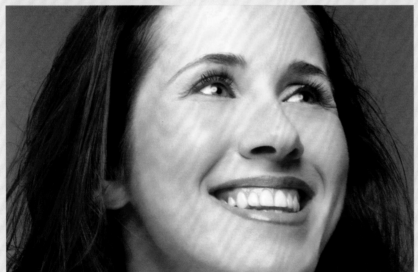

Beauty Comes from within
For a beautiful face, it is just as or even more effective to take care of the body's inner health than apply creams onto it.

Facts and Figures About the Face

5 to 6	Normal pH facial skin (pH under 7 is acidic). Soaps and creams should help maintain this level of skin acidity.
10 to 13%	Proportion of water that should be in the outer layer of skin (epidermis) on the face.
14	Number of bones that make up the face.
30	Number of muscles that participate in all of the face's expressions.

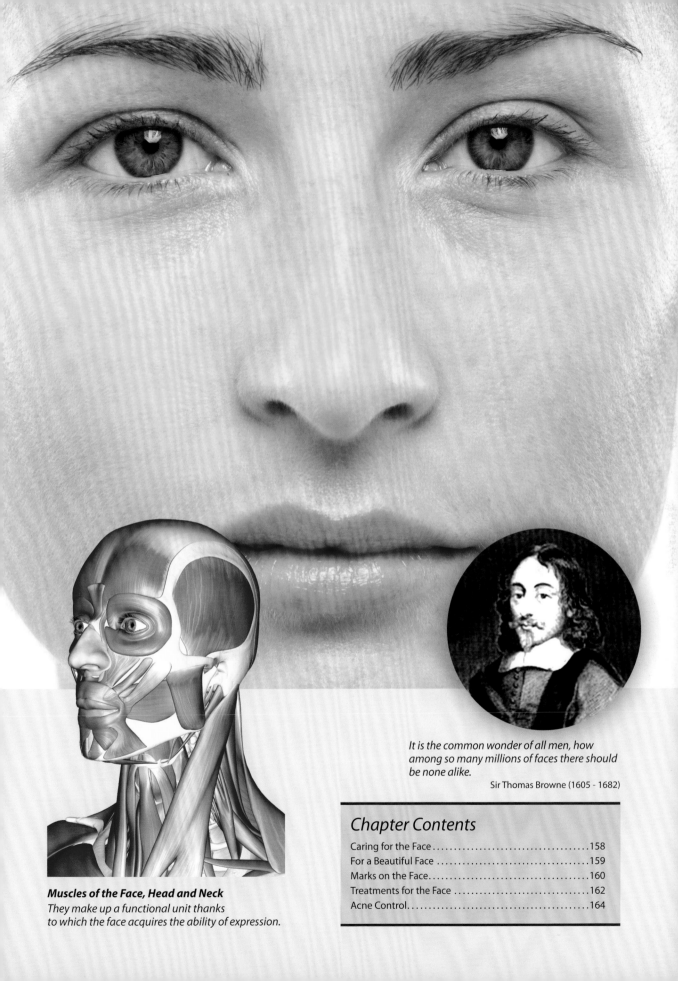

It is the common wonder of all men, how among so many millions of faces there should be none alike.

Sir Thomas Browne (1605 - 1682)

Muscles of the Face, Head and Neck
They make up a functional unit thanks to which the face acquires the ability of expression.

Chapter Contents

CARING FOR THE FACE

*The skin on the face requires more care than the skin on
any other part of the body, because most of the time it is uncovered.
In addition, there are a large number of sweat
and oil-producing glands concentrated on facial skin.*

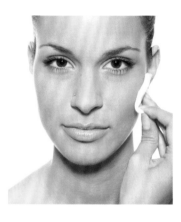

CLEANSING

Cleansing of
the facial skin
is the first step
before applying
any cream or
treatment. The
face is usually left
uncovered and in
contact with the
environment all
day long, which
means it can build
up foreign substances that should be eliminated
with good cleansing.

In addition, cleansing the face should eliminate
the skin's own secretions, such as sweat and
sebaceous secretions, as well as any traces of
make-up.

Recommended Products
- A cleansing milk or special soap for oily skin, if skin
  is oily.
- Facial toner or lotion.

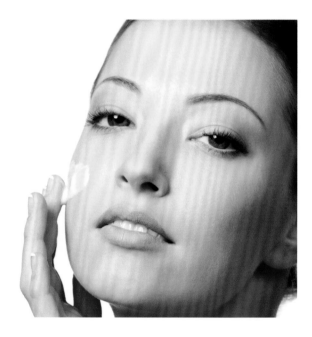

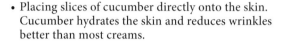

- Placing slices of cucumber directly onto the skin.
  Cucumber hydrates the skin and reduces wrinkles
  better than most creams.

HYDRATION

With exposure to sun and
air, skin cells on the face
quickly lose their water
content. With age, the skin
starts losing water and dries
out.

The use of tobacco, alcohol,
and other drugs, and a diet
low in natural products,
promotes water loss in skin
cells.

Recommended Products
- Hydrating creams, such as one made with cucumber
  juice.

NUTRITION

Applying creams with vegetable extracts rich in
protein, vitamins, and minerals, nourishes and
strengthens skin cells.

Recommended Product
- Nourishing cream for dry skin:
  – 4 tablespoons of almond oil.
  – Two tablespoons of rose water.
  – One tablespoon of beeswax.

Reasons You Must See a Doctor

- Non-healing wound on the facial skin.
- Reddish blotches on the face.
- Lump or hardening of any part of the face.

FOR A BEAUTIFUL FACE

The face is a reflection of the soul, and of the health of the rest of the body.

TAKE CARE OF FACIAL SKIN

Cleanliness, hydration and nutrition of the skin are essential to keeping it in good condition.

AVOID EXCESSIVE SUN

Excessive exposure to sunlight promotes wrinkles on the face and it also increases the risk of getting skin cancer. The most common location of this type of cancer is the facial skin in particular.

DO NOT SMOKE

The nicotine in tobacco has a vasoconstrictor effect (tightens the arteries), which reduces blood flow to the skin as well as to other parts of the body. The lack of blood flow wrinkles and dries out the skin.

REMOVE MAKE-UP BEFORE BEDTIME

Make-up clogs the skin's pores and hinders the airing out that they require.

WATCH DIGESTION

Dyspepsia (indigestion) and excess stomach acid quickly show up in facial expressions.

THINK POSITIVELY

Facial muscles contract involuntarily with negative thoughts, anguish or stress. This

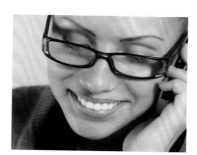

continuous muscle contraction reduces blood flow to the skin, and ages it.

Facial Skin Types

NORMAL
- Blushed color, looking like the skin of a healthy child.

DRY
- Taut skin lacking elasticity.
- Sebaceous glands produce little sebum, which predisposes to wrinkles.
- Dry skin could be due to nutrition deficiencies or a smoking habit.

OILY
- Shiny, sticky skin.
- Sebaceous glands produce excess sebum, which predisposes it to acne and pimples or blackheads.
- Oily skin is associated with hereditary factors, hormonal imbalance (such as occurs in adolescence), obesity, or a diet high in meat, fat, shellfish, or milk products.

COMBINATION
- Slightly oily on the forehead, nose, and chin, and somewhat dry everywhere else.

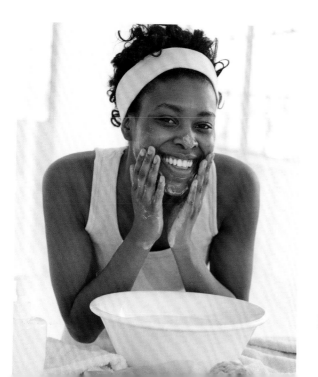

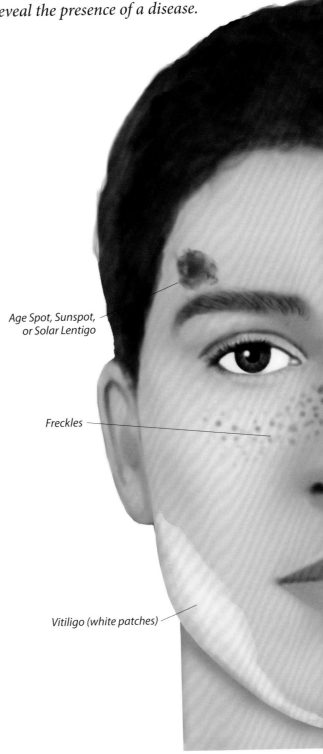

MARKS ON THE FACE

Marks are changes in skin color. In the majority of cases, marks on the face are only an aesthetic problem, but there are also disease-related marks that can reveal the presence of a disease.

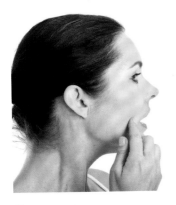

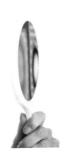

FRECKLES

Small, flat, brown spots that are hereditary, manifest in people with light skin and hair. They have no disease-related significance.

VITILIGO

Vitiligo is the presence of white, flat patches with irregular borders, due to a lack of the skin's natural pigment, melanin.

Vitiligo can appear due to a fungal infection, a nutritional deficiency or anxiety. In many cases, the cause is unknown.

Natural Remedies for Vitiligo
- Lotion made from tea tree oil or rose hip oil.
- B-group vitamin supplements taken by mouth.
- Between a half and a full glass of carrot juice daily, over one to two months.

AGE SPOTS , SUNSPOTS, OR SOLAR LENTIGO

These appear with age in people who have been exposed to the sun throughout their lives. They should be watched closely, as these sunspots can turn into melanoma, a type of skin cancer.

Malignant degeneration of a sunspot should be suspected when there is any change in their color, size or shape.

Age Spot, Sunspot, or Solar Lentigo

Freckles

Vitiligo (white patches)

DISEASE-RELATED MARKS

Several diseases can cause marks on facial skin, such as Addison's disease, hemochromatosis, leprosy, or lead poisoning.

Reddish blotches can be due to dermatitis (skin inflammation), angiomas (abnormal growth of the capillaries), purpura, or erythematosus lupus.

Chloasma

Reddish blotches on the face, typical to lupus erythematosus, an autoimmune disease that is difficult to treat.

Mole or Nevus

CHLOASMA

Chloasma (also, melasma) is the appearance of flat, light brown blotches, generally located on the cheeks, forehead or chin. They tend to appear in women beginning at age 20, almost always related to pregnancy or hormone treatments. They are due to a localized increase in melanin, the natural pigment that gives the skin its color.

Although chloasma presents an aesthetic problem, it rarely has disease-related significance.

How to Prevent Chloasma

- Protect facial skin with a factor 15 or higher sunscreen.
- Do not expose the face to sunbathing during pregnancy.
- Wear a cap or hat, especially in the middle of the day.
- Avoid direct exposure to the sun while under treatment with photosensitizing medications, such as:
  - Hormonal contraceptives, whether oral, patches, or vaginal ring.
  - Tetracyclines and their derivatives, as these antibiotics stimulate melanin production.
  - Certain anxiety medications, antidepressants and other psychoactive drugs.

MOLES OR NEVI

Dark brown isolated spots which are usually raised. They tend to be present from birth, although they sometimes appear with age.

Caution: Any change in a mole should be reported to a dermatologist, as it may be a melanoma; especially if it grows more than 6 mm in diameter, its borders become irregular, its surface becomes rugged, its coloring becomes uneven, or it bleeds.

Dermatological Treatments for Marks on the Face

- Laser: Usually done under local anesthesia, and does not leave a scar.
- Chemical exfoliation or "peeling": Usually done in weekly sessions, over several weeks.
- Vegetable-oil based lightening formulas with fruit vitamins and acids: Results achieved after a few months.
- Chemical lightening: Hydroquinone is one of the most effective, although because it can cause permanent depigmentation and darkening of the skin, its use has been limited.

TREATMENTS FOR THE FACE

The face very much welcomes the application of local treatments, such as oils, compresses, and lotions from medicinal herbs.

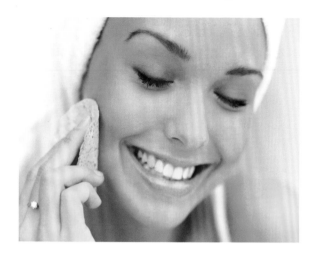

FACIAL MASSAGE

A facial massage is easy to do, even to oneself, and has these benefits:

- Improves blood flow to the skin and tissues.
- Tones facial muscles and improves facial expression.
- Promotes absorption of creams and lotions into the skin.

EXFOLIATION

Exfoliation is a skin treatment, generally of the face, that consists of eliminating the outer layer of the skin (epidermis) in a limited and controlled manner.

Goals of Exfoliation

- Speed up the natural process of skin peeling, and in this way promoting regeneration.
- Eliminate dead cells from the outer layers of skin.
- Open closed pores in cases of acne.

Types of Exfoliation

- Chemical exfoliation or peeling: Application of creams or lotions with exfoliating products.
- Mechanical exfoliation: Application of abrasive granules through massage.

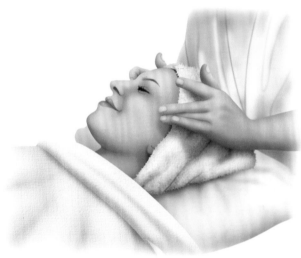

How to Do a Facial Massage
- *Use the fingertips.*
- *Massage in a circle around the eyes (without touching the eyelids) and around the mouth.*
- *Massage the forehead horizontally.*
- *Massage the cheeks downward.*

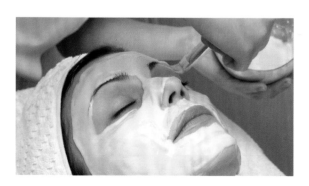

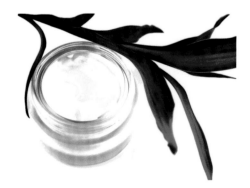

Botox®

Botox® is a medication obtained from a paralyzing toxin produced by the bacteria *Clostridium botulinum* (the cause of botulism). When injected into the face in low doses, the botulin toxin is able to relax the muscles responsible for a wrinkled brow and certain facial wrinkles.

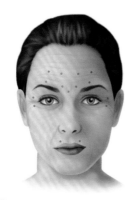

Botox® Injection Points

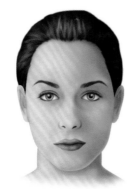

Eliminated Wrinkles
The face appears younger, but only for 4 months following the injection.

Caution

Despite the enthusiasm evoked by this medication, which was approved in the United States and Europe in 2004, there are certain precautions that must not be overlooked:

- Although it can smooth certain wrinkles, it also takes away from the facial expression by paralyzing the mimetic muscles.
- It only eliminates dynamic wrinkles caused by contraction of the mimetic muscles in the face, and not the fixed wrinkles caused by skin aging.
- It should be applied by only a plastic surgeon, dermatologist, neurologist or maxillofacial surgeon.
- The effect lasts between 4 and 6 months. After this time, a new dose must be injected if wishing to prolong the effect.
- It is not recommended during pregnancy and nursing.
- It should not be administered simultaneously with Aminoglycosidic antibiotics, antihypertensive calcium channel blockers or with anticoagulants.
- Side effects (generally rare): Droopy eyelids; asymmetrical facial movements; difficulty swallowing or speaking.

Natural Remedies to Minimize Marks and Imperfections on the Face

- **Rose Hip Oil**: The oil from the seeds of this plant, which belongs to the same genus as dog rose (*Rosa canina*), is very effective in redistributing skin pigmentation. It is applied with the fingertips over the mark, two or three times daily. It is also used to reduce the appearance of scars.
- **Tea Tree Oil** (*Melaleuca alternifolia*): This oil cleanses, reduces inflammation and regenerates the skin. It is applied over the affected area with the fingertips, two or three times daily.
- **Carrot Mask**: Shred a medium-sized carrot and apply it to the marks on the face like a mask for half an hour. Wash with water when finished.

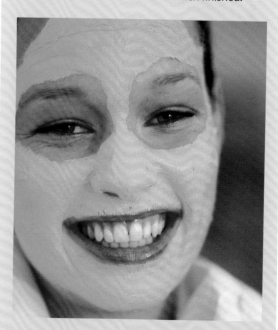

- **Lemon Juice Lotion**: Apply a few drops of pure lemon juice over the marks, several times per day.
- **Cucumber Lotion**: Liquefy a cucumber and apply the juice over the marks, several times per day.
- **Crushed Parsley Compresses**, applied with a pad over the marks for 15-30 minutes per day.
- **Gayuba Infusion Compresses** (*Arctostaphylos uva-ursi*): This plant decreases the synthesis of melanin. Its infusion is applied as a compress over the marks for half an hour per day.

ACNE CONTROL

Acne treatments should be complemented with diet and skin care.

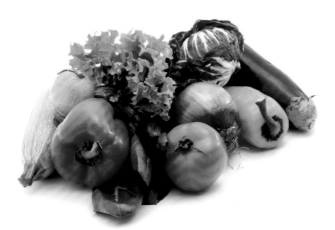

WATCH THE DIET

Although it depends mainly on hereditary and hormonal factors, the diet also influences the appearance of acne.

- **More Vitamin A**: Needed for good function of the sebaceous glands in the skin. Orange-colored fruits and vegetables, such as carrots, mangos, and apricots, provide beta-carotene, which converts to vitamin A in the body as it is needed.

- **More Zinc**: Needed for hormonal balance and for the immune system. Good diet sources are brewer's yeast, wheat germ, walnuts, and squash and sunflower seeds. It can also be taken as a supplement, 30-50 mg per day.

- **Fewer Fats**: Although there is no scientific proof to confirm it, there are fact-based suspicions that luncheon meats and pork in general, chocolate, butter and other high-fat animal products promote acne.

- **Less Cow's Milk**: A study by Harvard University shows that adolescents who consume more cow's milk, even if it is nonfat, are at higher risk of suffering acne.[a] The cause may be the metabolic effect of the milk proteins and the hormone residues that it tends to contain, which are present in whole milk as well as nonfat milk.

- **Less Sugar and Sweets**: A diet high in sugar and other high glycemic index products, such as white or refined flours, promote acne. On the other hand, regular consumption of whole grains and foods with a low glycemic load protect against acne, according to a study by RMIT Melbourne University (Australia).[b]

TAKE CARE OF THE SKIN

Taking care of facial skin, keeping these simple hygiene guidelines in mind can prevent acne from being triggered in predisposed skin.

- **Do not Touch Pimples**: Squeezing pimples can increase inflammation and spread infection.

- **Careful with Make-Up**: Greasy make-up made with oil or lanolin clog pores where the sebaceous glands come to the surface. This obstruction promotes the oil buildup in the glands, leading to acne's pimples. If make-up is used, no matter what it is, it must be removed at night.

- **Use Oil-Free Cosmetics**: Use as few skin products, cleansing creams, sun lotions and other cosmetics as possible. If they are used, they should be oil-free and water-based, so they do not clog pores. These products tend to be labeled "non-comedogenic" (do not produce comedones or pimples).

- **Wash the Face**: Gentle face cleansing (without rubbing the skin) two or three times per day with a mild soap, rinsing well with warm or cold water to completely rid it of soap.

a. High school dietary dairy intake and teenage acne. Adebamowo CA, Spiegelman D, Danby FW, Frazier AL, Willett WC, Holmes MD. J Am Acad Dermatol. 2005 Feb;52(2):207-14. PMID: 15692464

b. A low-glycemic-load diet improves symptoms in acne vulgaris patients: a randomized controlled trial. Smith RN, Mann NJ, Braue A, Mäkeläinen H, Varigos GA. Am J Clin Nutr. 2007 Jul;86(1):107-15.PMID: 17616769

Less Fats, Less Cow's Milk, and Less Candy

The skin, and especially facial skin, is very sensitive to what is eaten. There are scientific studies showing that the greater the intake of cow's milk and candy, the greater risk there is of acne.

On the other hand, whole grains and salads protect against acne.

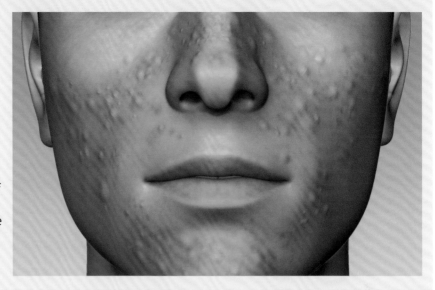

The Progression of Acne

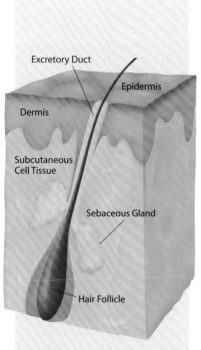

Excretory Duct
Epidermis
Dermis
Subcutaneous Cell Tissue
Sebaceous Gland
Hair Follicle

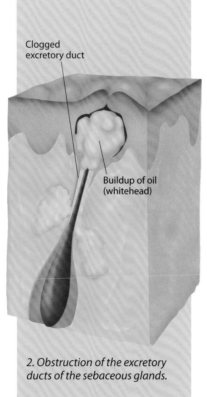

Clogged excretory duct
Buildup of oil (whitehead)

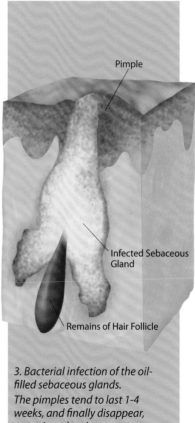

Pimple
Infected Sebaceous Gland
Remains of Hair Follicle

1. Overproduction of oil (grease) in the skin's sebaceous glands, caused generally by sex hormones.

2. Obstruction of the excretory ducts of the sebaceous glands.

3. Bacterial infection of the oil-filled sebaceous glands.

The pimples tend to last 1-4 weeks, and finally disappear, sometimes leaving a scar.

Mouth

Those wishing to eat, speak and kiss well should know their mouths, and how to take care of them.

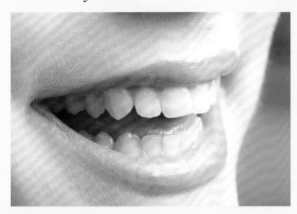

The joy of a smile is enough to make taking care of the mouth worthwhile.

*T*he mouth may well be the most versatile part of the human body, as it is capable of the most functions. First, the mouth is for eating and drinking, but it is also for speaking, breathing, gesturing and even kissing.

The mouth is a very special body part, due mainly to the following three characteristics:

- **Almost Constant Activity**: Throughout the day, the mouth is always doing something, due to the variety of functions it carries out. This constant activity requires high efficiency.

- **High Sensitivity**: The tongue, teeth and lips are, along with the cornea of the eye as well as the hands, the body parts that have the greatest number of sensitive nerve endings. Any injury or change in the mouth can cause severe pain.

- **Risk of Infection**: Due to its level of moisture and temperature, the mouth is an ideal place for the growth of all kinds of germs, due to which it is constantly under threat of infection. Despite its surprising design and its defense mechanisms, the mouth is where the most common infection occurs in humans: dental cavities, a disease that is infectious in origin, but promoted by today's bad eating habits.

The mouth, therefore, needs to be given special care. There are people who go their whole lives without needing to see a cardiologist or a urologist; but all of them, and surely more than once over their lifetimes, must see a dentist.

Facts and Figures About the Mouth

5	pH in the mouth after eating candy (acid).
7	pH in the mouth when it is empty (neutral).
20	Different types of bacteria found in the mouth.
20	Number of times saliva is swallowed every hour.
32	Number of teeth in a normal set.
32 to 37°C (89.6 to 100.4 °F)	Temperature inside the oral cavity.
200 cm² (31 sq in)	Surface of the oral mucosa.
100 000 000 (one hundred million)	Number of bacteria in one milliliter of saliva.
100 000 000 000 (one hundred billion)	Total number of bacteria living in the oral cavity.

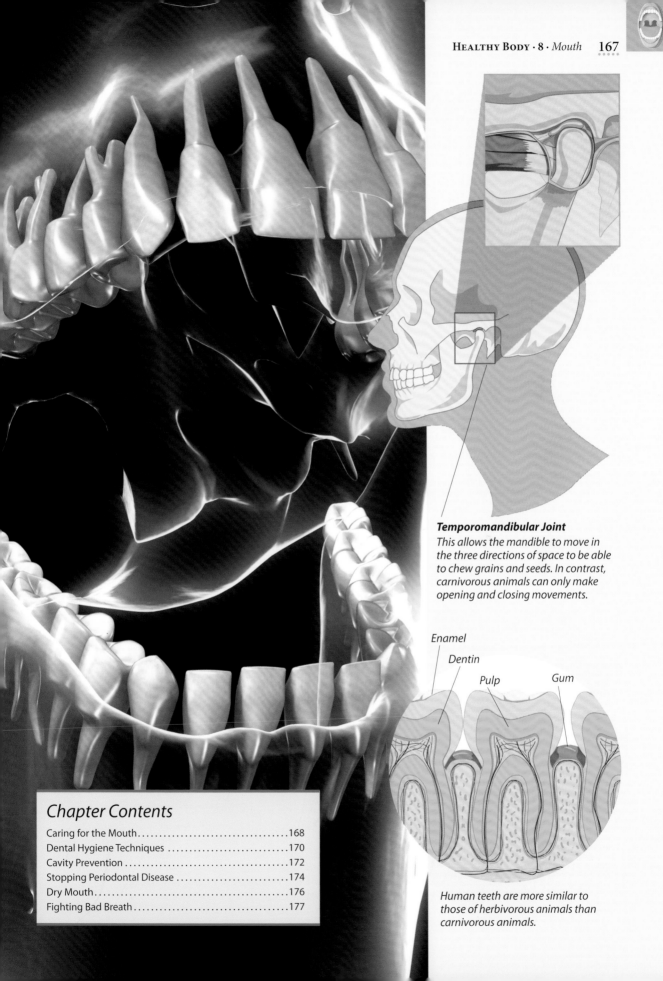

Temporomandibular Joint
This allows the mandible to move in the three directions of space to be able to chew grains and seeds. In contrast, carnivorous animals can only make opening and closing movements.

Enamel

Dentin

Pulp

Gum

Human teeth are more similar to those of herbivorous animals than carnivorous animals.

Chapter Contents

CARING FOR THE MOUTH

Proper oral hygiene requires much more than routine tooth brushing.

TOOTH BRUSHING

The teeth should be brushed after every meal, and always before going to bed.

Fluoride toothpastes offer additional protection against cavities.

See details on correct tooth brushing in "Dental Hygiene Techniques".

TONGUE BRUSHING

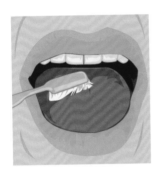

For good oral hygiene and to prevent halitosis, it is recommended to brush the tongue with a toothbrush at least once per day. Do not use toothpaste.

Tongue brushing can be accompanied by mouth rinses:
- With water,
- With antiseptic liquids, or
- With an infusion of medicinal herbs (see antiseptic herbs for the throat and mouth in the "Throat" chapter).

REGULAR DENTAL VISITS

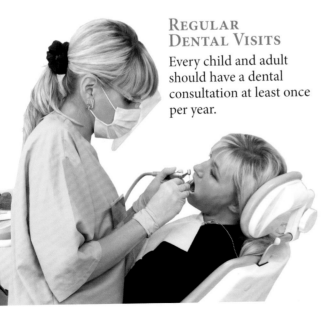

Every child and adult should have a dental consultation at least once per year.

FLOSSING

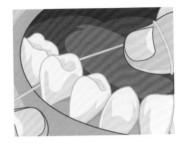

The toothbrush is unable to reach traces of food remaining between the teeth. These traces cause infection and cavities, and should be eliminated by flossing between the teeth at least once per day.

When the spaces between teeth are very wide, it is recommended to use an interdental brush after flossing (see "Dental Hygiene Techniques").

MOUTH RINSING

Rinsing the mouth with water after eating is a simple and effective oral hygiene habit. Rinsing the mouth is very necessary after eating candies, in order to eliminate the traces of sugar left over in the mouth.

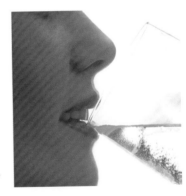

Caution: Liquids for rinsing the mouth containing alcohol can cause irritation of the mucosa and show up as a positive result on an alcohol breath test.

Antiseptic Rinses: Add a few drops of disinfecting essential oils to water to make rinses (3-4 drops per glass of water). These are the most recommended because of their antiseptic and refreshing effects:
- Essential Sage Oil *(Salvia officinalis)*.
- Essential Tea Tree Oil *(Melaleuca alternifolia)*.
- Essential Common Thyme Oil *(Thymus vulgaris)*.

DO NOT WEAR MOUTH PIERCINGS

Having pieces of metal in the mouth alters the balance in the oral mucosa, atrophies the gums and causes infections.

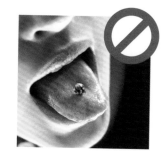

WEAR A MOUTHGUARD

When playing sports such as football, basketball or cycling, it is a good idea to wear a mouth protector made from flexible material in order to avoid injury to the teeth, lips or tongue.

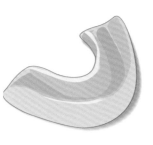

REDUCE SUGAR INTAKE

It has been well proven than the more sugar consumed, and the longer it remains in the mouth, the more cavities develop.

In order to stop cavities, it is essential to reduce or eliminate intake of confections, candies, sugared chocolate and other sweets. Brown sugar, syrup and refined products such as white bread and rolls also promote cavities.

Sweet and sticky foods, such as chocolate and rolls, promote cavities the most.

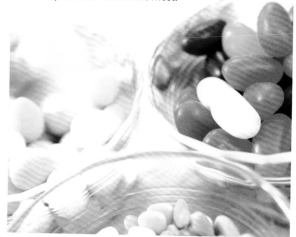

EXERCISE THE CHEWING MUSCLES

Chewing raw, crisp foods every day, such as carrots, cauliflower and other vegetables that require an effort to chew, strengthens teeth and gums. A plate of fresh salad each day contributes to the health of the mouth and teeth.

In order to keep the chewing mechanism in shape, at least 50% of the diet should consist of raw foods.

Chewing exercise is especially important in children, as it promotes correct development of the jaw and other facial bones.

Having at least one raw carrot per day helps keep the mouth healthy and to prevent cavities.

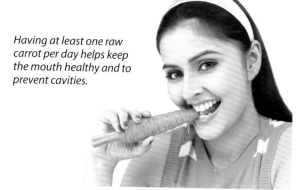

DO NOT SMOKE

Tobacco smoke not only affects the mouth's appearance, staining the teeth to a brown color, it is also a powerful gum irritant.

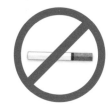

Smokers run a greater risk of having gingivitis (inflammation of the gums), tooth loss, oral infections and cancer of the mouth.

Reasons You Must See a Dentist

- Bleeding gums.
- Tartar on teeth.
- Sensitivity and pain in a tooth with cold or heat.
- Dry mouth sensation.
- White patches in the mouth (leukoplakia).
- Non-healing mouth ulcer.

DENTAL HYGIENE TECHNIQUES

Tooth brushing is the most simple and effective way to care for the teeth and gums. However, there are also other ways to keep them clean.

GOALS OF TOOTH BRUSHING

- Eliminate any traces of food remaining in teeth or gums. Food that remains in the mouth promotes the spread of tooth-destroying bacteria.
- Eliminate bacterial plaque, made up of traces of food and bacteria on the tooth surface.
- Clean and strengthen gums.

PRACTICAL TIPS FOR PROPER TOOTH BRUSHING

- The toothbrush should be in good condition, with firm bristles that are not warped or bent. Every 3 or 4 months, a new toothbrush is needed.

- Brush teeth at least twice daily, after the main meal of the day and especially before going to bed.
- After eating something sweet, rinse mouth and brush teeth as soon as possible. Sugar is the best nutrient for the growth of tooth-destroying bacteria.
- Avoid brushing too hard so the gums will not become injured.
- An electric toothbrush improves tooth cleanliness, eliminates bacterial plaque better and strengthens gums thanks to its massaging action. However, it is not necessary to use an electric toothbrush in order to have proper hygiene.
- To check whether the tooth brushing has been effective, use a plaque-coloring tablet or liquid. If the tooth surfaces change color, it means there is still bacterial plaque.

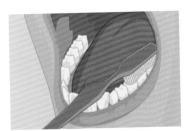

Hold the toothbrush with the fingers, not the palm of the hand. Toothpaste is optional.

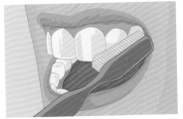

Start on the outer or vestibular surface of the teeth, making circular movements with the toothbrush slightly tipped.

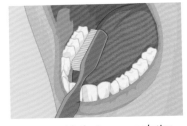

Continue with the inner or palatine surface, with front-to-back movements.

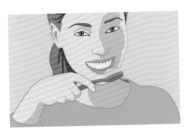

Then brush the chewing surface of the molars.

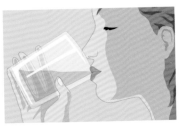

Rinse with an antiseptic liquid for mouthwashes, an antiseptic herbal infusion for the mouth, or plain water.

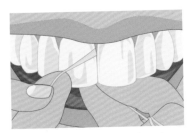

After brushing (or before), floss the spaces between teeth.

OTHER DENTAL HYGIENE TECHNIQUES

In addition to brushing and flossing, there are other techniques to prevent and stop the progression of periodontal disease.

Although these techniques can be applied at home, they should be recommended and under the supervision of an odontologist or dental hygienist.

Interdental Brushing

Interdental brushes, also called interproximal brushes, are better able to reach spaces between teeth.

Toothpicks

Toothpicks are made from balsa wood (there are also plastic-type). These are able to clean deeply between teeth. They should be used gently, once per week.

Gum Stimulator

Gum stimulators are usually cone-shaped and made of rubber. This device is used to massage the gums, which promotes their regeneration.

Dental Irrigators or Rinses

Irrigators spray a fine stream of water onto the gums, which eliminates food particles completely.

The water pressure should not be excessive, to avoid injury to the gums. Irrigators do not replace the need to brush and floss.

Bite Splint

This is a piece of flexible material placed between teeth at night to avoid bruxism (teeth grinding). The habit of nighttime teeth clenching can be a result of stress. Wearing a bite splint at night prevents dental abrasion or wear, and protects the jaw joint.

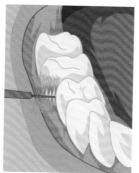

Interdental brush to clean the space between widely-spaced teeth.

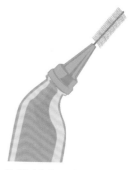

Refillable Interdental brush. Allows antiseptic liquid to be released around bridges, implants and orthodontic appliances.

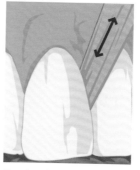

Toothpick made from balsa wood (a soft wood).

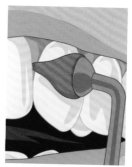

Gum stimulator, made of rubber.

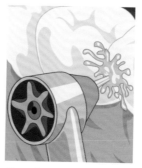

Dental pressure-irrigator or rinse.

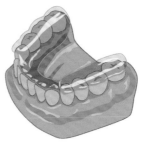

Bite splint for nighttime use.

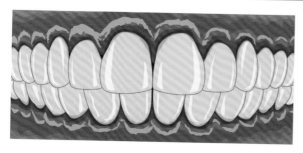

Bleeding Gums

If there is blood on gums or in saliva after brushing teeth, or after using a dental hygiene technique, it is a sign of gingivitis (inflammation of the gums).

Gingivitis is the first stage of periodontal disease, which eventually leads to tooth loss.

CAVITY PREVENTION

Having cavities is the most common disease in humans, along with the common cold. It is possible to prevent them, but action must be taken on the four causation factors.

The oral cavity is a warm, moist environment that is ideal for germ growth (bacteria, fungi, viruses…). In a healthy mouth, there can be about one hundred billion bacteria from about 20 different species.

As long as proper balance is maintained among the different species of germs and the oral mucosa's anti-infection defenses, infections do not occur. But if this balance is altered, periodontitis (pyorrhea), halitosis (bad breath) and different infections appear.

CAUSES OF ALTERATIONS IN THE BALANCE OF BACTERIAL FLORA IN THE MOUTH

- Traces of sweet foods left in the mouth.
- Traces of any food left in the mouth.
- Poor oral hygiene.
- Antibiotic abuse.
- Smoking.
- Injuries, tears, and ulcerations in the oral mucosa.

BACTERIAL PLAQUE

Traces of food left in the mouth, especially if they contain sugar, overfeed the enemy bacteria that cause cavities.

These traces of food left in the mouth, along with the bacteria and the saliva, form a sticky substance that adheres to tooth surfaces, called bacterial plaque. The presence of bacterial plaque on tooth surfaces promotes cavities, gingivitis, periodontitis (pyorrhea) and other oral infections.

Individual with his predisposing traits, such as the shape and alignment of teeth, composition of saliva and genetic predisposition.

Cariogenic *bacteria*, mainly from the genus Streptococcus, Lactobacilli and Actinomyces, making up a bacterial plaque on the surface of teeth.

Enamel

Cavity

Dentin

Pulp

Cavities are a result of a set of four factors: Individual, bacteria, time and substrate.

Bacteria

Individual

Cavities

Time

Substrate

Time the substrate (traces of sweet foods) remains in the mouth.

Substrate, that is, food for bacteria (mainly, sugar and white flour).

How to Prevent Cavities

Dental cavities are prevented by avoiding or minimizing the four individual causation factors, by following these recommendations:

- Brush teeth after every meal.
- Use a fluoride toothpaste.
- Floss once a day.
- Reduce or eliminate intake of sugar (candies, cakes, chocolate, sweets in general) and refined or white flour (rolls, cakes, white bread, etc.).
- Do not snack between meals.
- Reduce or eliminate intake of sweet and sticky foods that stick to teeth.
- Eat raw foods (at least 50% of daily intake).
- Reduce or eliminate sugary soft drinks, such as cola drinks.
- See a dentist regularly.

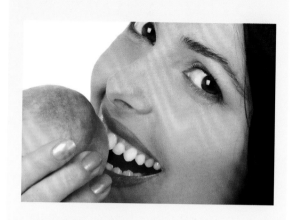

Eating an Apple Reduces Dental Bacterial Plaque

An experiment done in Germany[a] has shown that eating a raw apple reduces dental bacterial plaque by 15.9%, while tooth brushing reduces it by 14.9%.

According to these figures, this means that eating an apple is just as beneficial to dental hygiene as brushing teeth. The apple's high fiber content helps explain its anti-plaque effect.

---

a. Reduction of dental plaque by apples and chewing gum. Schneider HG, Knieknecht I. Nahrung. 1986;30(9):907-12.PMID: 3796719

Enamel

Bacterial Plaque
Thin layer around the tooth's surface, made up of accumulated bacteria, traces of food and saliva.

Acids produced by the bacteria of bacterial plaque go through the fine pores in the enamel and cause cavities.

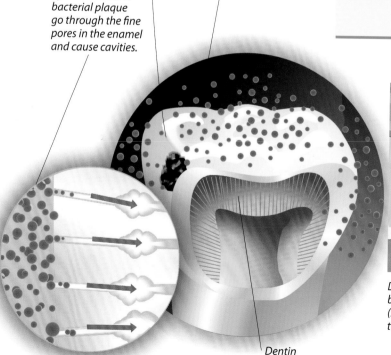

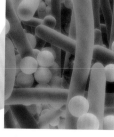

Chains of cavity-causing bacteria in dental plaque, as seen under a microscope.

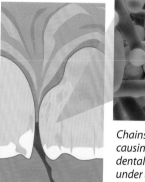

Dental bacterial plaque, colored by chewing a revealing tablet (sold in pharmacies). The brighter the color, the more bacterial plaque.

Dentin

STOPPING PERIODONTAL DISEASE

*Periodontal disease does not cause any pain,
and can therefore go unnoticed. But if it is not stopped,
it progresses in silence until it causes tooth loss.*

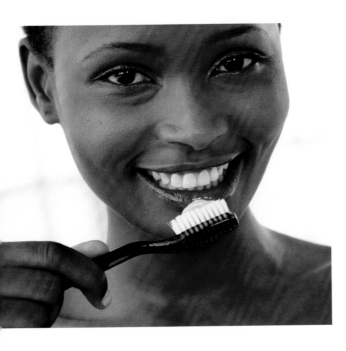

Periodontal disease, also known as periodontitis or pyorrhea, is the top cause of tooth loss. It is characterized by inflammation and weakening of the gums and the alveolar bone holding the teeth in place.

Periodontal disease can be prevented with good personal dental hygiene, and the professional care of a dentist.

If it is not properly stopped, periodontal disease progresses silently and painlessly over the years, destroying the alveolar bone holding the teeth in place.

Gum bleeding with tooth brushing is the first obvious manifestation of periodontitis.

DENTAL HYGIENE PRACTICES AGAINST PERIODONTAL DISEASE

These simple dental hygiene practices prevent periodontal disease from progressing and causing tooth loss.

- Brush teeth after every meal to really eliminate all of the remaining particles. An electric toothbrush strengthens the gums better than a manual toothbrush.
- Floss daily.
- Rinse the mouth with an aloe vera gel solution (a tablespoon in half a glass of water). The aloe vera gel can also be applied directly onto the gums.
- See a dentist or dental hygienist regularly. Eliminating tartar through dental cleaning is essential to stopping the progression of periodontal disease.
- Take a vitamin C supplement (500 - 1 000 mg per day).

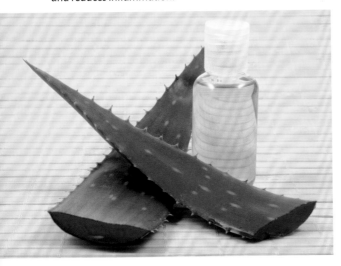

Aloe vera gel softens the gums and reduces inflammation.

Progression of Periodontal Disease

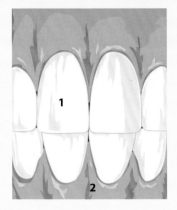 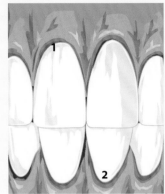 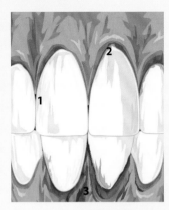

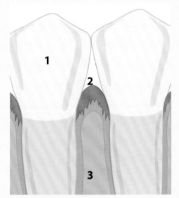 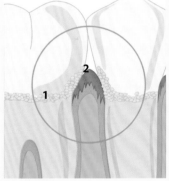 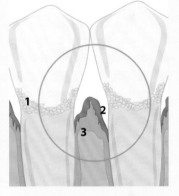

A. Healthy Teeth
(1) Clean teeth
(2) Healthy gums
(3) Healthy alveolar bone

B. Gingivitis
(1) Appearance of dental bacterial plaque on the edges of the gums.
(2) Inflamed gums that begin to bleed.
There is no pain, which is why gingivitis can go unnoticed.

C. Periodontitis (pyorrhea)
(1) Tartar formation over the dental plaque.
(2) Receding gums.
(3) Loss of alveolar bone
The teeth move and can fall out.

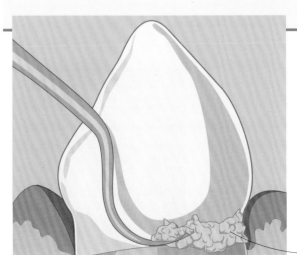

Tartar

Eliminating Tartar
Tartar is the substance that forms over dental bacterial plaque. It must be eliminated, as it causes gingivitis (inflammation of the gums).

Dental cleaning by a hygienist or odontologist eliminates tartar. As a home remedy, green clay can be applied onto the gums with a gentle massage every night after dinner.

DRY MOUTH

A disorder that is becoming more common,
and which predisposes to dental cavities and periodontitis.

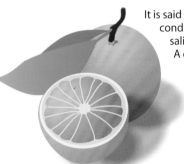

It is said that a dry mouth is the condition of not having enough saliva to keep the mouth wet.. A dry mouth interferes with speaking and chewing, as well as predisposes to dental cavities and oral infections, especially gingivitis and periodontitis.

WHY SALIVA IS IMPORTANT

- In addition to providing moisture for the mouth, saliva has many functions. When not enough saliva is produced, the risk of several oral diseases increases.
- It keeps the mouth moist and lubricated to make chewing and swallowing easier.
- It starts the digestion process of foods, especially those rich in carbohydrates, thanks to the enzyme ptyalin.
- It protects the teeth, creating a protective film around them.
- It prevents many oral infections, thanks to the antibodies and anti-infective proteins it contains.
- It helps maintain the necessary balance among the various microorganisms normally living in the oral cavity (bacteria, fungi and viruses), preventing their overgrowth.

FREQUENT CAUSES OF DRY MOUTH

- Diseases such as Sjögren's syndrome (dry mouth, dry eyes and arthritis, affecting mainly women), Parkinson's, uncontrolled diabetes or AIDS.
- Medication: There are over 400 types of medication that reduce saliva production, among which are certain antidepressives and antihypertensives.
- Chemotherapy and radiation therapy.
- Injuries to facial nerves due to wounds or trauma.

ADVICE FOR A DRY MOUTH

- Follow meticulous dental hygiene: brushing after every meal, avoiding sugary products, and using oral rinses with fluoride.
- Avoid tobacco, coffee and alcoholic beverages, because nicotine as well as coffee and alcohol reduce saliva production and dry the mouth.
- Sip small amounts of water or non-sugary liquids often.
- Chew sugarless gum.
- Suck on hard, sugarless candies with essence of lemon, cinnamon or mint.
- Lemons, oranges and other citrus fruits are highly recommended because they stimulate saliva production.
- Use a room humidifier in the bedroom, especially at night.
- When having dry foods, such as bread, dip them in water first, or sip water while chewing.
- Reduce the dose, avoid or replace medications that cause dry mouth as a side effect.
- Consult with a doctor or dentist about using the medication pilocarpine, which increases the secretion of saliva. Pilocarpine has side effects, such as increased perspiration, hypotension and difficulty breathing.

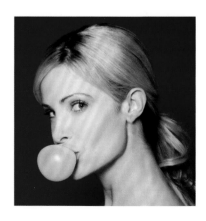

FIGHTING BAD BREATH

*Bad breath, or halitosis, is due to the presence of sulfurated substances
in the air exhaled through the nose or mouth.*

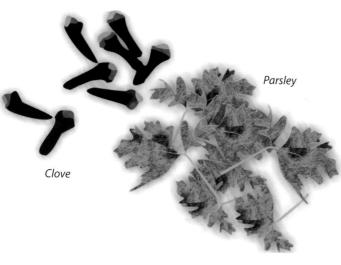

Parsley

Clove

The most important part of fighting bad breath
is identifying its cause. This can be found in both
local infections of the mouth, throat or paranasal
sinuses (sinusitis) and in disorders of the bronchi,
stomach or even the bowel (constipation). It
is always a good idea to see the dentist for the
correction of any issue with the mouth or teeth.

- Drink enough water to keep well hydrated and
  to produce enough saliva (6-8 glasses per day).
  Mild dehydration, such as what occurs when
  sleeping, can cause halitosis, as it reduces the
  flow of saliva. When there is little saliva, there is
  a greater tendency toward bad breath.
- Avoid eating garlic and onion.
- Avoid constipation.
- Eliminate tobacco, coffee, and alcoholic
  beverages.
- Put some drops of lemon onto the tongue
  several times per day in order to increase saliva
  production.
- Suck on chlorophyll tablets or chew parsley
  leaves.
- Chew on fennel or anise leaves.
- Suck on a piece of ginger root (*Zingiber
  officinale*).
- Suck on a clove (*Eugenia caryophyllata*), an oral
  antiseptic and anti-inflammatory herb.

HOME REMEDIES FOR BAD BREATH

- When a clear cause cannot be found, these
  remedies are helpful:
- Be meticulous about oral hygiene, with
  brushing and flossing (see "Dental Hygiene
  Techniques"), especially before going to bed.
- Brush the tongue from front to back with a
  toothbrush, preferably before going to bed.
  Brushing eliminates traces of food and bacteria.
- Do mouth rinses with oral antiseptics. A good
  antiseptic rinse can be made by adding 3-4
  drops of essential sage oil (*Salvia officinalis*),
  essential tea tree oil (*Melaleuca alternifolia*) r
  essential common thyme oil (*Thymus vulgaris*),
  to a glass of water.

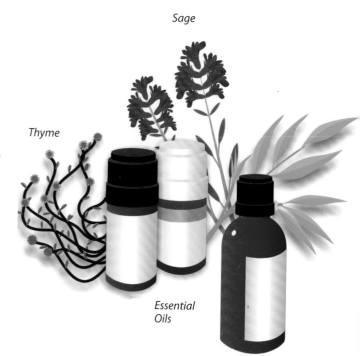

Sage

Thyme

*Essential
Oils*

Throat

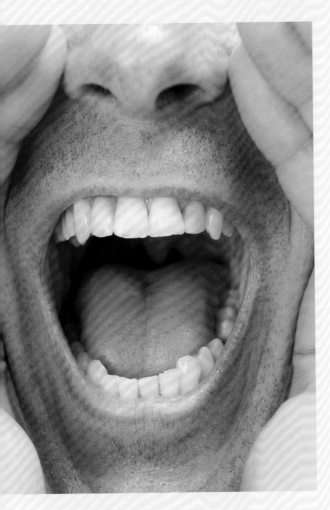

A complex, bidirectional transportation system for gases, liquids and solids, that is able to differentiate each from the other.

When we speak of the throat, we are referring to the anatomical space extending from the uvula all the way to the trachea. It has an upper part, the pharynx, and a lower part, the larynx.

The throat is located between the head and the neck. Its extremely sensitive interior protects the airways, preventing solids or liquids from getting into the trachea and lungs, which could cause asphyxia.

The throat is also the entrance into the body. The tonsils guard the entrance, preventing the passage of infectious agents.

A few decades ago, the tonsils were considered an evolutionary leftover –a vestigial organ that should be removed as soon as it became enlarged and inflamed. Today, however, modern medicine recognizes that more respiratory infections occur after removal of the tonsils than before their removal. Fortunately, their removal is becoming less and less common.

Through the air we breathe and the foods we eat, the throat is in constant contact with infectious agents –true invaders that must be detected and eliminated.

Facts and Figures About the Throat

15 mm (0.59 in)	Length of a woman's vocal cords.
20 mm (0.79 in)	Length of a man's vocal cords.
70 to 200	Number of times the vocal cords move every second in order to produce the voice.
320 km/hour (200 mph)	Speed of expelled air and saliva droplets during a cough.

The Tonsils Have Their Function

We should see the tonsils as friends, not enemies. Many infectious agents become trapped in their crypts (small folds); without tonsils, these would get into the airways or the blood.

When tonsils are enlarged and inflamed, it is because they are overloaded trying to fight off bacteria and other infectious agents. Instead of removing them, we should help strengthen them so they can carry out their important function.

The tonsils should only be removed when there have been more than five episodes of tonsillitis over a period of a year, or in the case of recurring abscesses.

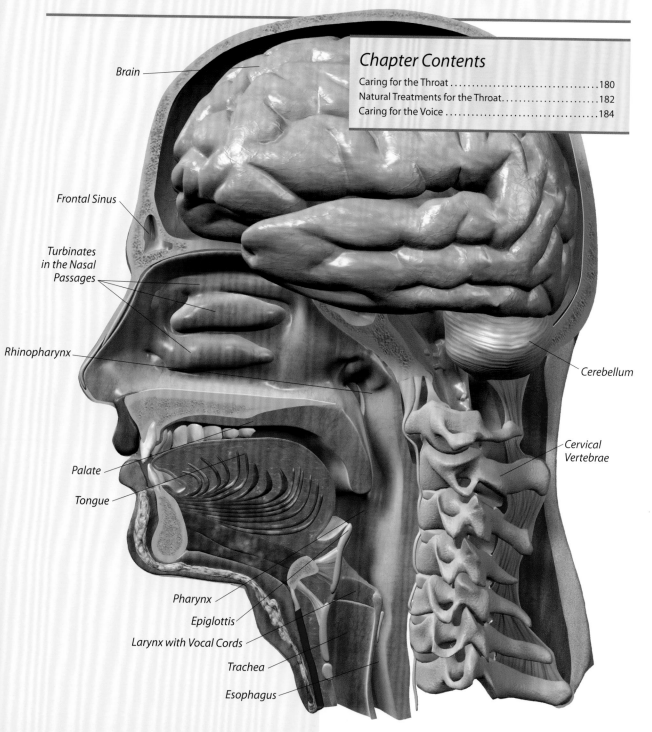

Brain

Frontal Sinus

Turbinates in the Nasal Passages

Rhinopharynx

Palate

Tongue

Pharynx

Epiglottis

Larynx with Vocal Cords

Trachea

Esophagus

Cerebellum

Cervical Vertebrae

Chapter Contents

CARING FOR THE THROAT

The mucosa lining the inside of the throat is especially sensitive to cold, whether from the environment, inhaled air or swallowed drinks. A scratchy throat, cough and voice changes are signs that the throat is not being properly cared for.

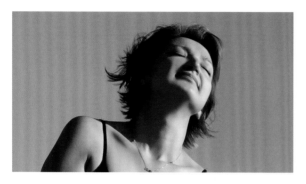

BREATHE THROUGH THE NOSE

The nostrils are anatomically equipped to receive cold air. Thanks to the chambers and spongy mucosa inside the nasal passages, air inhaled through the nose is warmed, moistened and filtered of impurities.

However, the throat does not have defenses against cold air, and cannot heat, filter or moisten the air entering it. For this reason, mouth breathing affects the throat mucosa, making it dry and irritated.

USE A ROOM HUMIDIFIER

Warm, dry air, such as the air that is breathed in a heated bedroom, causes the throat mucosa to become dry. A room humidifier helps soothe the throat, especially in wintertime.

After using the humidifier for several hours, windows should be opened for a few minutes for ventilation.

BREATHE FRESH AIR

Contaminated air and tobacco smoke in particular irritate the delicate mucosa lining the throat. Living in a smoke-free environment far away from contamination prevents throat conditions.

DO NOT SMOKE

Contrary to what some smokers think, tobacco smoke does not strengthen the throat or the lungs whatsoever. In fact, it causes chronic irritation and inflammation of the mucosa, promoting infection and cancer.

KEEP FEET WARM

Having cold feet predisposes the throat to infections due to a reflex mechanism that causes vasoconstriction in the throat and nose.

To take care of the throat, having cold feet must be avoided, especially in wintertime.

AVOID VERY COLD DRINKS

Cold is a big enemy of the throat. On a hot day, an overly cold drink can represent an attack on the delicate mucosa of the pharynx.

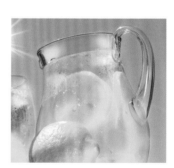

Reasons You Must See a Doctor

- Difficulty breathing or swallowing.
- Dysphonia (hoarseness) lasting more than a week.
- Persistent dry cough lasting more than a week.
- Streaks of blood in saliva or mucus.
- A persistent bulge in the throat.

The Organs of Speech

Along with the opposable thumb, the ability to produce the voice and speak is one of the characteristics most specific to humankind. Although the voice is produced in a part of the throat called the larynx, it must be controlled by the brain in order to result in speech. Without control from the brain, the larynx is like a musical instrument without a musician.

CAUSES OF DYSPHONIA (VOICE CONDITIONS)

Dysphonia is a condition that affects the normal characteristics of the voice. Dysphonia can manifest as hoarseness, softness, cracking, or a complete absence of the voice. If dysphonia persists for more than a week, a physician specializing in otolaryngology should be consulted.

Some causes of dysphonia include:
• Laryngitis (laryngeal infection), generally viral.
• Respiratory allergy.
• Polyps on the vocal cords.
• Gastroesophageal reflux (due to irritation caused by gastric juices entering the throat).
• Laryngeal cancer (common among smokers).
• Parkinson's disease.
• *Miastenia gravis* (muscle weakness).
• Multiple sclerosis.

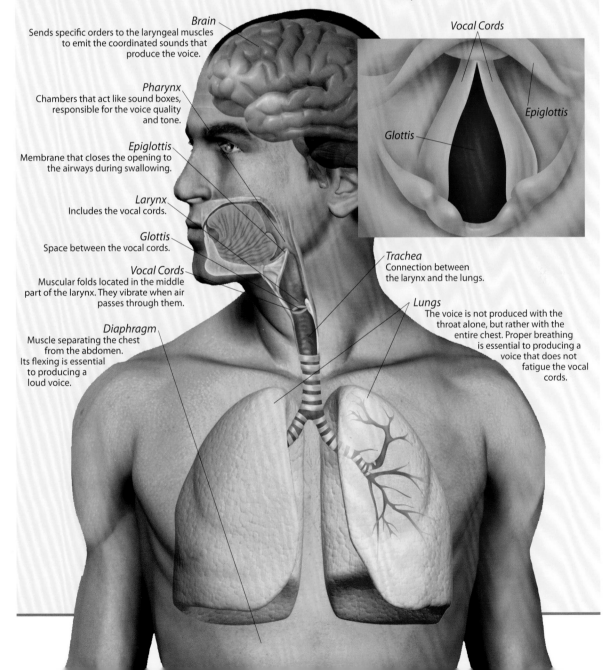

Brain
Sends specific orders to the laryngeal muscles to emit the coordinated sounds that produce the voice.

Pharynx
Chambers that act like sound boxes, responsible for the voice quality and tone.

Epiglottis
Membrane that closes the opening to the airways during swallowing.

Larynx
Includes the vocal cords.

Glottis
Space between the vocal cords.

Vocal Cords
Muscular folds located in the middle part of the larynx. They vibrate when air passes through them.

Diaphragm
Muscle separating the chest from the abdomen. Its flexing is essential to producing a loud voice.

Vocal Cords

Epiglottis

Glottis

Trachea
Connection between the larynx and the lungs.

Lungs
The voice is not produced with the throat alone, but rather with the entire chest. Proper breathing is essential to producing a voice that does not fatigue the vocal cords.

182

NATURAL TREATMENTS FOR THE THROAT

These simple home remedies are effective in relieving tonsillitis as well as pharyngitis.

INCREASING TEMPERATURE FOOT BATH

An increasing temperature foot bath has a stronger decongestive effect for the throat than the typical foot bath (see the latter technique in "Natural Treatments for the Nose", Ch. 5). The stimulus produced by the hot water on the feet triggers a nerve reflex that relieves throat inflammation and congestion.

Water Temperature: Begin at 30 ˚C (86 ˚F), gradually adding hot water until reaching 42 ˚C (108 ˚F).

Duration: 15-20 minutes.

Afterward: Apply a cold rinse or rub on both feet, put on wool socks and keep bundled up.

Frequency: Once or twice per day. To treat throat infections, this should be done over at least a week.

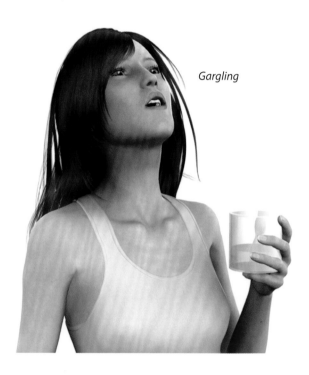

Gargling

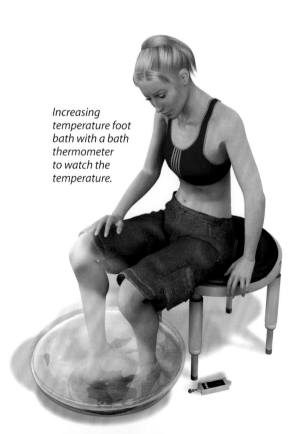

Increasing temperature foot bath with a bath thermometer to watch the temperature.

GARGLING

Gargling clears the throat of mucus, germs and remains of dead cells due to infection.

Plain warm water gargling is effective enough. For a stronger effect, one of the following liquids can be used, always warm:

• Water with lemon juice (optional to add honey, but not for children under a year old).

• Water with salt (a dessert spoon, which is about 5 grams of salt per cup of water).

• Ginger infusion (*Zingiber officinale*).

• Common agrimony infusion (*Agrimonia eupatoria*).

• Aromatic herbal infusion, such as lavender (*Lavandula angustifolia*) or common thyme (*Thymus vulgaris*).

Liquid Temperature: Lukewarm or warm.

Duration: About 5 minutes.

Afterward: Spit liquid out without swallowing.

Frequency: One to three times per day.

WARM COMPRESS ON THE THROAT

Heat applied to the skin causes dilation of superficial blood vessels. This way, throat and laryngeal congestion are relieved.

Water Temperature: Dip a cotton cloth in warm water, 30-40 ˚C (86-104 ˚F). Drain the cloth well.

Duration: The compress can be left in place for one or two hours continuously. It should be changed every 15 or 20 minutes, soaking it in warm water again.

Afterward: After removing the compress, replace it with a scarf or wool cloth, covering the throat.

Frequency: One to three times per day.

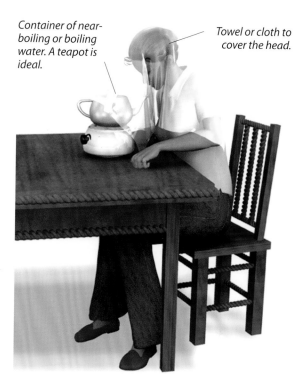

Container of near-boiling or boiling water. A teapot is ideal.

Towel or cloth to cover the head.

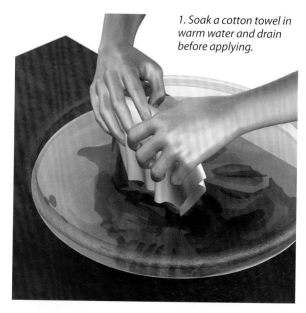

1. Soak a cotton towel in warm water and drain before applying.

STEAM INHALATION

Moisture is essential to keeping the throat mucosa in good condition. The combination of moisture and heat is especially beneficial for throat irritation.

Beneficial Effects of Steam Inhalation

- Improves the defense mechanisms of throat mucosa.
- Facilitates expectoration of mucus and impurities.
- Soothes the throat.
- Relieves cough.

For a stronger effect, a few drops of an antiseptic essential oil from medicinal herbs should be added, such as:
- Essential Sage Oil (*Salvia officinalis*).
- Essential Tea Tree Oil (*Melaleuca alternifolia*).
- Essential Common Thyme Oil (*Thymus vulgaris*).

Water Temperature: As hot as possible, in order to produce steam. Ideally, it should be near-boiling.

Duration: 5-10 minutes.

Afterward: Rub the face and neck with cold water, to close skin pores.

Frequency: One to three times per day, while throat irritation persists.

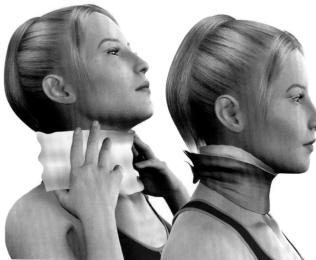

2. Place the cloth on the throat.

3. Place a wool cloth or scarf over it.

CARING FOR THE VOICE

The voice is a reflection of the personality, and its tone identifies each human being. When hearing somebody speak, one can learn about their mood: happiness and sadness, trust and worry, pleasure and pain, can all be identified depending on the tone of the voice. Taking care of our voices is worthwhile, as it can be used to benefit others.

MAINTAIN PROPER POSTURE

In order for the voice to be produced with clarity and without fatiguing the throat, the neck must be extended and the chest must be kept erect.

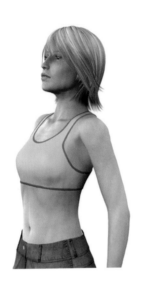

USE THE DIAPHRAGM AND THE ABDOMINAL MUSCLES

When needing to raise voice intensity, using the throat alone should be avoided because it causes vocal cord fatigue. To increase voice power, flex the diaphragm by pushing out the belly, like babies do when they cry.

Singers, teachers and conference speakers must learn to speak with their bellies in order to completely fill their lungs with air, and thereby sustain voice performance.

BREATHE DEEPLY

Teachers, professors, conference speakers, singers and anyone who uses their voice extensively need to learn to breathe deeply when speaking. This facilitates voice production and alleviates stress on the vocal cords..

PRACTICE ABDOMINAL BREATHING

In order to fill the lungs with air, it is just as important to fill the chest as it is to flex the diaphragm downward. To achieve this, the belly must be pressed outward.

DO NOT STRAIN THE VOICE

Avoid speaking in noisy places, as this causes a tendency to strain the voice without realizing it. Speak softly when noticing a hoarse or fatigued voice. Consider using a microphone with a sound amplification system (some are portable).

WATCH OUT FOR AIR CONDITIONING

The drastic change in temperature occuring when coming into a cold place from a hot outside environment can be a cause of aphonia. The cold air entering the throat causes vasoconstriction (tightening of blood vessels) in the vocal cords, including decreased blood flow and stiffness. The result is softening or loss of the voice.

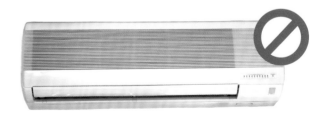

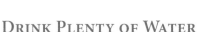

DRINK PLENTY OF WATER

It is well known that drinking water clears the voice; this is not only due to the rinsing mechanism of secretions produced by drinking, but also because when the vocal cord mucosa is well hydrated, they vibrate better.

DRINK A WARM INFUSION

When the voice is fatigued, a warm infusion of medicinal herbs improves blood flow to the larynx and contributes to clearing the voice. These are some of the recommended herbs:

- Hedge mustard (*Sisymbrium officinale = Erysimum officinale*).
- Licorice (*Glycyrrhiza glabra*).
- Oregano (*Origanum vulgare*)
- Chamomile (*Matricaria chamomilla*) with anise (*Pimpinella anisum*).

Lemon juice diluted with honey or sugarcane is also a good remedy for clearing the voice and relieving a sore throat.

INHALE AROMATIC ESSENCES

Inhaling essence of common thyme (*Thymus vulgaris*), lavender (*Lavandula angustifolia*), rosemary (*Rosmarinus officinalis*) or other aromatic herbs has a disinfecting and anti-inflammatory effect on the vocal cords.

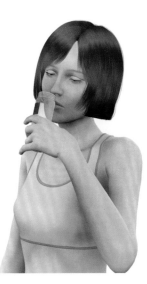

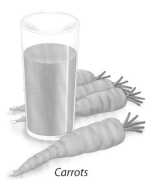

DRINK CARROT JUICE

Due to its high beta-carotene content that converts to vitamin A, carrot juice contributes to reinforcing the mucosa of the vocal cords and strengthening the voice.

Carrots

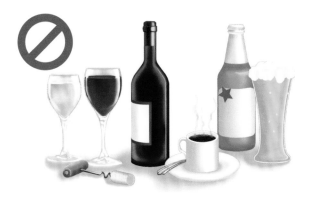

LIMIT CERTAIN PRODUCTS

Singers and speakers know that drinking alcoholic beverages or eating certain foods reduces voice quality.

Some of products and foods most affecting the voice are:

- **Alcoholic beverages**, due to the irritating effect of alcohol.
- **Cold drinks.**
- **Coffee**, possibly because caffeine promotes reflux of the stomach contents toward the esophagus and throat.
- **Milk**, possibly because it increases mucus secretion in the airways.
- **Ice cream**, due to its dairy content and low temperature.
- **Spicy condiments**, which also promotes acid reflux toward the esophagus and throat.

KEEP GENERAL THROAT CARE IN MIND

Breathe through the nose, use a room humidifier, breathe fresh air, do not smoke and keep feet warm (see earlier units).

USE NATURAL TREATMENTS FOR THE THROAT

Increasing temperature foot baths, gargling, warm compresses on the throat and steam inhalation (see prior units) are very effective for improving and preserving the voice.

CONSULT A SPECIALIST

If voice fatigue or weakness continues, a laryngologist or speech pathologist should be consulted.

Neck

Strong, yet flexible.

The neck's strength and resistance are surprising, yet so is its flexibility. The cervical vertebrae are not in straight alignment, like a column; they have a curvature called lordosis. This supports the weight of the head better than if they were simply stacked atop each other. Many consider this natural neck curvature as evidence of intelligent design, since mathematically an arch is more weight resistant than a straight line.

The neck needs this curve, and when it disappears due to the muscle stiffness that goes along with stress, pain and discomfort ensue.

A healthy neck is both strong and flexible, and can painlessly perform a wide variety of movements. The neck has four primary functions:

- Supports the weight of the head.
- Allows the head to move.
- A passageway for arteries and veins feeding the head and neck; for lymph vessels; for the trachea, which carries air to the lings; for the esophagus, which carries food to the stomach; and for the spinal cord, which connects the brain to the rest of the body.
- Physical protection for the spinal cord passing through the vertebrae. Together with the brain, the spinal cord is part of the nervous system. Numerous motor and sensory nerves extend out from it.

In addition to all of this, the neck is the anatomical site of an important endocrine gland: the thyroid. The hormones produced in the thyroid gland regulate metabolism for the entire body as well as promote a child's intellectual development.

Facts and Figures About the Neck

4 to 5 kg (8.8 to 11 lb)	Weight of the head, supported by the neck.
6	Number of movements that the neck can carry out.
7	Number of cervical vertebrae.
12	Number of joints between the cervical vertebrae (2 between each vertebra).
15	Number of muscles on each side involved in neck movement.
20 g (0.7 oz)	Weight of the thyroid gland.
100 kg (220.5 lb)	Weight in kilos that the neck can support.

Intervertebral Disk

The disks separating the vertebrae seem to be simply padding for cushioning the impact of the weight they support. However, they are really very delicate structures. Over the years, the gelatin-like elastic tissue making up the intervertebral disks becomes dry and loses its ability to cushion the pressure between the vertebrae. Due to this wear and tear, the vertebrae become inflamed and degenerated (known as cervical osteoarthritis or spondylosis) and the nerves become compressed.

Intervertebral disk disease is the primary cause of neck pain. Taking care of the neck by following the advice offered on these pages can stop the process of intervertebral disk degeneration that comes with aging.

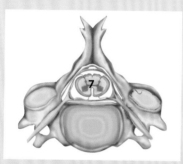

Cervical vertebra as seen from above.

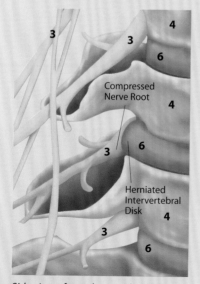

Compressed Nerve Root

Herniated Intervertebral Disk

Side view of vertebrae with a herniated intervertebral disk.

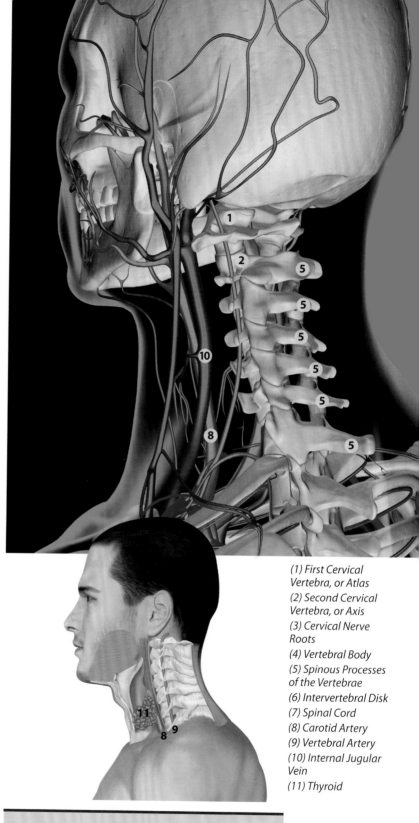

(1) First Cervical Vertebra, or Atlas
(2) Second Cervical Vertebra, or Axis
(3) Cervical Nerve Roots
(4) Vertebral Body
(5) Spinous Processes of the Vertebrae
(6) Intervertebral Disk
(7) Spinal Cord
(8) Carotid Artery
(9) Vertebral Artery
(10) Internal Jugular Vein
(11) Thyroid

Chapter Contents

CARING FOR THE NECK

*Keeping the neck flexible and avoiding muscle spasms
and intervertebral disk deterioration are the primary challenges
to caring for the neck.*

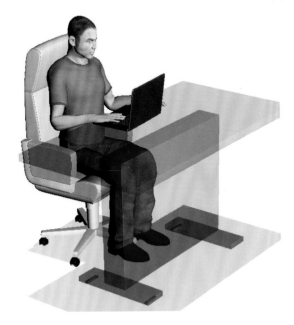

SIT CORRECTLY

Bad posture while seated is the primary cause of neck pain. When reading, writing or working on the computer:

- Avoid bending the neck toward the chest.
- Keep the neck erect, without thrusting the head forward.
- The chin should be kept up and away from the chest.
- Adjust the back so that it is properly supported by the chair's backrest.
- Rest the forearms on the table.

AVOID STRAINED POSITIONS AT WORK

The sedentary work so common to modern life requires long hours of sitting in front of a computer screen or at a desk. Without correct posture, muscle contractures and pain occur in the neck.

- Keep the head erect and properly positioned.
- Avoid spending too much time with the head in the same position. About every hour, do neck relaxation exercises.
- Do not hold the telephone between the head and shoulder.

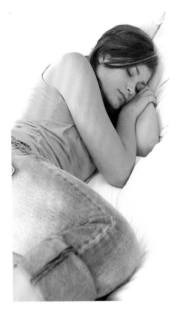

MAINTAIN A GOOD SLEEPING POSITION

If neck pain and stiffness are worse in the morning than at night, it is very likely that the cause is a bad nighttime resting position.

- The best position is on the side, with the legs slightly bent (fetal position).
- Avoid sleeping face-down, as this position strains the position of the cervical spine.
- The pillow should be made of down or pieces of foam for proper adaptation to neck curvature without being too high.

AVOID DRAFTS ON THE NECK

When cold air hits the neck, especially after having perspired, it can cause a painful neck spasm.

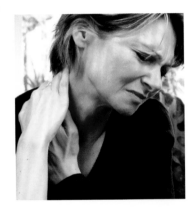

Some common causes of exposure to cold air are:

- Driving with the car window down.
- Staying near an air conditioning unit.

CORRECT USE OF AN AUTOMOTIVE HEADREST

All automobile seats must now have headrests, neck rests or cervical support. But in order for these to provide the necessary protection in case of a head-on collision or rear impact, these devices must be positioned close to the neck.

Some automobiles have active headrests. These move forward in a collision, thereby offering supplemental protection.

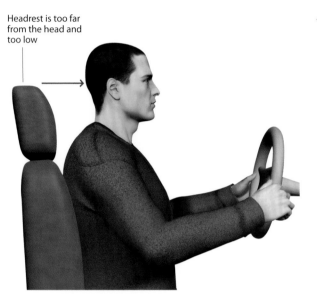

Headrest is too far from the head and too low

Poorly Adjusted Headrest.

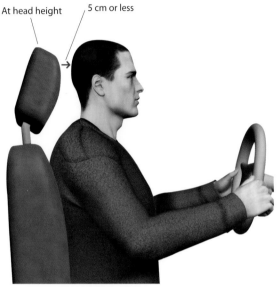

At head height   5 cm or less

Properly Adjusted Headrest.

DO NECK EXERCISES

Every day, all neck muscles should be moved in order to avoid stiffness and contractures. The most recommended exercises for keeping the neck flexible can be found on the pages that follow.

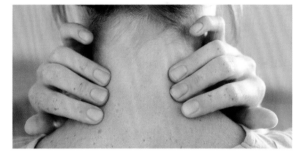

USE A CERVICAL PILLOW

When sitting for long periods, such as on long flights, use a cervical pillow or cushion for neck support.

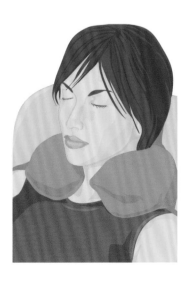

Reasons You Must See a Doctor

- Neck pain accompanied by disorientation.
- Neck pain accompanied with loss of balance or visual disturbances.
- Neck pain accompanied with pain, loss of strength, or numbness in the arms or hands.

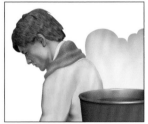

NATURAL TREATMENTS FOR THE NECK

Heat and muscle relaxation are the primary healing factors for regaining neck flexibility. All of these treatments are effective against neck spasms and other types of neck pain.

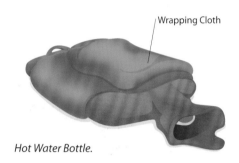

Wrapping Cloth

Hot Water Bottle.

DRY HEAT ON THE NECK

Dry heat is effective in relieving neck pain, although to a lesser degree than moist heat.

Dry heat is applied with a heating pad or a hot water bottle wrapped with a cloth.

Caution: Do not sleep with the heating pad plugged into an outlet.

Temperature: 30-36 ˚C (86-97 ˚F). Avoid higher temperatures that could cause burns to the skin.

Duration: 10-30 minutes or more.

Afterward: Cover the neck with a wool scarf or cloth.

Frequency: Several times per day.

WARM STREAM OR SHOWER ON THE NECK

The combination of heat and water pressure on the neck muscles produces a pleasant relaxing and analgesic effect for stiff neck muscles.

Water Temperature: Start at 30 ˚C (86 ˚F) and increase the temperature of the stream or shower of water gradually until it reaches 42 ˚C (108 ˚F).

Duration: 3-5 minutes.

Afterward: Dry and cover the neck with a wool scarf or cloth.

Frequency: One to three times a day.

NECK COMPRESSES

Compresses consist of applying moist heat by way of a cloth soaked in water as hot as the skin can tolerate. Its effect is very intense and effective, relieving pain and relaxing tight muscles.

Water Temperature: As hot as possible, so steam is produced. Ideally, it should be near-boiling.

Duration: 10-15 minutes. When the moist cloth loses its heat (usually after two or three minutes), soak it in hot water again.

Afterward: Dry the neck and cover with a wool scarf or cloth.

Frequency: Once or twice per day.

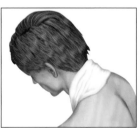

1. Protect skin with a dry cotton cloth.

2. Soak and drain a towel in very hot water, and place it over the dry protective cloth.

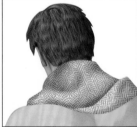

3. Cover these two cloths with a wool blanket.

NECK BRACE

A neck brace provides stability and support for the cervical vertebrae. It must be used after trauma or injury to the neck.

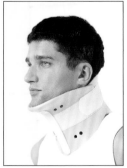

NECK MASSAGE

A neck massage is very effective for relaxing muscles and improving circulation.

It can be done in a seated position, with head support, as well as lying down.

Cuando existe rigidez y dolor, el masaje debe ser aplicado por un fisioterapeuta.

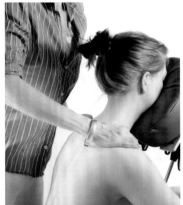

Neck massage, seated position with head support.

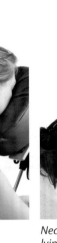

Neck massage, lying position.

NECK TRACTION

Neck traction relaxes muscles and relieves pain caused by radiculitis (nerve root inflammation, usually due to a herniated intervertebral disk). It is also effective for neck pain due to spasm or other causes.

Neck traction should be under the supervision of a physical therapist.

How to Perform: It usually begins with hanging 2 kg (about 4.5 pounds) for 10 minutes, increasing as tolerated up to 10 kg of weight (= 22 pounds). The counterweight is usually a hanging bag of water or, in more modern equipment, an electronic device.

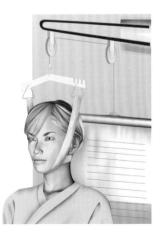

Home device for neck traction, using a bag of water as a counterweight.

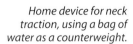

Exercises for the Neck

The monotony of activities of modern life keeps the neck stiff for many hours, causing it to lose its flexibility. These exercises are designed to restore normal neck movements, avoid neck contractures and relieve pain.

General Recommendations

- Never start exercise when having severe pain.
- Whenever possible, and especially if there is stiffness, apply mild heat to the neck for five or ten minutes prior to starting exercises. Then, massage gently. This allows exercise to be better tolerated and have more beneficial results.
- For each exercise, push to but not past the point of pain.
- To keep the neck in good condition, perform stretching and resistance strengthening exercises at least once per day, using each one of the neck's six movements. Between 5 and 10 minutes per day is enough.

Stretching Exercises

These are for increasing the range of every movement, with a little extra push at the end.

- Do each of the 6 movements of the neck.
- Upon reaching the end of the movement, apply a little extra pressure in order to achieve an effective stretch.

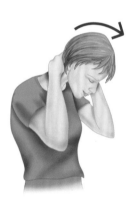

Flexion movement stretching.

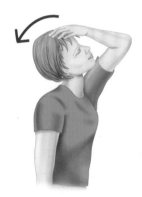

Extension movement stretching.

The 6 Movements of the Neck

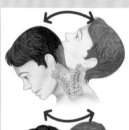

Flexion and Extension
Normal range:
90 degrees

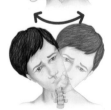

Right and Left Ear-to-Shoulder
Normal range:
120 degrees

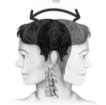

Right and Left Rotation
Normal range:
180 degrees

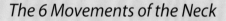

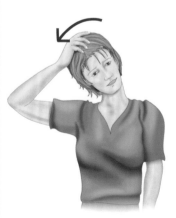

Left ear-to-shoulder movement stretching (repeat toward the right).

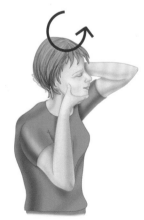

Left rotation movement stretching (repeat toward the right).

RESISTANCE STRENGTHENING EXERCISES

These are designed to strengthen the neck muscles.

- Doe each of the 6 movements of the neck.

- While performing each movement, use the hand to provide counter-resistance.

Rotation movement strengthening (rotate toward the left and right).

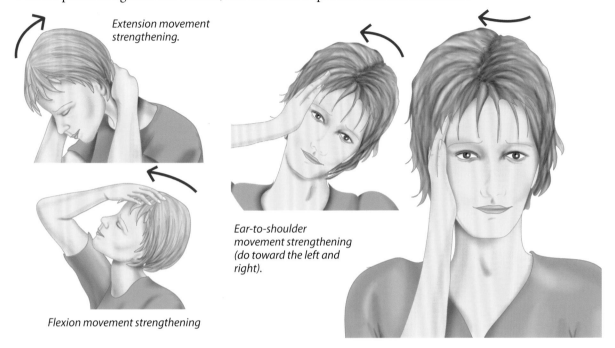

Extension movement strengthening.

Ear-to-shoulder movement strengthening (do toward the left and right).

Flexion movement strengthening

Whiplash

The neck is the most commonly injured body part in automobile accidents. As low as 20 km/h (= 12.5 mph), a head-on crash or a rear impact can cause a neck injury known as whiplash.

The jerking motion overstretches the neck, damaging its joints and ligaments. The pain and contracture can last several weeks.

WHIPLASH PREVENTION

Properly use the seat's headrests, positioning them close to the head (preferably at less than 5 cm, about 2 inches).

TREATMENT

- Ice pack on the neck for the first 2 days to reduce inflammation (about 10 minutes every hour).

- Immobilization with a neck brace: Continuously for a week. Every other day for 10 more days. Prolonged neck immobilization has undesirable effects, as muscles become atrophied and weaken even further.

- Neck exercises after the 7th day post-accident, for at least two weeks. The exercises should be moderate in order to strengthen the neck muscles, and should include stretching and resistance strengthening.

- Heat with a heating pad, hot stream of water or shower, or hot packs (see previous pages).

- Anti-inflammatories and muscle relaxers.

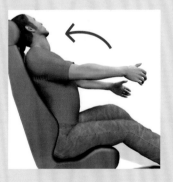

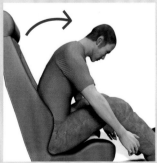

CARING FOR THE THYROID

The thyroid gland, located at the front of the neck, works silently and inconspicuously. But just like other more notable body parts, the thyroid also needs care to promote good functioning.

DIET

The diet is the primary source of iodine for the body. In order to function properly, the thyroid needs 150 μg of iodine every day (220 μg for pregnant women). Between 2-3 g of iodized salt per day provide this amount of iodine.

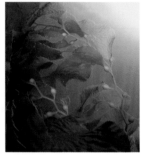

Kelp seaweed, one of the richest in iodine.

Both an insufficient level and an excess of iodine in the diet can cause thyroid disorders:

- Iodine deficient diet: In adults, this manifests as goiter (increase in the size of the thyroid). In children, serious deficiency slows growth and mental development.

- Excessive iodine in the diet: When the thyroid is working well, it is able to assimilate only the iodine it needs, and the excess of iodine does not cause any disorders. But when there is a certain level of thyroiditis (thyroid inflammation), an excess of iodine can cause hyperthyroidism.

Foods Rich in Iodine: Kelp, other seaweed and fish. In some countries, salt, milk and bread are enriched with iodine.

Foods Low in Iodine: All foods raised in mountainous areas where the ground has low iodine levels.

Foods that Reduce Iodine Absorption: Cabbage, cauliflower, broccoli and other vegetables in the crucifer family, manioc or cassava, yams, taro and bamboo shoots contain substances that reduce iodine absorption in the intestines. However, in order for these foods to produce an iodine deficiency they would need to be consumed regularly and in very high amounts.

Foods that Promote Iodine Absorption: Foods rich in vitamin A and vitamin E.

AVOID RADIATION

Exposure of the head or neck to ionizing radiation especially during childhood is a risk factor for thyroid cancer. Thyroid-damaging radiation can come from:

- Radioactive rain, like after the 1986 Chernobyl (Ukraine) accident, or after an atomic bomb attack.
  - In case of a nuclear accident with radioactive iodine emissions, potassium iodide pills should be taken to protect the thyroid gland. The recommended daily dose is 130 mg for teens, adults and pregnant women, 65 mg for children from 3-11 years of age, and 32 mg for 3 years of age and under.

- Radiation therapy given for another type of cancer without protecting the thyroid area. In the middle of last century, children and young people received radiation therapy for treatment of acne, tonsillitis, growths and ringworm. Children who were exposed to this radiation have a higher risk of developing thyroid cancer as adults.

- X-Rays: Radiation doses are usually low, but cumulative. It is estimated that after ten panoramic x-rays of the jaw (orthopanto-mography) without protection, the risk of thyroid cancer increases significantly.

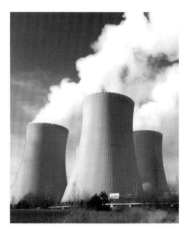

AVOID TOBACCO

It has been shown that tobacco use promotes the development of hyperthyroidism (Graves' disease) in people with genetic predisposition.

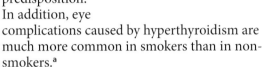

In addition, eye complications caused by hyperthyroidism are much more common in smokers than in non-smokers.[a]

a. Relationship between cigarette smoking and Graves' ophthalmopathy. Hegediüs L, Brix TH, Vestergaard P. J Endocrinol Invest. 2004 Mar;27(3):265-71. Review. PMID: 15165003

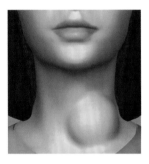

Goiter is enlargement of the thyroid gland. In many cases, it is the result of a diet low in iodine.

WATCH OUT FOR CERTAIN MEDICATIONS

Some medications can affect thyroid function as a side effect:

- **Lithium Salts**: These are used to treat manic-depressive bipolar disorder. Over the long term, they decrease thyroid hormone production (hypothyroidism).

- **Amiodarone**: Used to treat of cardiac arrhythmias, but can cause hypothyroidism or hyperthyroidism.

- **Interferon or Interleukin**: Medications used to treat hepatitis, multiple sclerosis and some types of cancer can affect thyroid function.

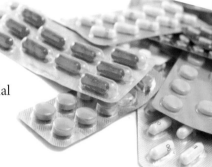

If any of these medications are required, their potential side effects on the thyroid must be considered.

Main Thyroid Diseases

- **Goiter**: Enlarged thyroid gland, accompanied by hypo- or hyperthyroidism. Can be caused by an iodine-deficient diet.

- **Hyperthyroidism**: Excessive hormone production in the thyroid gland. In 75% of cases, hyperthyroidism is the result of hereditary Graves' disease. It manifests as anxiety, tachycardia, trembling, hair loss and bulging eyes. It is most common in women between the ages of 40-50.

- **Hypothyroidism**: Insufficient hormone production in the thyroid gland. It manifests as fatigue, weight gain, depression and increased cholesterol levels. It is most common in women beginning at 55 years of age.

- **Hashimoto's Thyroiditis**: Autoimmune thyroid inflammation. It manifests as a slow-growing goiter and hypothyroidism alternating with phases of hyperthyroidism.

- **De Quervain's Thyroiditis**: Inflammation of the thyroid due to a viral infection. It manifests as cold symptoms accompanied by neck soreness and hyperthyroidism. It tends to resolve after a few weeks without any need for treatment.

- **Thyroid Cancer**: It can manifest as a lump on the thyroid that is usually painless. Diagnostic testing determines if the nodule is benign or malignant (cancerous). Surgical treatment yields good results.

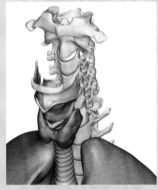

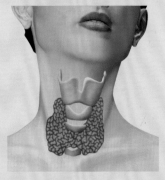

Upper Limbs

Serving the hands, from shoulder to wrist.

The upper limbs make up a functional unit endowed with amazing abilities. The shoulder joint stands out among these, with its ability to perform the skeleton's most ample and varied movements; the arm, endowed with powerful biceps and triceps; the elbow, with its strength and stability; and the wrist, with its flexibility and resistance. All of these work together in harmony to allow each hand to have a broad range of motion, allowing them to reach nearly anything within a shoulder-centered sphere measuring about 120 cm (3.9 ft) in diameter. The arm also contributes to the hand being able to perform a wide variety of tasks with a surprising combination of strength and grace, power and precision. Thanks to the arm, the hand can reach just about anywhere on the body to do just about anything.

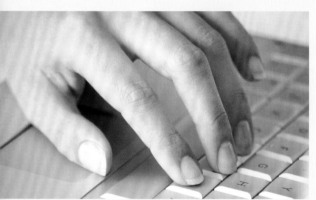

What is amazing about the hands is all that can be done with them.

It has been said that the hand is an extension of the brain. Brain and hand make up an extraordinary tandem, with the ability to carry out the greatest awe-inspiring works and actions, such as creating, caressing or healing; but also the vilest of acts, including destruction, abuse or injury.

Both the brain and the hand have the anatomical traits that are most specific to humankind; these represent the major difference from animals, making us a unique species.

Cancer is not common in the upper limbs; however, trauma and inflammation are indeed common. Avoiding accidents and relieving inflammation requires the specific care and attention described in this chapter.

Facts and Figures About the Upper Limbs

5%	Percentage of left-handed people among the general population.
9	Number of muscles acting in conjunction to perform the pincer grasp between the thumb and forefinger.
19	Number of precision muscles in the arm and forearm.
20 cm (7.87 in)	Average length of the palm of the hand, measured from the tip of the thumb to the tip of the pinky finger, with the hand fully extended.
30	Number of bones in each upper limb (27 in the hand and wrist, 2 in the forearm and 1 in the arm).
40 kg (88.19 lb)	A man's average grip strength.
25 000	Number of sweat glands in each armpit.

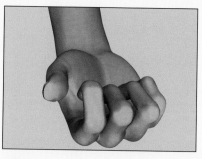

Grip

In addition to humans, apes and other animals can do this.

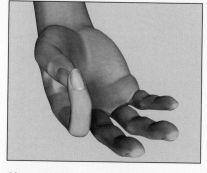

Pincer Grasp

Only human beings can perform the complex movement of touching thumb to forefinger with precision; to do so requires nine muscles to work together.

Thanks to this anatomical feature, human hands can perform extremely fine movements and develop skills to an advanced level.

Some animals appear to have an opposable thumb, but without the functionality and skills of the human thumb. In pandas, for example, the opposition is not done by the thumb, but rather by a hypertrophied sesamoid bone.

In the absence of any other proof, the thumb alone would convince me of God's existence.

Sir Isaac Newton (1643-1727)

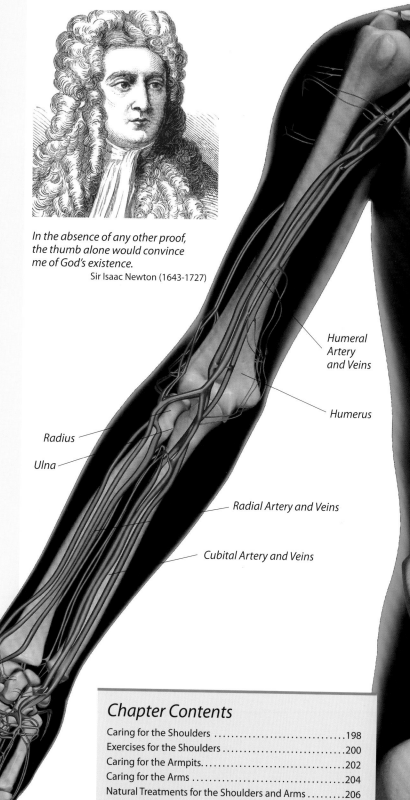

Humeral Artery and Veins

Humerus

Radius

Ulna

Radial Artery and Veins

Cubital Artery and Veins

Chapter Contents

CARING FOR THE SHOULDERS

The shoulder joint is the most mobile of the entire skeleton. However, the cost of such range of motion is decreased stability. For this reason, the shoulder is the joint that is the most delicate and in need of care.

USE AN ERGONOMIC PILLOW

An ergonomic pillow promotes proper posture of the cervical spine and shoulders. The pillow should not elevate the shoulders, but instead allow them to stay in contact with the bed, whether in the supine decubitus (face up) or lateral decubitus (on the side) position.

Considering we spend nearly a third of our lives in bed, it is very important to have proper sleeping posture.

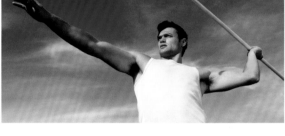

Sports requiring the arms to be raised, such as javelin throwing, cause wear and tear of the shoulders.

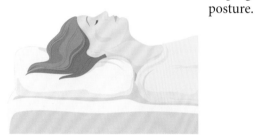

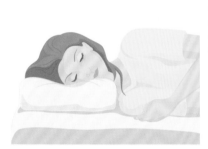

Ergonomic Pillow
Should allow shoulders to rest on the bed and not on the pillow. To that end, it must have an indentation in which to place the head.

CAUTION WHEN PLAYING SPORTS

Playing certain sports is very strenuous on the shoulder. Sports that require raising the arm above the head are especially hard on the shoulders, such as:

- Swimming.
- Baseball.
- Weightlifting.
- Shot putting, discus and javelin throwing.
- Basketball.
- Tennis and ping-pong.

Preventing Sports Injuries to the Shoulder

- Keep sports training sessions to a moderate level.
- Do warm-up exercises.
- Schedule a rest period.
- Avoid any intense and unusual straining of the shoulder, such as a "weekend sailor" would do by hoisting a sail. Extremely strenuous tasks can cause tearing of the tendons that make up the rotator cuff.
- If exercise causes pain, the activity should be discontinued until the pain resolves. Continuing with exercise when there is shoulder pain can cause tendinitis (inflammation of the rotator cuff or other shoulder tendons) as well as tendon tears.
- Wear shoulder pads when playing certain sports, such as rugby.

Reasons You Must See a Doctor

- Shoulder pain that does not improve with rest. It could be heart-related (if pain is on the left), liver-related (if pain is on the right), or related to the lungs or abdomen.
- Pain in the left shoulder radiating or traveling toward the arm (could be heart-related).
- Inability to raise the arm.
- Redness and inflammation of the shoulder.

CAUTION WHEN WORKING WITH THE ARMS

Repetitive and strenuous shoulder movements eventually cause pain and inflammation in this complex joint.

Some jobs that put the shoulder at risk are:

- Carrying a load on the shoulders.
- Painting.
- Steering a vehicle.
- Any type of manual labor that requires arm raising.

Preventing Work Injuries to the Shoulder

- Do not strain the shoulder while working.

- If there is shoulder pain, discontinue the related task until the pain resolves. It can be helpful to apply something cold to the shoulder and do stretching exercises.

- If there is a shoulder injury, reduce or avoid the triggering activity until the inflammation resolves.

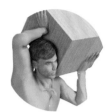

The Rotator Cuff

The rotator cuff is an important structure in the shoulder, and is made up of the tendons of four muscles: the supraspinatus, infraspinatus, subscapularis and teres minor. The cuff surrounds and secures the primary joint of the shoulder (glenohumeral joint) in place; this gives it the stability needed so the humeral head does not come out of the glenoid cavity of the scapula.

When the shoulder is exercised extensively, the rotator cuff has to endure a great amount of stress. Because of this, it is prone to suffer inflammation and tears. Repeatedly raising the arm over shoulder level is the movement that most affects this important shoulder-securing structure.

ROTATOR CUFF TENDINITIS

- **Symptoms**: Pain and inability to raise the arm.
- **Treatment**: Ice pack to the shoulder the first few days, shoulder immobilization for about two weeks (not too long, in order to prevent adhesions and a "frozen shoulder"), stretching and strengthening exercises, anti-inflammatories and application of short waves or ultrasound, all under the supervision of a physical therapy professional. In more difficult cases, corticosteroid injections may be used.

ROTATOR CUFF TEAR

- **Symptoms**: Pain and inability to raise the arm.
- **Treatment**: A rotator cuff tear should be repaired surgically, either by open surgery or arthroscopy (a tiny tube inserted into the joint).

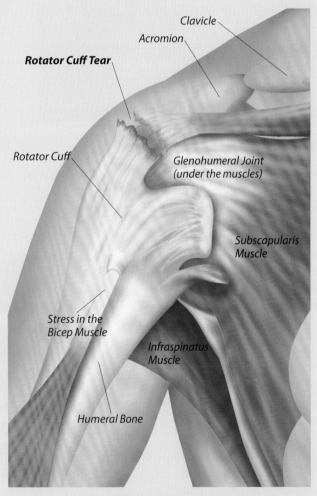

Rotator cuff tendinitis (inflammation) or tearing is the most common injury in people who strain the shoulder.

EXERCISES FOR THE SHOULDERS

Performing these exercises contributes to recovery from shoulder injuries; they also help keep the shoulders in good condition to prevent injury. Remember, rehabilitation after a shoulder injury requires a great deal of consistency and the supervision of a physical therapy professional.

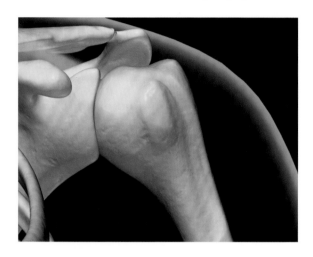

GENERAL RECOMMENDATIONS

- If pain is severe, exercise should never be started.
- Each stretching, strengthening or maintenance exercise (depending on the shoulder's condition) should be repeated 5 times, two or three times per day.
- Each exercise is taken only to the point of pain, and no farther.

STRETCHING EXERCISES

- Because they are the most gentle, these should be done first, once the most acute phase of tendinitis or other shoulder injury has passed.
- Their goal is to increase shoulder flexibility.

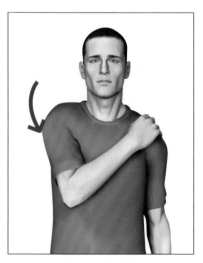

1. Touch the front of the unaffected shoulder with the other hand.

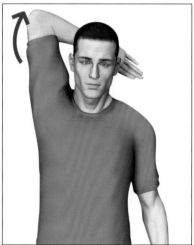

2. Raise the affected arm above the head and touch the back of the unaffected shoulder. Force the elbow backward.

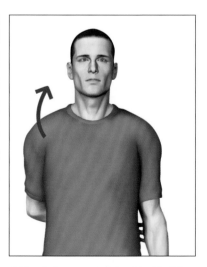

3. Touch the scapula (shoulder blade) on the back on the unaffected side, keeping the affected arm next to the body. Move the shoulder and elbow of the unaffected side backward.

STRENGTHENING EXERCISES

- Because these are the most difficult, they should be done after getting past the acute inflammatory phase.
- Their goal is to strengthen shoulder tendons and ligaments in order to achieve greater joint stability.

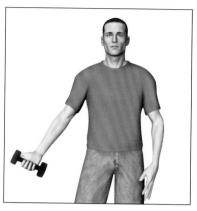

1. Without bending the elbow, raise the arm to a 45-degree angle to the body, or as tolerated depending on pain. A progressively heavier weight should be held in the hand, with the thumb pointing upward.
Lifting weights in this way strengthens the rotator cuff.

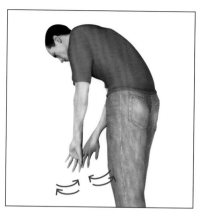

2. While standing, bend forward, with the arms hanging. Make twisting movements with the hands while holding a weighted object.

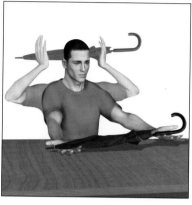

3. Sit at a table with the back straight. Hold a stick (an umbrella would work) with both hands, and place it behind the neck. Lift it above the head and put it on the table as far away from the body as possible.

MAINTENANCE EXERCISES

- These are recommended as a daily activity for keeping the shoulders in good condition.
- They can also be done in the recovery phase after a shoulder injury.

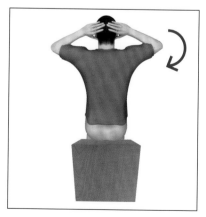

1. Place both hands on the back of the neck and force the elbows backward, while inhaling deeply.

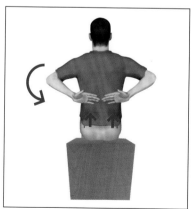

2. Put both hands behind the back, keeping it straight, then raise and lower the hands.

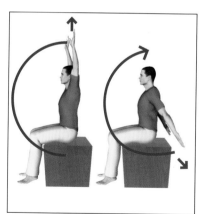

3. Lift the arms up vertically until they touch the ears, inhaling deeply. Keep them there for 10-20 seconds.
Next, lower the arms, swinging them backward and exhaling deeply.

CARING FOR THE ARMPITS

A warm, moist environment such as that of the armpits promotes bacterial and fungal growth. Taking care of the armpits is essential to body hygiene.

ARMPIT HYGIENE

- **Wash with Soap and Water**: This is the most simple and effective method for armpit hygiene. Even if deodorants or antiperspirants are used, the armpits should be washed with soap and water at least once per day. This eliminates the bacteria that ferment sweat and cause bad odor.

- **Deodorants**: These contain bactericidal (bacteria-killing) substances that eliminate the bacteria living in the armpits; in turn, the sweat that is still being produced is prevented from acquiring a bad odor.

- **Odor Absorbers**: These are substances that retain the molecules responsible for body odor, which are mostly produced by bacteria present on the skin.

- **Antiperspirants**: Substances that reduce sweat production by blocking the pores that drain to the skin. Their chemical makeup is based on aluminum salts, a metal that damages the sweat gland excretion ducts, causing their blockage. Antiperspirant use has not been shown to be associated with breast cancer (see facing table), but it does appear to promote armpit infections, such as hydrosadenitis: an armpit abscess.

SPECIAL CARE FOR DIABETICS

Diabetics should be strict about armpit hygiene, due to their greater risk of bacterial infection (such as boils), fungal infection (such as candidiasis and erythrasma). The following care methods can prevent many infections:

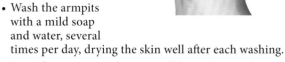

- Wash the armpits with a mild soap and water, several times per day, drying the skin well after each washing.

- Keep the armpits as dry as possible, applying talcum powder or drying them with a cotton cloth.

- Wear absorbent undergarments, preferably made of cotton, and change them at least once per day.

- Avoid excessive heat and humidity.

- Keep a proper body weight, avoiding obesity.

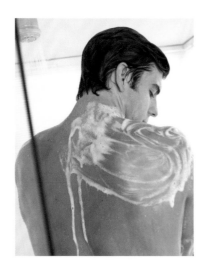

The best standard of hygiene is more soap and water, and less antiperspirant.

Reasons You Must See a Doctor

- Lump or node deep in the armpit. This could be adenopathy or a lymph node related to a breast or chest tumor.

- Superficial red bump in the armpit: This is typically due to a benign infection of some skin structure, usually a hair follicle (boil) or a sweat gland (hydrosadenitis or armpit abscess).

HAIR REMOVAL

Armpit hair removal helps reduce odor, as it decreases the amount of sweat retained in the armpit. Armpit hair can be removed by:

- Cutting the hairs (regular shaving).
- Pulling the hairs out with wax.
- Hair elimination by chemical hair removal creams or lotions. Chemical hair removers can cause skin allergies and photosensitivity (appearance of blotches on the skin after sun exposure).
- Hair follicle (hair root) elimination by laser. Although it can cause mild skin irritation, this method has the fewest undesirable effects.

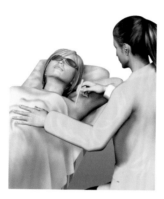

Laser removal of armpit hair.

ALTERNATIVES TO DEODORANTS

Deodorants, and especially antiperspirants, have undesirable effects such as skin irritation and allergic reactions to their ingredients. The following alternatives may prove useful:

- Using an antibacterial soap.
- Changing clothes at least once daily.
- Shaving or removing hair from armpits.
- Applying a cold compress to each armpit, soaking a cloth in hydrogen peroxide. Lower the arms to hold the compress in each armpit for at least one minute.
- Applying a pinch or two of baking soda to each armpit. Baking soda prevents the development of bacteria in armpit perspiration.
- Using a deodorant crystal made of natural aluminum mineral salts. It does not contain alcohol or irritating chemicals, and does not stain clothing.
- Reducing intake of meat and spicy foods, as they increase body odor; increase consumption of fresh fruits and vegetables.

Antiperspirants and Breast Cancer

Because many breast cancers are located in the breast's supero-external quadrant, close to the armpit, it is thought that armpit antiperspirant use could promote breast cancer. It has been argued that because antiperspirants block sweat elimination (unlike deodorants, which only change their odor), they block the elimination of toxins. Some of these toxins that are said to be retained with the remaining sweat circulate throughout the lymph glands in the armpits and breasts, causing cancerous cell mutations.

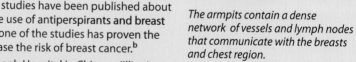

The armpits contain a dense network of vessels and lymph nodes that communicate with the breasts and chest region.

Since the year 2000, several scientific studies have been published about the possible relationship between the use of antiperspirants and breast cancer.[a] It is important to note that none of the studies has proven the hypothesis that antiperspirants increase the risk of breast cancer.[b]

However, in a study done by Saint Joseph Hospital in Chicago (Illinois, United States) with 437 women diagnosed with breast cancer, those who shaved armpits and used antiperspirants and deodorants more often were found to be diagnosed with breast cancer at an earlier age than the others.[c] This finding could be explained by the fact that women who dedicate more time and care to armpit hygiene are more likely to have early detection of any node or lump appearing in armpits or breasts.

Although there has been no direct association shown between the use of antiperspirants and breast cancer, care should be taken with these products that change a physiological function such as perspiration.

a. http://www.cancer.gov/espanol/cancer/hojas-informativas/antitranspirantes-desodorantes/
b. The use of deodorants/antiperspirants does not constitute a risk factor for breast cancer. Namer M, Luporsi E, Gligorov J, Lokiec F, Spielmann M. Bull Cancer. 2008 Sep;95(9):871-80. Review. PMID: 18829420
c. An earlier age of breast cancer diagnosis related to more frequent use of antiperspirants/deodorants and underarm shaving. McGrath KG. Eur J Cancer Prev. 2003 Dec;12(6):479-85. PMID: 14639125

CARING FOR THE ARMS

Two anatomical sections make up what is commonly known as the arm:
The arm itself (from the shoulder to the elbow) and the forearms
(from the elbow to the wrist). Because the majority of work and sports
are done with the arms, care must be taken to prevent overload.

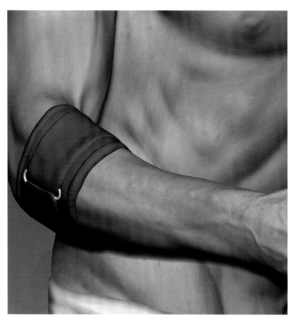

To protect the elbow and forearm, one should place a brace or band 5 to 10 cm (2 to 4 inches) below the elbow.

Do Not Overload the Arms

When working with the hands or playing certain sports, there is a risk of overloading forearm muscles, which carry out the majority of hand movements. With the following recommendations, the forearms can be protected from excessive overload:

Reasons You Must See a Doctor

- Elbow or forearm pain not subsiding after rest.
- Numbness or limpness of the arm or forearm.
- Loss of strength in the arm or forearm.

- Avoid repetitive and prolonged movements of the forearm or wrist. The movements that most overload the forearm muscles, capable of causing "tennis elbow", are twisting combined with grasping an object, such as:
  – Playing tennis, ping-pong or golf.
  – Turning a screwdriver.
  – Painting with a brush.
  – Ironing.
  – Cutting objects with a knife.
- Try to make sure that work tools and instruments are light and gripped firmly.
- Take short breaks, at least once an hour.
- Do forearm stretching exercises after work, followed by strengthening exercises.
- Stop any exercise when any pain appears.

Do Natural Treatments

Some helpful home remedies for the arms are detailed in "Natural Treatments for the Shoulders and Arms".

Caution When Playing Tennis

Playing tennis and ping-pong subject the elbow and forearm to continuous strain. As a result, players often suffer tennis elbow. The following recommendations can help prevent it:

- Try to be sure the racket is light and grasp it firmly.
- Do forearm stretching exercises after a game, then do strengthening exercises.
- Do not strain the elbow when doing a backhand.
- Avoid playing with balls that are wet or too heavy.
- Pause the game if there is pain.

FOREARM STRETCHING EXERCISES

These exercises distend and relax contracted muscles after intense forearm muscle exercise. Each exercise is done at least 5 times after working with the forearm.

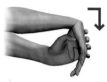

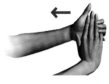

2. Try to flex or move the hand down while placing resistance on it with the other hand.

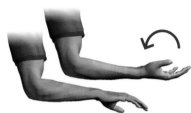

3. With the elbow flexed 90 degrees, twist the hand upward and downward.

1. Try to extend or raise the hand while placing resistance on it with the other hand.

FOREARM STRENGTHENING EXERCISES

These exercises strengthen the forearm muscles, preparing them to better withstand the efforts made during work or sports. Repeat each at least 5 times before working or playing sports involving the forearm.

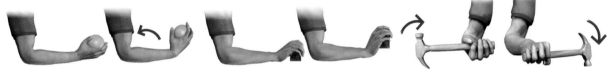

1. Flexor muscle strengthening: Take a weight in the hand and raise it with the palm facing upward.

2. Extensor muscle strengthening: Take a weight in the hand and raise it with the palm facing downward.

3. Prono-supinator muscle strengthening: Take a hammer or another long, heavy object and twist forward upward and downward, keeping the elbow flexed at a 90-degree angle.

Tennis Elbow

Tennis elbow is overload of the forearm and hand muscles from strenuous twisting. Despite its name, it does not only affect tennis players, but also those who subject the elbow and forearm to prolonged straining.

TREATMENT

- Apply cold with an ice pack on the elbow and forearm, in 20-minute sessions, 6 times per day for the first two or three days (see "Natural Treatments for the Shoulders and Arms").
- Discontinue the exercise that caused the muscle inflammation.
- Local immobilization with splints or bandages.
- Stretching and strengthening exercises of the forearm and wrist muscles.
- Use a band when resuming play or work.
- Physical therapy.
- Anti-inflammatory medication, infiltrations with local anesthesia or corticosteroids.
- Surgery in recurring cases.

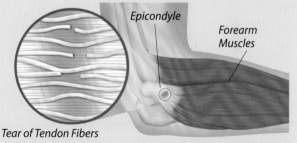

Epicondyle

Forearm Muscles

Tear of Tendon Fibers

The cause of pain in tennis elbow is lateral epicondylitis (inflammation of the muscles and tendons that insert into the lateral epicondyle of the humerus, a protrusion on this bone).

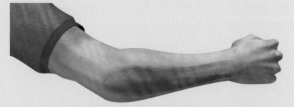

Elbow or forearm pain is an indication that the exercise should be discontinued. This way, progression to lateral epicondylitis or tennis elbow is prevented.

Natural Treatments for the Shoulders and Arms

In general, cold should be applied the first few days after an injury.
Once the acute phase has ended, heat is better.

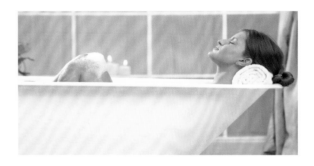

Hot Bath Up to the Neck

In addition to the torso and legs, a hot bath up to the neck should include the arms and shoulders.

This bath relaxes back, shoulder, and arm muscles, which relieves pain and improves blood flow to the upper limbs.

Water Temperature: 36-40 ˚C (97-104 ˚F).

Duration: 10-20 minutes.

Afterward: Dry the body well, put on warm clothing and rest for half an hour in bed or on the sofa.

Frequency: Once or twice per day.

Hot Arm Bath

A hot arm bath should be done with both arms at the same time. It relaxes the arm and forearm muscles while increasing circulation.

This is good whenever the arms are fatigued or heavy after strenuous work or sports, and after the acute phase of shoulder or elbow injuries.

Water Temperature: 36-40 ˚C (97-104 ˚F). Hot water can be added gradually until the temperature reaches 44 ˚C (111 ˚F).

Duration: 10-15 minutes.

Afterward: Dry the body well, put on warm clothing and rest for a few minutes.

Frequency: Once or twice per day.

Clay Compress on the Shoulder or Elbow

A clay compress is an interesting alternative to an ice pack. Just like the ice pack, it should be used for the first few days of acute shoulder or elbow inflammation. The anti-inflammatory effect of the ice combines with by the same effect of the clay.

A clay poultice is a variation of the compress. The clay paste is thickened and applied directly over the skin, then covered with a cloth.

Temperature: The water used to make the clay mixture should be room temperature or cold.

Duration: 20-30 minutes.

Afterward: Rinse remaining clay from the skin with water and cover with something warm.

Frequency: Once or twice per day.

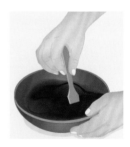

1. Add clay to a container of water, making a light, even paste.

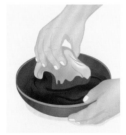

2. Dip a cloth or gauze pad into the clay.

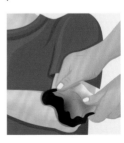

3. Place the clay-soaked cloth or gauze pad onto the affected shoulder or elbow.

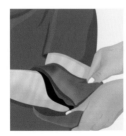

4. Cover with a wool wrap.

ICE PACK ON THE SHOULDER OR ELBOW

Cold on the shoulder is indicated during the first days of acute shoulder joint inflammation, such as in rotator cuff tendinitis (see "Caring for the Shoulders"), or elbow inflammation, such as in tennis elbow (see "Caring for the Arms").

Temperature: Under 0 ˚C (32 ˚F).

Duration: 15-20 minutes.

Afterward: Remove the ice and cover.

Frequency: Up to 6 times per day (every 2 or 3 hours).

PARAFFIN BATH FOR THE ELBOW

A paraffin bath for the elbow is done just like the paraffin bath for the hands (see "Natural Treatments for the Hands").

This should be done in the recovery phase of lateral epicondylitis or tennis elbow, and for elbow joint inflammation.

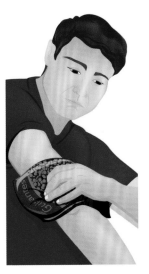

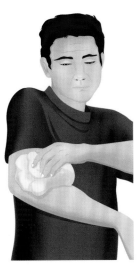

Place crushed ice into a plastic bag. Wrap the ice pack with a towel or cloth and place it onto the affected area. Avoid direct contact between the ice and the skin.

A bag of frozen peas can also be used, as it molds well to the shoulder and elbow surfaces, and can be re-frozen and used again.

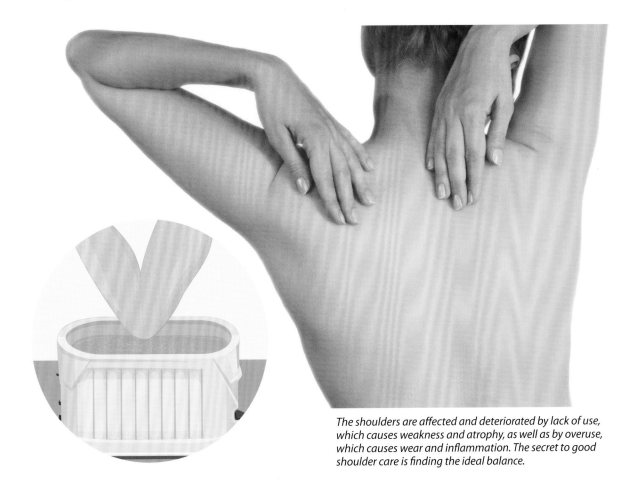

The shoulders are affected and deteriorated by lack of use, which causes weakness and atrophy, as well as by overuse, which causes wear and inflammation. The secret to good shoulder care is finding the ideal balance.

CARING FOR THE HANDS

Along with the face, the hands are a personal business card.
Hands that are well-cared for say a lot about their owner.

BASIC HAND CARE

- Avoid excessive sun exposure to the hands.
- Use a moisturizer, especially on the back of the hands.
- Care for the nails by filing rough edges and trimming with suitable nail clippers.
- Do not tear off the cuticles growing around the nails.
- Do not bite nails.
- Get a manicure by a trained professional.

A GOOD WORKING POSTURE

Do not support the wrist directly on the table when using a computer mouse or keyboard, as this promotes joint inflammation as well as carpal tunnel syndrome.

Placing a pillow under the wrist when using a mouse can provide a more ergonomic position and allows the hand to rest.

PROPER PROTECTION FOR THE HANDS

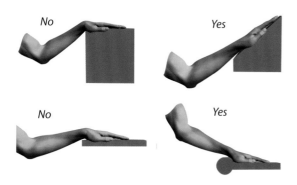

Because the majority of work and home accidents affect the hands, before working with them, their protection must be considered.

- Wear work gloves whenever possible, especially in the shop, garden and kitchen.
- Do not touch the following with the bare hands: chemicals, cement, animal carcasses or any harsh or contaminated substance.

REST FOR THE HANDS

When working with the hands, they should be given a little rest. Raising the fatigued hand above shoulder level and moving the wrist around for one minute improves blood circulation to the hands and rests them.

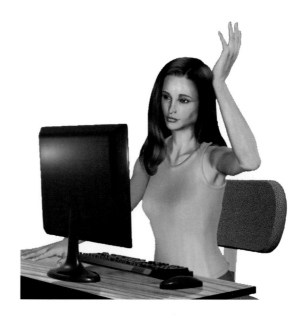

LOOK OUT FOR COMMON HAND CONDITIONS

The hands are constantly active throughout the day and can suffer conditions that require attention and care. These are the most common:

- **Sweaty Hands**: Along with the armpits and soles of the feet, the palms are the area with the most sweat-producing glands. Excessive perspiration can be bothersome and require specific care:
  - Use of antiperspirants, like those used for the armpits.
  - Iontophoresis: Applying certain medications through a low-voltage electrical current that closes sweat glands.
  - Stress control.

- **Dry or Cracked Hands**: These are due to loss of the protective oil layer normally covering the skin of the hands.
  - Do not wash hands excessively. Soap and detergents damage the protective layer of skin.
  - Whenever possible, wash hands with a suitable lotion, cleaning them afterward with a disposable cloth or towel.
  - Do not dry hands with air dryers.
  - Apply a moisturizer several times per day, rubbing hands together. Glycerin with a few drops of essential lemon oil is a good skin moisturizer.
  - Wear cotton gloves for tasks at home or at work. Cotton allows the skin to breathe while retaining moisture. By wearing gloves, hands can be washed less frequently.
  - Wear rubber gloves for touching water or liquids, but protect the skin by wearing cotton gloves under the rubber gloves.
  - Rub hands with oatmeal powder (see "Natural Treatments for the Hands").
  - Apply urea and/or cortisone creams when dryness is excessive and accompanied by eczema or dermatitis.

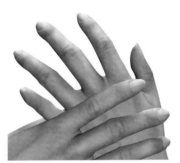

Reasons You Must See a Doctor

- Numbness or tingling in the fingers.
- Loss of strength in the fingers.
- Chilblains with blisters or blue-colored areas on the fingers.
- Pain due to chilblains that does not resolve within a few hours.

- **Cold Hands**: This can be due to circulation disorders such as Raynaud's syndrome (spasm of finger arteries), hypothyroidism and even iron deficiency. The following recommendations also help prevent chilblains:
  - Wear gloves or mittens.
  - Do not expose hands to cold wind or cold water.
  - When hands get cold, warm them up by putting them under the armpits, or dipping them in a tub of lukewarm water (never near an open flame or sources of intense heat).
  - Drink plenty of water.
  - Do not breathe in tobacco smoke, not even second-hand, as nicotine narrows the arteries.
  - Avoid coffee, which also narrows the arteries.
  - Take ginkgo leaf (*Ginkgo biloba*) extracts for their dilator effect on the blood vessels.

Carpal Tunnel

Carpal tunnel syndrome is compression of the median nerve where it passes through the wrist. It manifests as cramping and numbness of the fingers innervated by this nerve (thumb, index, middle, and half of the ring finger) as well as reduced grip strength.

It is promoted by repetitive wrist movement, pregnancy, menopause, oral contraceptives and diabetes.

Treatment

- Rest the wrist and hand.
- Wear a wrist brace or resting splint, mainly at night.
- Eat foods rich in vitamin B_6 (wheat germ, brewer's yeast, sesame, legumes, avocado) and/or B_6 supplements.
- Physical therapy.
- Anti-inflammatory and diuretic medications.
- Surgery, in recurring cases.

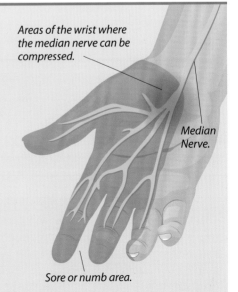

Areas of the wrist where the median nerve can be compressed.

Median Nerve.

Sore or numb area.

HAND WASHING

Caring for the hands is caring for the rest of the body. Simple hand washing continues to be the simplest, most effective way to prevent infection –especially colds, flu, diarrhea and skin infections.

WHY WASH THE HANDS?

- The hands can transmit many infectious agents. By touching the mouth, nose, eyes or any other part of the body with contaminated hands, germs enter the body and can cause infection.
- Eighty per cent of common infections are transmitted through contact with the hands.
- Children who wash their hands frequently get sick less often.

ALWAYS WASH HANDS BEFORE:

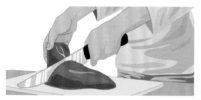
1. Handling or preparing food.

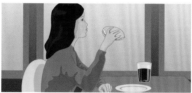
2. Eating.

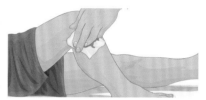
3. Treating a cut or wound on the skin.

ALWAYS WASH HANDS AFTER:

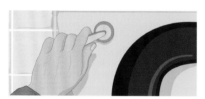
1. Using the bathroom.

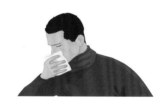
2. Sneezing, coughing or blowing the nose.

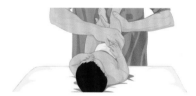
3. Changing a baby's diaper.

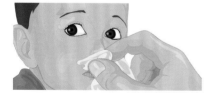
4. Wiping a child's nose.

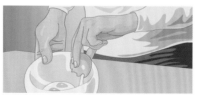
5. Touching raw meat or eggs in the kitchen.

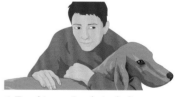
6. Touching animals, including pets, or their waste products.

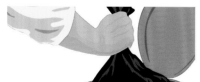
7. Touching trash.

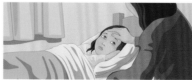
8. Caring for a sick person.

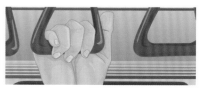
9. Being in a crowd, especially public transportation or events.

HOW TO WASH HANDS

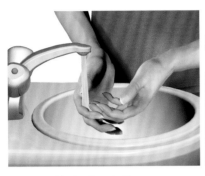

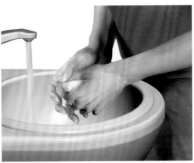

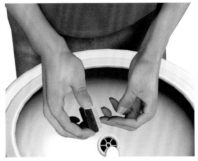

1. Wet and lather hands. Try to use warm or lukewarm water.
Adjust the stream to prevent it from coming out too fast and splattering.

2. Rub the hands together for at least 10 seconds, including the palms, backs of hands, between the fingers and the wrists.

3. It is very helpful to use a nail brush or an old toothbrush to clean under and around the nails.

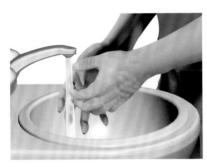

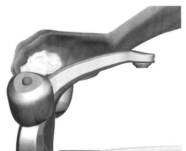

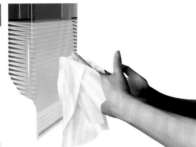

4. Rinse the hands with warm or lukewarm water, preferably.

5. Shut off the faucet without touching it, as it could be contaminated. In order to do this, use a paper or cloth towel or, if possible, shut it off using the elbow.

6. Dry the hands with a clean cloth or towel, or use a warm air dryer.

HAND WASHING WITH ALCOHOL-BASED SANITIZERS

Alcohol-based hand sanitizers are an appealing alternative to traditional washing with soap and water.

When the hands are not excessively soiled, an alcohol-based sanitizer can be used. Alcohol concentrations of 60-95% achieve the highest sanitizing strength and are available in liquid, gel or foam.

Advantages of Alcohol-Based Hand Sanitizers:

- They only take 10-15 seconds to use, which is less than traditional washing with soap and water.
- They do not require towel drying, as the alcohol evaporates on its own.
- They dry and irritate the skin less than traditional washing.

How to Use Alcohol-Based Hand Sanitizers:

- Apply an amount of alcohol-based sanitizer onto the hands.
- Rub the liquid vigorously in both hands, paying special attention to fingertips, between the fingers and the thumbs.
- Continue rubbing until the liquid evaporates. It is not necessary to dry the hands. The hands should not be shaken to speed up evaporation, since the alcohol must act on the skin for at least 10 seconds.

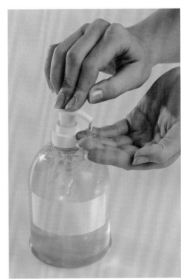

Natural Treatments for the Hands

The hands are an easily accessible body part for the application of physical agents and natural products. With these treatments, many anti-inflammatory medications can be avoided.

Hand Bathing

Hand bathing is dipping the hands in a liquid, which may be:

- Plain water.
- Water with salt or seawater.
- Water with seaweed.
- Infusion or preparation of medicinal anti-inflammatory herbs, such as rosemary (*Rosmarinus officinalis*), black mustard seed (*Brassica nigra*), meadowsweet leaves (*Filipendula ulmaria*), walnut leaves (*Juglans regia*) or others.

Hand baths relieve the pain and inflammation caused by arthritis of the hands. They are a simple remedy and have no undesirable effects, allowing the use of anti-inflammatory medication to be reduced or avoided.

Temperature: 36-40 °C (97-104 °F).

Duration: 2-5 minutes.

Afterward: Dip the hands in cold water and cover them with mittens.

Frequency: Several times per day.

Rubbing Hands with Oatmeal Powder

Oatmeal is an excellent skin softener and protector. For use on the hands, crush a cup 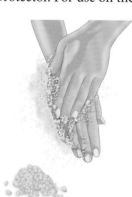 of raw oats into a powder. Place the oatmeal powder into a container and put the hands in it, rubbing. After a few minutes, wash the hands with water, then dry. Apply a moisturizer.

Clay Bath for the Hands

A clay or fango bath has an anti-inflammatory effect for the joints and tendons, improves circulation and tones connective tissue. All of this is good for inflammation, pain and deformity of the hands due to rheumatoid arthritis.

Temperature: The water and clay can be at room temperature or even slightly warm.

Duration: 5-10 minutes.

Afterward: Rinse the clay off the hands, dry, apply a moisturizer and put on some mittens.

Frequency: Once or twice per day.

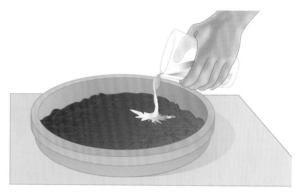

1. Mix the clay with water in a container, making an even paste into which the hands can be placed.

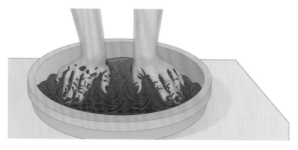

2. Place the hands in the clay paste for a few minutes. If the clay dries the skin too much, apply a moisturizer before putting the hands in, and put on some cotton gloves.

PARAFFIN BATH FOR THE HANDS

Paraffin is a substance derived from petroleum, made of a mixture of hydrocarbons.

Paraffin has the property of molding to body shapes, conserving heat. Heat is the therapeutic agent of paraffin baths.

Paraffin baths relieve pain and stiffness, without the need to take medication.

Effects

• Relief of pain and inflammation caused by arthritis in the joints.

• Improves joint mobility in cases of stiffness due to sprains or fractures.

• Relieves pain in cases of tendosynovitis (inflammation of tendons and their sheaths) and bursitis (inflammation of the fluid-filled sacs).

• Relaxes muscles and relieves spasms and contractures.

• Softens dry, cracked skin.

Paraffin Temperature: 50-54 °C (122-130 °F).

Duration: After dipping the hand fully or partially 6-12 times for a few seconds, allow the paraffin to act for 15-20 minutes.

Afterward: Remove the paraffin from the treated area and rub with alcohol.

Frequency: Once or twice per day.

Caution

• Do not use the paraffin bath if there are wounds or ulcers on the skin of the hands.

• Do not use the paraffin bath when there is acute inflammation of tendons or joints, presenting as redness and swelling. This initial phase must be over first.

• To avoid burns, do not use the paraffin bath when skin sensitivity is decreased due to diabetes or neurologic disorders.

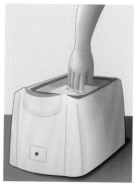

1. Place the hand in the paraffin bath for a few seconds.

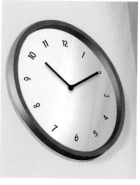

2. Remove the hand from the bath and wait for paraffin to cool and form a solid layer.

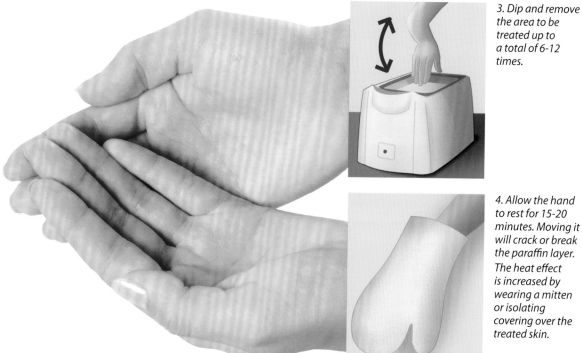

3. Dip and remove the area to be treated up to a total of 6-12 times.

4. Allow the hand to rest for 15-20 minutes. Moving it will crack or break the paraffin layer. The heat effect is increased by wearing a mitten or isolating covering over the treated skin.

Breasts

The breast symbolizes so much for a woman: from a life-giving organ for her baby, to a body part associated with cancer and with death, as well a symbol of femininity and sex appeal. These are more than enough reasons to give special attention to this delicate body part.

Life-giving organs for a baby and the symbol of feminine identity.

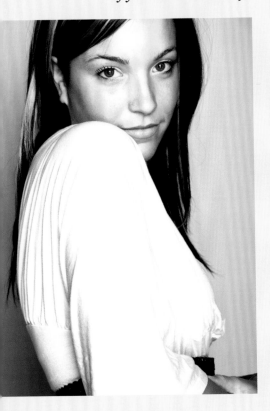

CANCER

The most common type of cancer in women is found in the mammary glands. It is estimated that one out of every eleven women who currently live in developed countries will have a cancer at some point in her life. The breast is the body part most likely to undergo cancerous changes.

Prevention of breast cancer is possible, thanks to discoveries made in the field of epidemiology in recent decades. There are many conclusive studies on the risk factors that promote breast cancer, and the factors that prevent it. Among all of them, nutrition stands out as increasingly significant.

The breast is also the location of benign pathologies, called this because they are non-life-threatening for women, such as occurs in the malignant pathology represented by cancer. These are known as "breast lumps", usually fibromas and cysts, as well as infections. It is estimated that for every ten benign breast tumors ("breast lumps"), only one becomes malignant.

THE MALE BREAST

Male breasts remain like girls' prepubescent breasts all throughout life.

Men should not ignore breasts because, although male breast cancer is 100 times less common than in women, it is usually very malignant and aggressive.

Facts and Figures about Breasts

2 mm (0.078 in)	Size of the smallest tumor that can be detected by mammography.
90%	Percentage of breast tumors that are non-cancerous (fibromas, cysts, lipomas, etc.).
10 seconds	Time it takes for milk to get to the nipple after a stimulus occurs in a lactating woman.
15 to 20	Number of divisions in each breast (lobules), the same as the number of openings in each nipple. Each lobule drains milk through an opening in the nipple.
500 ml (about 1 US pt)	Volume of milk normally produced by each breast during lactation.
20 billion	Number of milk-producing cells in each breast.

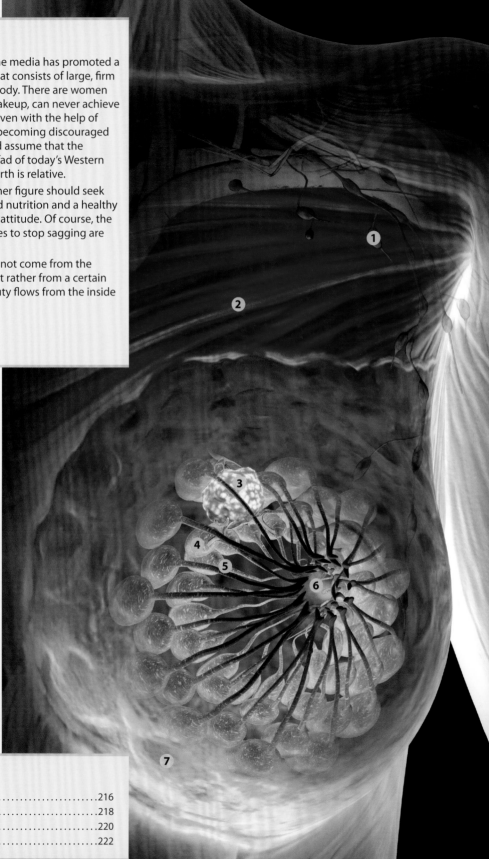

Breast and Beauty

Over the last few decades, the media has promoted a model of feminine beauty that consists of large, firm breasts and a slim, shapely body. There are women that, due to their physical makeup, can never achieve this pattern of beauty –not even with the help of plastic surgery. Rather than becoming discouraged or depressed, women should assume that the voluminous, firm breast is a fad of today's Western society and, therefore, its worth is relative.

A woman concerned about her figure should seek overall health based on good nutrition and a healthy lifestyle, as well as a positive attitude. Of course, the tips presented on these pages to stop sagging are helpful.

After all, attractiveness does not come from the body's geometric shapes, but rather from a certain attitude about life. True beauty flows from the inside out.

(1) Lymph Nodes

(2) Greater Pectoral Muscle

(3) Mammary Nodule
Benign tumor or "breast lump". Approximately one out of every ten breast nodules can be cancerous.

(4) Mammary Lobules
These contain milk-producing cells. All of the lobules together constitute the mammary gland.

(5) Milk Duct
Carries the milk from the lobules to the nipple.

(6) Nipple

(7) Fat Tissue
Surrounds the breast and helps keep gland tissue in place.

Chapter Contents

CARING FOR THE BREASTS

Due to a lack of bony protection and muscles of its own, the breast is an especially vulnerable part of the body. Consequently, the firmness and good condition of the breast depend on the care given to the skin that surrounds it.

DO NOT WEAR A TIGHT BRA

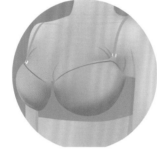

A bra should support, not constrict. Bras that are too tight are usually padded with synthetic knits, which restrict circulation and weaken breast tissue.

A bra is too tight when any part of it causes redness or chafing of the skin.

For sleeping, remove the bra or, in the case of large breasts, wear one that is softer.

AVOID MOISTURE UNDER THE BREASTS

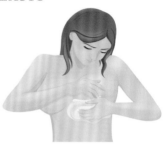

The breast crease (the space underneath the breasts when they are large or sagging) should always be kept dry, especially in the summertime. Moisture caused by perspiration can lead to fungal and bacterial growth in the area, especially among diabetic women, appearing as redness and burning.

To avoid moisture underneath the breasts, one should:
- Use an appropriate bra that lifts the breasts.
- Eliminate sweat with a gauze or cotton cloth.
- Apply talcum powders and clean the area several times a day, thoroughly drying it with a towel.

AVOID EXCESSIVE EXPOSURE OF THE BREASTS TO SUNLIGHT

Breast skin is very sensitive, and when it is exposed excessively to sunlight, it loses its elasticity, promoting breast sagging.

Excessive exposure means spending more than one hour in the sun with the skin exposed.

Reasons You Must See a Doctor

- Abnormal discharge of milk, blood or pus from the nipple.
- Retraction, scabbing or itching of the nipple.
- Asymmetrical appearance of the breasts.
- Creasing, dimpling or orange-rind appearance of the breast.

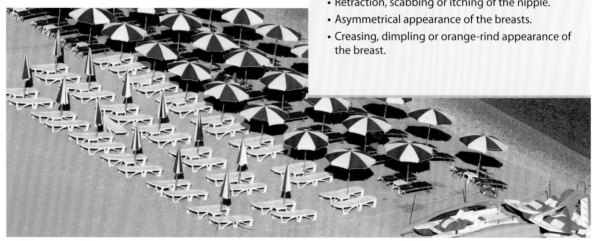

FOLLOW A DIET LOW IN ANIMAL FAT

Animal fat is the breasts' biggest enemy. In addition to promoting breast cancer, animal fat is also associated with fibrocystic breast disease (appearance of painful nodules in the breasts).

Following a diet low in animal fat means reducing or eliminating the following foods:
- Meats, especially bacon and sausage.
- Cured cheese (contains up to 60% fat).
- Butter, cream, and milk skin.
- Pastries and cakes.

NUTRITIONAL SUPPLEMENTS

Vitamin E supplements and primrose and borage oils relieve premenstrual breast pain and the discomfort associated with fibrocystic breast disease.

STOP THE SAGGING

Breast sagging is a physiological process that increases with age, as the milk-producing glandular mammary tissue is replaced by softer fatty tissue.

The following tips may help stop breast sagging:
- Do not expose the breasts to too much sunlight.
- Strengthen the pectoral muscles with physical exercise and sports such as swimming and rowing. Although exercise by itself does not strengthen the breasts, due to their lack of muscle, it does contribute to better posture and helps elevate the ribcage, making the breasts appear more firm.
- Avoid obesity, since increased fat in the breasts causes them to sag more.
- Maintain good posture when walking and sitting, since the collapsing of the ribcage and curving of the back promote breast sagging.
- Use a moisturizing cream to care for breast skin.
- Do not smoke, as nicotine narrows arteries and causes skin dryness and atrophy, especially of the face and breasts.
- Take 4-6 capsules of primrose or borage oil per day.
- Apply warm compresses on the breasts with seawater or medicinal herbs (see "Natural Treatments for Breasts").

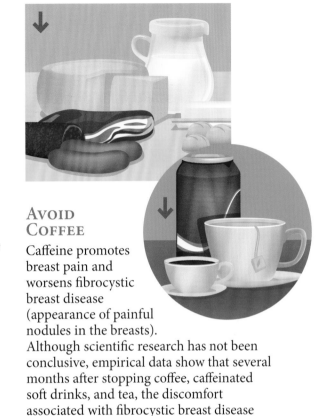

AVOID COFFEE

Caffeine promotes breast pain and worsens fibrocystic breast disease (appearance of painful nodules in the breasts). Although scientific research has not been conclusive, empirical data show that several months after stopping coffee, caffeinated soft drinks, and tea, the discomfort associated with fibrocystic breast disease improves.

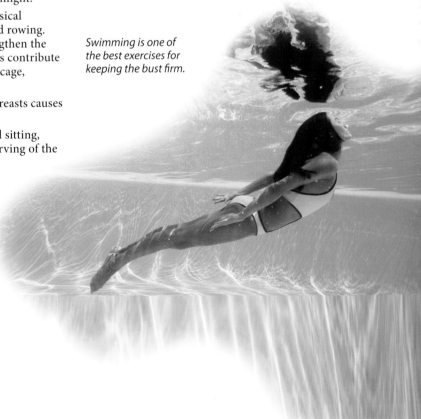

Swimming is one of the best exercises for keeping the bust firm.

Natural Treatments for the Breasts

Breasts benefit from physical agents such as heat, cold or massage. Before opting for plastic surgery, it is worthwhile to try natural treatments for the breasts.

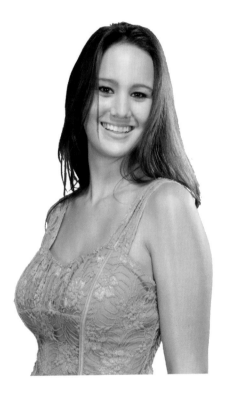

Liquid for the compress

The compress is made by soaking a cloth or gauze pad in a warm liquid, which may be:

- Seawater, or salt water (9 grams of salt per liter of water, equivalent to about two heaping teaspoons of coffee).

- Horsetail (*Equisetum arvense*) preparation, made with 100 to 150 g of the herb per liter of water. The horsetail is rich in silicon, a mineral that stimulates the regeneration of the skins collagen fibers.

- Witch hazel (*Hamamelis virginiana*) preparation, with 30 g of leaves per liter of water. Improves circulation and tones breast tissue.

Temperature: The water or preparation should be lukewarm or slightly warm, or 30-40 ºC (86-104 ºF).

Duration: 10-15 minutes.

Afterward: Dry the breasts and apply a softening cream onto the skin.

Frequency: Once or twice per day.

Compress on the Breasts

The effects of breast compresses depend on the temperature.

- **Warm Compress**: Has a mild anti-inflammatory effect. It is recommended pain relief in fibrocystic disease (breast lumps).

- **Cold Compress**: Recommended for stopping sagging. Promotes turgency of the mammary glands, tones the elastic fibers and strengthens the surrounding skin tissue.

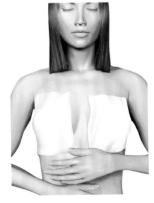

Cold-Water Shower for the Breasts

A cold-water shower on the breasts tones mammary tissues and promotes smoothness.

This should be done in the morning by directing the stream of cold water at each breast, making circular movements.

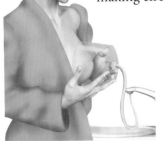

Device for the breast shower that helps avoid wetting the rest of the body. If this device is not available, use the stream of water directly from the showerhead.

Temperature: Cold, just as it comes out of the shower without heating.

Duration: 1-2 minutes.

Afterward: Dry breasts well and apply a softening cream onto the skin.

Frequency: Once or twice per day.

BREAST MASSAGE

As with any other type of massage, a breast massage promotes the drainage of blood circulating through the veins and lymph drainage. In this way, it improves tissue nutrition and firmness.

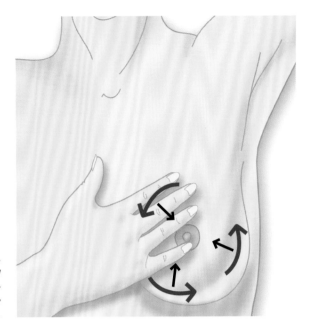

Breast massages should be done with gentle movements toward the armpit. Both the veins and the lymphatic ducts drain toward the armpit.

Breast Augmentation Surgery

Augmentation mammoplasty consists of inserting a breast implant or prosthesis filled with saline solution or silicone gel. The implant or prosthesis may be placed in front of the pectoral muscle or behind it, each location having its own advantages and drawbacks.

In some cases, breast augmentation surgery is performed to reconstruct a breast after removal due to cancer, or to correct atrophy (breasts that are too small) due to hereditary or hormonal factors.

However, the majority of breast augmentations are performed for purely aesthetic reasons. In these cases, although the results achieved are generally quite good, there can be undesirable complications and consequences that should be known before opting for the procedure.

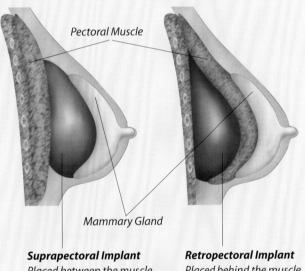

Suprapectoral Implant
Placed between the muscle and the mammary gland.

Retropectoral Implant
Placed behind the muscle.

POTENTIAL COMPLICATIONS AND UNWANTED EFFECTS OF BREAST AUGMENTATION SURGERY

• **Capsular retraction**: Abnormal thickening of the fibrous layer that normally forms around the implant. This manifests as hardness and stiffness of the breast and, sometimes, deformities. This happens in up to 15% of cases, and starts to become noticeable a few months after the procedure.

• **Difficult natural breastfeeding**, since placement of a prosthesis requires sectioning of some galactophorous ducts, which decreases milk production.

• Formation of unsightly **scarring** or keloids.

• **Changes in sensitivity** of the nipple and areola, which may be permanent.

• **Difficult breast exams**: Breast implants make breast self-exams difficult. They also decrease the clarity of mammography images. Women who have a breast implant must inform the diagnostic imaging technician prior to having a mammogram.

• **Anesthesia**-related complications.

BREAST CANCER PREVENTION

Out of the entire female body, the breast cells are the most likely to degenerate and become cancerous. It is therefore important to know the factors increasing the risk of breast cancer and those reducing it.

FACTORS THAT INCREASE THE RISK

- **Genetic mutations**: It is estimated that 5% of all breast cancers are related to a hereditary change in these two genes, which are charged with stopping cell growth: BRCA1 (found on chromosome 17) and BRCA2 (found on chromosome 13).

- **Hormones**: Hormone replacement therapy, usually given as patches after menopause (especially the combination of estrogens and progesterone) increase the risk of breast cancer. Taking oral contraceptives (the pill) over long periods of time also increases the risk, although to a lesser degree than hormones for menopause.

- **Alcohol consumption**: Even in socially acceptable low doses, alcohol increases the risk of cancer. It has been shown that for every 10 g of alcohol (half a glass of wine) per day, the risk of breast cancer increases by 7%. Women who drink 35-44 g of alcohol per day (considered a moderate dose) have a 32% greater risk of breast cancer than those who do not drink.

- **Obesity**: The higher the body mass index (BMI), the greater the risk of breast cancer, especially after menopause. It is estimated that women who weigh more than 82.2 kg (181 pounds) have nearly triple the possibility of developing breast cancer as compared to those who weigh less than 58.7 kg (129 pounds).

- **Breast size**: Women who have larger breasts should dedicate more care to breast cancer prevention, due to their increased risk of having it before menopause.[a]

- **Exposure to ionizing radiation**, such as radiation therapy used for acne treatment, hypertrophy of the thymus or Hodgkin's lymphoma. When radiation exposure occurs before the age of 20, the risk is greater. However, there is research that shows that radiation therapy used for breast cancer treatment does not increase the risk of the healthy breast becoming malignant.
  - Electromagnetic (non-ionizing) radiation should also be avoided, such as that given off by electric blankets for heating a bed, when they are plugged in. According to a study by the University of Pennsylvania (United States)[b], these devices can promote breast cancer in premenopausal women.
  -
  -

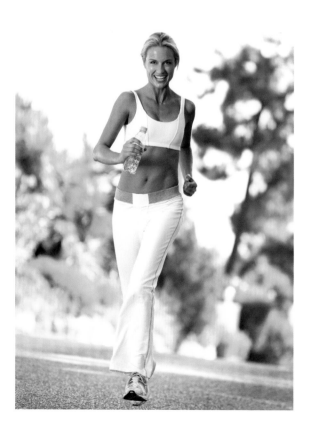

---

a. A prospective study of breast size and premenopausal breast cancer incidence. Kusano AS, Trichopoulos D, Terry KL, Chen WY, Willett WC, Michels KB. Int J Cancer. 2006 Apr 15;118(8):2031-4. PMID: 16284954

b. Use of electric bedding devices and risk of breast cancer in African-American women. Zhu K, Hunter S, Payne-Wilks K, Roland CL, Forbes DS. Am J Epidemiol. 2003 Oct 15;158(8):798-806. PMID: 14561670

RISK REDUCING FACTORS

• **Physical Activity**: Getting at least 4 hours of aerobic exercise per week reduces the risk of breast cancer by 30%.

• Less time exposed to natural estrogens: Throughout her lifetime, a woman is exposed to estrogens produced in her ovaries. The less time the breast cells are subjected to the estrogens' action, the lower the risk of developing a cancer. The following life events reduce exposure time to natural estrogens:

– Pregnancy: During gestation, estrogen production in the ovaries decreases. The more the number of pregnancies, the less the risk. In addition, it has been shown that having a first full-term gestation before the age of 20 reduces the likelihood of premenopausal breast cancer.
– Breastfeeding.
– Delayed menarche (first period) and early menopause.

• **Diet Low in Fat and Meat**: Despite the fact that some research has had questionable results, a relationship between breast cancer and certain types of diets, such as those high in fat and meat, is currently well demonstrated. More details are given about this interesting topic on the next page.

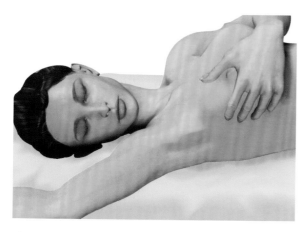

There is currently controversy among the experts about the helpfulness of breast self-exams. For some, it continues to be useful for early diagnosis; for others, it unnecessarily increases a woman's worry and the number of breast biopsies performed, without statistically contributing to decreasing mortality rates.

REGULAR BREAST EXAMS

Several medical organizations propose different guidelines for exams for breast cancer screening. In the adjacent table, the recommendations of three organizations are shown: the European Union,[a] the National Cancer Institute (United States)[b] and the National Health Service (Great Britain).[c]

a. http://ec.europa.eu/health/ph_projects/2002/cancer/fp_cancer_2002_ext_guid_01.pdf
b. http://www.cancer.gov/espanol/cancer/hojas-informativas/mamografia-respuestas
c. http://www.cancerscreening.nhs.uk/breastscreen/ publications/nhsbsp-pocket-guide-2008.pdf

Recommendations for Breast Cancer Screening

Organization	Breast Self-Exam	Clinical Breast Exam (by a physician)	Mammography
European Union	• A regular monthly self-exam is not considered necessary.	• As needed.	• Between age 50-69: Mammogram every two years.
National Cancer Institute (United States)	• Starting at age 20: monthly.	• Between age 20-40: Every three years. • Starting at age 40: Every year.	• Between age 40-50: Every one or two years. • Starting at age 50: Every year.
National Health Service (Great Britain)	• A regular monthly self-exam is not considered necessary.	• Starting at age 50: Every three years.	• Starting at age 50: Every three years.

DIET FOR BREAST CANCER PREVENTION

*After many scientific controversies, it is now clear that diet is one
of the factors most influencing breast cancer –its development
as well as its prevention.*

THE PRICE OF PROSPERITY

Because it is more and more common in developed countries, and practically unheard of in poor countries, it is said that breast cancer is the price that must be paid for prosperity.

In 1975, United States researchers Armstrong and Doll showed statistically for the first time that there is a link between diet and breast cancer.[a] They showed that there is a direct correlation between consumption of animal fat and meat *per capita* among the inhabitants of a country and the incidence and mortality of cancer, including of the breast. The higher the consumption of animal fat and meat, like in wealthy countries, the greater the risk of breast cancer.

Although some researchers asserted that the association between eating animal fat and meat could be coincidence, a number of later studies confirmed it. There are certain types of meat that increase the risk of hormone-dependant breast cancer even more (see the table on the facing page) according to a study by Harvard University (United States).[b] The risk of premenopausal breast cancer is greater among women who consumed more red meat during adolescence.

Immigration and Cancer

The role of diet and general lifestyle in breast cancer has also been shown by studying different groups of immigrants. For example, when Japanese people immigrate to the United States and change their diet, mortality rates from breast cancer increases over two to three generations, equaling that of their new country.

YOUNG WOMEN AND MEAT CONSUMPTION

Adolescents and young women who eat more red meat increase their risk of premenopausal hormone-dependant breast cancer. For every additional 100 g (3.5 oz) of red meat consumed per day, the risk of breast cancer increases by 20%[c].

Processed meats such as sausage and ham, pork and hamburger are the most linked to the higher risk of breast cancer.

INCREASE CONSUMPTION OF THESE FOODS

- Olive oil and avocado, due to the beneficial effect of monounsaturated fatty acids.
- Walnuts and seeds in general, good sources of polyunsaturated alpha-linolenic acid (ALA).
- Soy, tofu and soy drink, due to their high isoflavone content (vegetable estrogens that act like partial antiestrogens). Many studies confirm the protective role that soy and soy products play in fighting breast cancer, especially when they are consumed during adolescence.
- Fruits and vegetables, carrots, and spinach. For cancer prevention, fresh fruits are preferred over vitamin supplements.
- Raw garlic or deodorized garlic extracts.
- Nonfat yogurt.

a. Environmental factors and cancer incidence and mortality in different countries, with special reference to dietary practices. Armstrong B, Doll R. Int J Cancer. 1975 Apr 15;15(4):617-31. PMID: 1140864
b. Red meat intake and risk of breast cancer among premenopausal women. Cho E, Chen WY, Hunter DJ, Stampfer MJ, Colditz GA, Hankinson SE, Willett WC. Arch Intern Med. 2006 Nov 13;166(20):2253-9. PMID: 17101944
c. Red meat consumption during adolescence among premenopausal women and risk of breast cancer. Linos E, Willett WC, Cho E, Colditz G, Frazier LA. Cancer Epidemiol Biomarkers Prev. 2008

Type of Meat and Breast Cancer

Type of Meat	Relative Hormone-Dependant* Breast Cancer Risk when Consumed Regularly
Processed meats, such as sausage and ham	2.34
Pork	1.81
Hamburger	1.71
Hot Dogs	1.43

* The fact that meat usually has residue from hormones used for bulking livestock can be one of the causes of the association between consumption of meat and breast cancer.

The bibliographic reference for table data appears in the main text on the previous page.

REDUCE CONSUMPTION OF THESE FOODS OR PRODUCTS

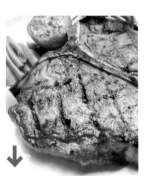

• **Meat in general**, and especially animal fats. Fatty meats, sausage, cheese and butter are the main sources of animal fat in the Western diet.

• **Meat**, especially processed red meat (see table).

• Dietary sources of **trans-fatty acids** or hydrogenated fatty acids, such as fried foods and margarines (also available without trans-fatty acids).

• Products with a **high glycemic index** (refined sugars, white bread, pastries, cakes and other products made with white flour and white sugar).

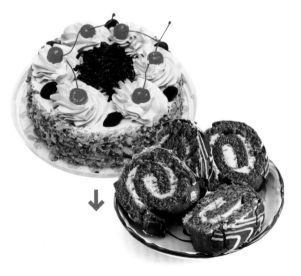

Can Women Who Have Survived Breast Cancer Eat Soy?

Women who have survived breast cancer, or those who still have it, often ask themselves if they can eat soy products or soy extracts, such as isoflavones.

It is no surprise that there is a widespread debate about the role of soy isoflavones. Like other phytoestrogens (vegetable hormones), isoflavones act like antiestrogens that protect against cancer and, at the same time, like weak estrogens that can promote cancer when in very high doses.

These conclusions can be drawn from the variety of research published on the subject:

• The consumption of foods rich in phytoestrogens (soy and soy products, flax, seeds, whole grains) in similar amounts consumed regularly by Asian populations does not stimulate tumor growth in breast cells. Therefore, women who are breast cancer survivors can consume moderate amounts of these foods without any risk whatsoever.[a]

• Avoid soy extracts, generally in pill form, which are high in isoflavones.

• Women who are undergoing treatment with tamoxifen (an antiestrogen hormone used to fight breast cancer) should avoid isoflavone extracts and foods high in phytoestrogens (soy and flax, primarily) because they interfere with the effect of this medication.

a. Epidemiology of soy exposures and breast cancer risk. Wu AH, Yu MC, Tseng CC, Pike MC. Br J Cancer. 2008 Jan 15;98(1):9-14. Epub 2008 Jan 8. PMID: 18182974

Lungs

Two organs in continuous contact with the outside and with the air we have them breathe.

The lungs make up the most important part of the respiratory system. Their primary function is to inhale a vital element, oxygen, and incorporate it into the blood for distribution to all the body's cells.

Our body's cells, especially those hardest at work –the neurons of the brain or the heart's muscle cells– require a continuous supply of oxygen. After just a few minutes without this gas, they die without hope of recovery.

The body's cells depend primarily on the lungs to maintain the continuous supply of oxygen keeping them alive. These spongy organs carry enormous responsibility, as a few minutes without their function results in death.

In addition to taking in the necessary oxygen supply, the lungs carry out another equally important function: elimination of the gas waste produced by cells as a result of their vital activity. If the lungs do not eliminate this carbon dioxide gas, the self-poisoning that occurs is just as incompatible with life as the resulting lack of oxygen. Taking in oxygen with every inhalation and eliminating carbon dioxide with every exhalation: two life-sustaining functions that the lungs must carry out continuously from the moment a human enters this world.

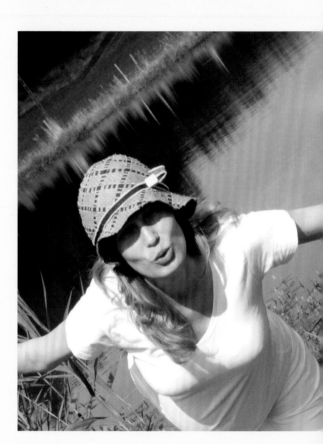

Facts and Figures About the Lungs

0.2 - 0.5 μm	Thickness of the alveolar wall.
0.1 - 0.3 mm	Diameter of a pulmonary alveolus.
2 liters (4.23 US pt)	Volume of air inhaled per minute, at rest.
12 liters (25.36 US pt)	Volume of air inhaled per minute, while running.
140 m2 (507 square feet)	Surface area of all of the alveoli in both lungs, spread out.
500 ml (1.05 US pt)	Volume of air entering the lungs with every breath.
23 040	Average number of breaths in 24 hours.
300 million	Number of alveoli in both lungs.

The lungs are pink-colored, but after more than eight and a half million breaths of urban air every year, even without smoking, the lungs start turning a dark color.

(1) Bronchial Cilia
Microscopic hairs anchored into a special type of bronchial cells. In a coordinated movement, the cilia carry a rolling layer of mucus lining the inside of the bronchial passages toward the throat. There, the impurity-filled mucus is swallowed or forced out by coughing.
Each cilia moves back and forth about 12 times per second. The millions of cilia in each lung move in a coordinated manner to carry the mucus layer toward the outside.

(2) Mucus
Sticky substance lining the bronchial passages and trapping entering dust particles and microorganisms suspended in the air.
(3) Bronchial Mucosa Cells
(4) Trachea
(5) Primary Bronchi

Chapter Contents

Caring for the Lungs

The lungs are permanently open to the world, exposed to the effects of the environment and to contaminants in the air. Due to this and because of their vital function, they deserve special attention.

Breathe Clean Air

The best way to care for the lungs is to allow them to breathe clean air that is free of the tobacco smoke, chemical contaminants, and germs present in the air in large urban areas.

Avoid Cold, Dry Air

In order for the lungs to carry out their function properly, air needs to get to the alveola with a certain amount of moisture and temperature. The nose and bronchial passages contribute to this by moistening and warming the air.

But when air is very cold and dry, moisture and temperature regulators are unable to condition the air; this irritates the bronchial passages and weakens the lungs, promoting respiratory infections.

Breathe Through the Nose

Upon passing through the cavities of the nasal passages, air becomes conditioned and prepared to enter into the lungs at the proper temperature and moisture levels. Breathing through the mouth, however, results in colder, drier air entering the airways and decreasing their resistance to infection.

Do Deep Breathing with the Abdomen

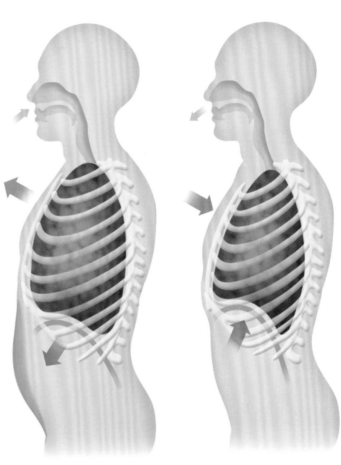

Deep Inhalation
Fill the lungs by pushing the belly outward.

Complete Exhalation
Empty the lungs by pushing the belly inward.

Reasons You Must See a Doctor

- Sharp chest pain.
- Coughing that does not improve after 3 or 4 days.
- Wheezing.
- Difficulty breathing.
- Streaks of blood in sputum.

At least 10 deep breaths should be taken every day to cleanse and strengthen the lungs.

In order to fill the lungs completely with air, it is as important to inflate the chest as it is to use the abdominal muscles to contract the diaphragm downward. In order for this to occur, the belly has to be pushed outward, just as babies do when they cry.

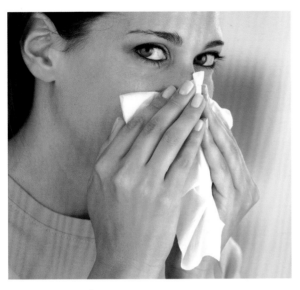

PREVENT COLDS

Colds can be the beginning of a case of bronchitis or pneumonia. Preventing and treating colds properly from the start is very important to prevent the complication from spreading to the lungs (see "Cold Prevention" in Chapter 5, which is dedicated to the nose).

INCREASE BETA-CAROTENE INTAKE

Beta-carotene is the primary yellow or orange-colored pigment found in fruits and vegetables. Dark green leaves are also good sources of beta-carotene. The following foods are known for their beta-carotene content:

– Carrots
– Chard and spinach
– Mango
– Apricots
– Pumpkin or squash
– Sweet potatoes or yams

Beta-carotene protects the lungs through at least three mechanisms:

• It is a powerful antioxidant capable of neutralizing free radicals or toxins present in the contaminated air of urban areas.

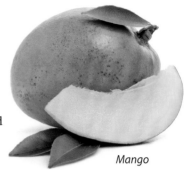

Mango

• It is the main source of vitamin A, needed for keeping the mucus layer lining the airways, both inside and outside the lungs, in good condition.

• It protects against lung cancer, which is still one of the most common types of cancer.

It should be noted that the beneficial effects of beta-carotene, especially protection against cancer, are obtained from naturally occurring beta-carotene in fruits and vegetables. On the other hand, synthetic beta-carotene obtained artificially in a laboratory, although appearing to have the same chemical composition (it is really an isomer), does not achieve the same results; it can even be counter-productive, according to some studies.[a]

EAT MORE BROCCOLI

Broccoli consumption can stop the progression of chronic obstructive pulmonary disease (COPD) and regenerate lung tissue damaged by tobacco or chronic infections. This beneficial effect of broccoli on the lungs is due to its level of sulforaphane, a powerful antioxidant that is also anticarcinogenic.[b]

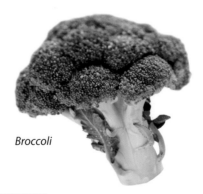

Broccoli

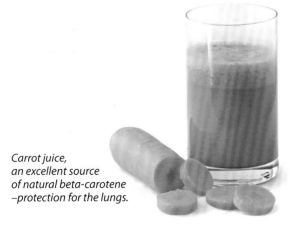

*Carrot juice,
an excellent source
of natural beta-carotene
–protection for the lungs.*

a. Chemoprevention of lung cancers: lessons from CARET, the beta-carotene and retinol efficacy trial, and prospects for the future. Omenn GS. Eur J Cancer Prev. 2007 Jun;16(3):184-91. PMID: 17415088
b. The role of oxidative stress in chronic obstructive pulmonary disease. Bowler RP, Barnes PJ, Crapo JD. COPD. 2004;1(2):255-77. PMID: 17136992

NATURAL TREATMENTS FOR THE LUNGS - 1

The lungs are endowed with a sophisticated cleansing mechanism. However, smoke, dust, chemicals and aggressive germs can overload the lungs' self-cleansing ability. Heat and moisture are great friends to the lungs.

STEAM INHALATION

Moisture and heat are the best gifts we can offer the bronchial passages. For this, there is nothing better than steam inhalation.

Beneficial Effects of Steam for the Lungs

- Mucolytic: Mucus becomes more fluid, making it easier to eliminate.
- Antitussive: Relieves coughing.
- Immunostimulant: Heat increases blood flow to the bronchial passages, which improves defenses against infection.

Water Temperature: As hot as possible to promote steam production. Ideally, it should be near-boiling.

Duration: 5-10 minutes.

Afterward: Rub the face, neck and chest with cold water to close the skin's pores.

Frequency: One to three times per day.

Other Ways to Inhale Steam

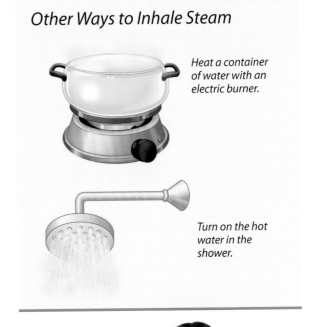

Heat a container of water with an electric burner.

Turn on the hot water in the shower.

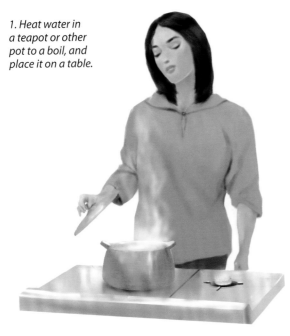

1. Heat water in a teapot or other pot to a boil, and place it on a table.

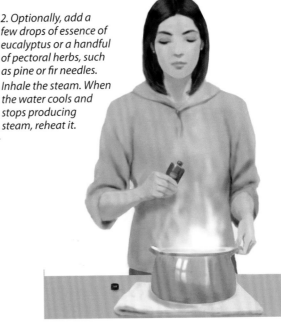

2. Optionally, add a few drops of essence of eucalyptus or a handful of pectoral herbs, such as pine or fir needles. Inhale the steam. When the water cools and stops producing steam, reheat it.

CHEST COMPRESSES

Compresses consist of applying moist heat by way of a cloth soaked in water as hot as the skin will tolerate. These can be applied onto the chest (anterior aspect of the thorax) or the side.

Beneficial Effects of Chest Compresses

• They decongest the lungs.
• They dilate the bronchial passages.
• They stimulate the immune system.
• They promote the elimination of toxins through the skin.

Water Temperature: As hot as possible. Ideally, it should be near-boiling.

Duration: 10-15 minutes. When the moist towel loses its heat (usually after two or three minutes), soak it in hot water again.

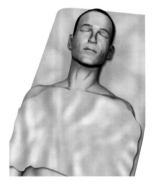

1. Protect the skin with a dry cotton cloth.

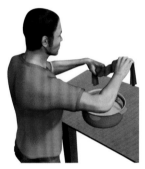

2. Soak a towel in very hot water, drain.

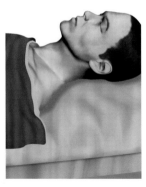

3. Place the hot towel over the dry protective cloth.

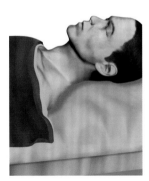

4. Cover these two cloths with a wool blanket. After a few minutes, soak the towel again in hot water and drain.

Caution: *Careful not to get burned, both when wetting the towel and when placing it on the chest.*

Afterward: Dry the skin on the chest and cover up with wool blankets.

Frequency: One or two times per day.

RESPIRATORY CLAPPING

Clapping is a type of physical therapy. Its goal is to dislodge mucus from the inside of the bronchial passages to make it easier to expel, through expectoration.

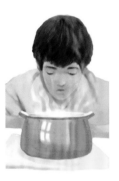
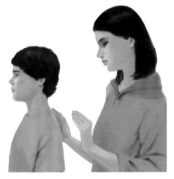

1. Before beginning clapping, steam should be inhaled to make the mucus more fluid and facilitate expulsion. It is not good to do this after eating.

2. With hands cupped, pat toward the throat, first on the chest, then on the back.

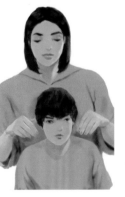
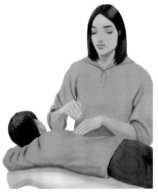

3. While doing the clapping, the patient should be breathing deeply and trying to expectorate.

4. The patient can be placed in different positions to facilitate mucus drainage.

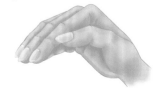

Correct hand position for clapping.

NATURAL TREATMENTS FOR THE LUNGS - 2

The lungs respond well to herbal essences, whether inhaled or ingested orally. In addition, antioxidant vitamins protect against free radicals generated by contamination.

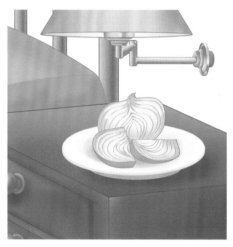

ONION INHALATION

The essence given off spontaneously by onions has a very beneficial mucolytic (breaks up mucus) and bronchodilator effect for the lungs.

An onion cut into pieces and left on the nightstand can quiet nighttime coughing and relieve asthma.

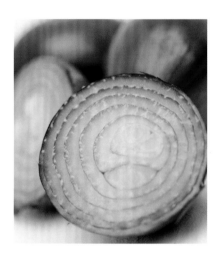

ONION SYRUP

Onions have a sulfurated essence that disinfects and reduces inflammation of airway mucosa and improves lung function. In order to take full advantage of the properties of onions for the respiratory system, it should be used raw. However, children and others find it easier taking this onion syrup than eating it raw.

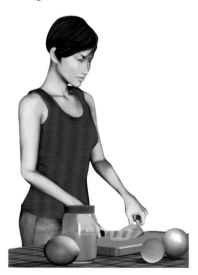

1. Cut an onion or two into pieces and add 6-8 tablespoons of honey and lemon juice.

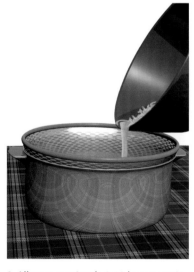

2. Allow to marinade 8-12 hours; strain.

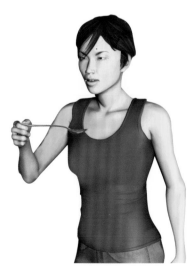

3. Take 2-3 tablespoons of the strained liquid about 6 times per day.

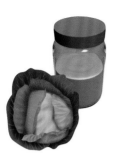

1. Blend all or several cabbage leaves and add 5-6 tablespoons of honey for every cup.

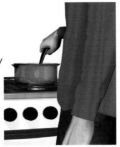

2. Heat on low, stirring, until an even syrup forms. Store in refrigerator.

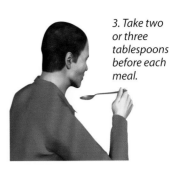

3. Take two or three tablespoons before each meal.

CABBAGE SYRUP

Cabbage has an antiseptic and mucolytic (breaks up mucus, allowing it to be expelled) essence which is very recommendable in bronchitis, asthma or pneumonia.

EAT RAW GARLIC

Chewing raw garlic breaks up its cells and releases their volatile essence. This essence is antibiotic, mucolytic (breaks up mucus) and soothing for airway mucosa. The medicinal essence of garlic passes quickly from the stomach into the blood, and from there it is eliminated by the lungs, disinfecting and reducing inflamed airways along the way.

Cooked garlic does not have a direct medicinal effect on the lungs.

ANTIOXIDANT VITAMINS

Antioxidant vitamins strengthen the immune system and fight free radicals in environmental contaminants. Ideally, supplements made from natural vitamin sources should be taken. The recommended doses are:

- **Provitamin A (beta-carotene)**: 7 000 µg of RE (Retinol Equivalents) per day, which can be obtained, for example, by consuming about 250 g (= 0.55 pounds) of carrots or their juice.

- **Vitamin C**: 500 mg per day, which can be obtained by consuming 5 medium oranges or their juice.

- **Vitamin E**: 200 IU per day, which can be obtained by, for example, consuming a handful of sunflower or pumpkin seeds, a handful of almonds or walnuts, two tablespoons of wheat germ and 4 tablespoons of olive or seed oil.

Acid Reflux from the Stomach Attacks the Lungs

The sensation of heartburn is caused by reflux of acidy stomach juices upward, that is, toward the esophagus.

When stomach acid irritates the nerve endings in the esophagus, a nerve reflex is produced toward the bronchial passages. These react by narrowing their lumen, which can cause aphonia, promote asthma and make breathing difficult.

If the acid goes up the esophagus and enters the airways, which can happen when lying down, aspiration pneumonia ensues.

To prevent the consequences that acid reflux in the esophagus has for the lungs, the following is recommended:

- Skip the late-evening meal, or have something very light.
- Go to bed at least two or three hours after having last eaten.
- Raise the head of the bed with bricks or stands.
- Decrease intake of fat, white flour and sugar.
- Take medication to reduce stomach acid secretion.

Aorta

Airways
These become inflamed and narrowed when stomach acid enters the esophagus.

Acid Reflux from the Stomach
The presence of acid in the esophagus triggers a nerve reflex that narrows the bronchial passages.

Esophagus

Stomach with Acidic Gastric Juices

Diaphragm

ASTHMA PREVENTION

These simple suggestions can prevent asthma attacks,
greatly improving quality of life for asthmatics.

AVOID ASTHMA ATTACK TRIGGERS

Some of the most common are:

- Aspirin.
- Smoke from firewood or tobacco (careful with second-hand smoke, especially children).
- Smoke from fryer grease in the kitchen.
- Cold air.
- Volatile chemicals (which evaporate spontaneously) such as paint, solvents, perfumes, air fresheners, certain cleaning products and ammonia.
- Talcum powders.

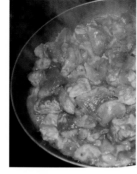

Smoke can trigger
an asthma attack.

AVOID ENVIRONMENTAL CONTAMINATION

Asthmatics living in large urban or industrial areas should pay attention to air quality reports issued by the environmental or health authorities. If contamination levels rise, it is recommended to stay home with the windows closed and the air conditioner running with filters in good condition.

The effects of environmental contamination on the bronchial passages do not tend to be immediate. Sometimes, asthma reactivates several days after a rise in contamination levels.

PREVENT ACID REFLUX FROM THE STOMACH

Acid reflux from the stomach upward –that is, toward the esophagus– can irritate the bronchial passages and promote asthma attacks. Reflux prevention reduces the risk of asthma. Find suggestions for preventing acid reflux in "Caring for the Lungs".

AVOID DUST

Household dust contains mites, which are tiny arthropods (about 0.5 mm) whose microscopic feces cause allergies and asthma. Dust and moisture promote multiplication of the mite population.

In order to reduce the population of mites living in a home, consider the following recommendations:

- Eliminate dust by cleaning thoroughly. Sweeping and dusting are inappropriate methods, as they only stir up dust and change its location, at best. The correct ways to eliminate dust are:
  – Use a vacuum cleaner, changing the bag before it becomes full.
  – Use a moist cloth for cleaning.
- Avoid moisture in the environment, especially in home carpeting and fabrics.
- Wash bed linens often, at a temperature above 55 ˚C (130 ˚F).
- Avoid carpeting, curtains and tapestries, as they tend to harbor household dust.
- Avoid pets or companion animals with hair.

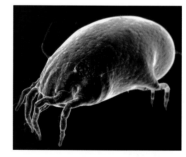

Mite seen through a microscope.

WATCH THE DIET

- Increase consumption of raw fruits and vegetables, and nuts. All of these provide antioxidant vitamins A, C and E that fight the free radicals and other contaminants that can worsen asthma.
- Reduce dairy consumption, especially milk. Asthma can be relieved or eliminated by replacing cow's milk and with a soy drink (preferably calcium-enriched).

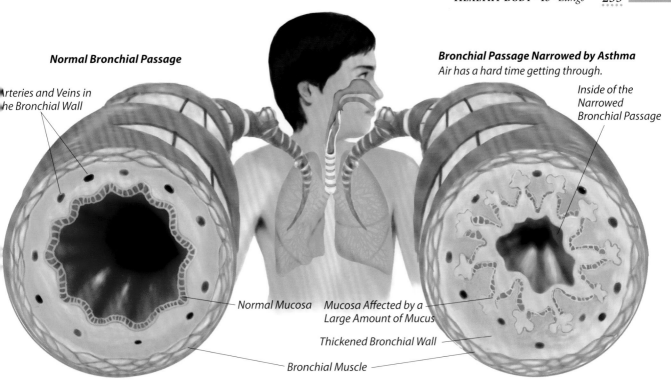

Normal Bronchial Passage

Arteries and Veins in the Bronchial Wall

Bronchial Passage Narrowed by Asthma
Air has a hard time getting through.

Inside of the Narrowed Bronchial Passage

Normal Mucosa

Mucosa Affected by a Large Amount of Mucus

Thickened Bronchial Wall

Bronchial Muscle

IDENTIFY FOOD ALLERGIES

Many cases of asthma, both in childhood and adulthood, are due to allergies to certain foods or food ingredients,[a] such as additives. Their consumption by sensitive children or adults can trigger asthma attacks.

In many cases, cutting out the allergy-causing foods or products from the diet relieves or eliminates asthma.

Allergists can identify which foods are responsible for the allergic asthma through allergy testing. As an alternative to testing, progressively eliminate the foods or products that most frequently cause allergy sensitivity, which are shown in the table on the right.

MAGNESIUM SUPPLEMENTS

One of the actions of magnesium is relaxation and dilation of the bronchial passages. Magnesium deficiency can be predisposing to asthma attacks. To prevent this, 250-500 mg of magnesium chloride should be taken per day as a mineral supplement.

Most Common Causes of Asthma-Related Food Allergies

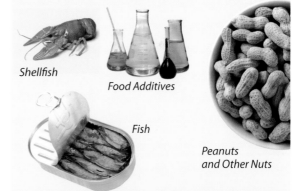

Shellfish

Food Additives

Fish

Peanuts and Other Nuts

Cow's Milk

This is the main cause of food allergies in children,[a] as well as a significant cause in adults. Therefore, without specific testing, the first foods that should be eliminated from the diet for asthma are milk and dairy products.

It is interesting to note that breastfeeding reduces a child's risk of asthma and other manifestations of allergies in later years.

a. Food allergy as a risk factor for asthma morbidity in adults. Berns SH, Halm EA, Sampson HA, Sicherer SH, Busse PJ, Wisnivesky JP. J Asthma. 2007 Jun;44(5):377-81. PMID: 17613633

a. The natural history of IgE-mediated cow's milk allergy. Skripak JM, Matsui EC, Mudd K, Wood RA. J Allergy Clin Immunol. 2007 Nov;120(5):1172-7. Epub 2007 Nov 1. PMID: 17935766

COUGH RELIEF

*Because coughing is a defense and cleansing mechanism
for the airways, it is not always good to fight it with an antitussive.
The following remedies help the cough to be productive,
which eventually serves to relieve it.*

LOOK FOR THE CAUSE

Coughing is always a response to a cause that one should attempt to discover. Sometimes, complex medical examinations are needed. A physician should be consulted if coughing does not improve after 3-4 days. The most common causes of a cough are:

- Airway **infections:** These tend to be accompanied by mucus and expectoration.
- **Exposure to smoke** or gas that cause irritation (such as tobacco smoke).
- Respiratory **allergy**.
- **Foreign objects** in the airways.
- **Pulmonary tuberculosis**.
- **Lung cancer**.
- **Medications**: Certain medications can cause coughing as a side effect. These are the most common:
  - Angiotensin converting enzyme (ACE) inhibitors, such as captopril and enalapril, which are used in arterial hypertension and heart failure.
  - Beta-blockers, such as propanolol (used as an antihypertensive) or timolol (used as eye drops for treating glaucoma).

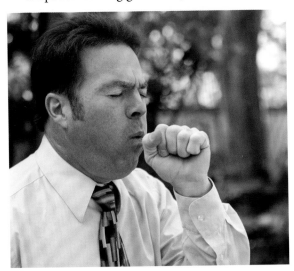

INHALE STEAM

Steam from hot water relaxes and reduces the inflammation in irritated bronchial passages that causes coughing. A balsamic or antiseptic essence can be added to the steam (see "Natural Treatments for the Lungs").

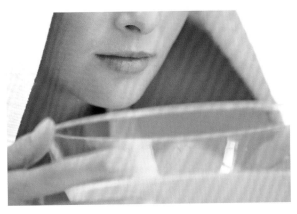

DRINK HOT HERBAL TEA

An herbal tea made from medicinal herbs relieves coughing by way of the heat's relaxing effect. If the throat is itchy, honey can be added for its antiseptic effect. Because of their soothing effect on the bronchial passages, the most recommended plants for herbal tea are:

- Eucalyptus (*Eucalyptus globulus*), an expectorant.
- Licorice (*Glycyrrhiza glabra*), an anti-inflammatory.
- Common plantain (*Plantago major*), has a soothing effect.
- Mallow (*Malva officinalis*), an expectorant and antitussive.

HUMIDIFY THE ENVIRONMENT

Dry air can irritate delicate bronchial mucosa. Use of a humidifier in a bedroom, placing moist cloths over a heating unit in wintertime, or taking a hot shower help increase the proportion of water vapor in inhaled air, and relieves coughing.

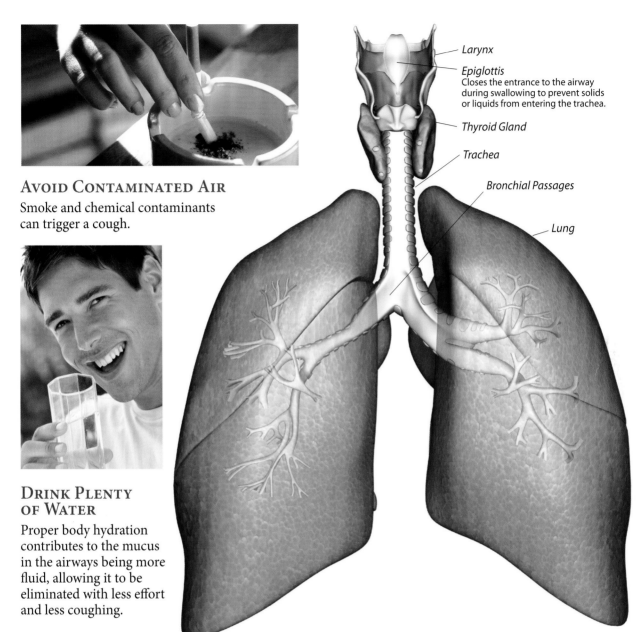

AVOID CONTAMINATED AIR

Smoke and chemical contaminants can trigger a cough.

Larynx

Epiglottis
Closes the entrance to the airway during swallowing to prevent solids or liquids from entering the trachea.

Thyroid Gland

Trachea

Bronchial Passages

Lung

DRINK PLENTY OF WATER

Proper body hydration contributes to the mucus in the airways being more fluid, allowing it to be eliminated with less effort and less coughing.

Tobacco: A Poisoned Gift

Smokers well know that inhaling cigarette smoke relieves a cough. This is a strange paradox that some smokers consider as the gift of smoking.

It is true that tobacco smoke can relieve a smoker's cough. But it is a poisoned gift because it eventually destroys the lungs.

Cough is relieved because the nicotine in smoke paralyzes the movements of cleansing cilia. When mucus does not enter the upper airways, no coughing reflex is triggered.

But when the cleansing hairs stop working, mucus loaded with impurities begins to accumulate in the bronchial passages and also in the alveoli, destroying them and causing pulmonary emphysema.

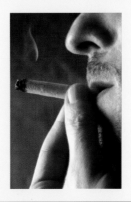

TUBERCULOSIS PREVENTION

Tuberculosis (TB) in general, and specifically pulmonary tuberculosis, is considered an emergent disease; that is, it worsens after it is believed to be under control. Therefore, it is unwise to let one's guard down and become lax in TB preventive measures and screening.

AVOID CLOSED ENVIRONMENTS

Avoid spending time in closed or poorly ventilated environments without air conditioning or air purifiers, especially when they are filled with people who could have TB.

AVOID SMOKE

Inhaling tobacco smoke and other types of smoke causes the mucus layer lining the bronchial passages to become inflamed. This weakens natural defenses against TB bacilli infection.

VENTILATION

Ensure that rooms and living areas are well ventilated at least a few hours each day. Remember: saliva droplets with TB bacilli can remain suspended in the air for several days.

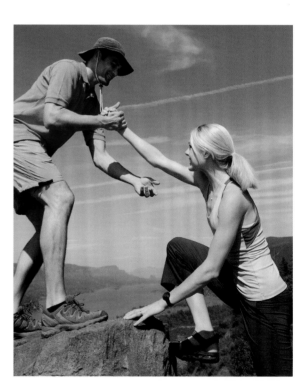

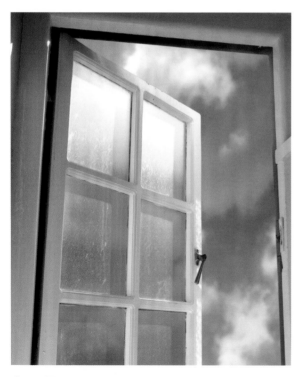

HEALTHY LIFESTYLE

This is summed up by the "Eight Health Factors": Fresh air, water inside and out, sunlight, a healthy diet, physical activity, regular periods of rest, abstinence from toxins and a positive mental attitude.

Practicing these eight health factors puts the body in good condition so it can fight TB bacilli and many other infectious agents.

SUN EXPOSURE

Open windows in rooms and living areas to let in sunlight. The sun's ultraviolet rays are effective in destroying TB bacilli.

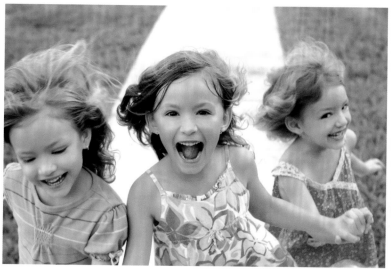

TB is spread primarily through saliva droplets that come out of the mouth with speaking, coughing or sneezing.

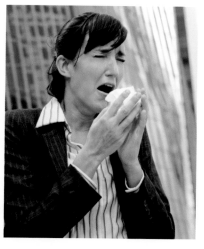

When coughing or sneezing, saliva droplets loaded with a person's germs shoot out at a speed of over 120 km/h (= 74.5 miles per hour).

TUBERCULOSIS (TB) PREVENTION IN CHILDHOOD

Children are especially susceptible to TB when living in environments with poor hygiene, inadequate diet, lack of fresh air and sun exposure, or insufficient rest.

Due to the immaturity of a child's immune system, pulmonary TB in children often spreads to other organs outside the lungs. Spread of TB to the brain's meninges, causing TB meningitis, is especially serious due to its consequences.

In addition to general recommendations, TB prevention during childhood also requires the following to be kept in mind:

- Avoid direct contact with adults who could be sick with TB.

- Do not use the plates, cups and cutlery of a family member who has TB, even if these have been washed.

- If drinking cow's milk, be sure it is sterilized or fully boiled.

- Exercise and play outdoors in the sunshine.

- Follow a healthy and plentiful diet.

- Sleep enough hours each day.

- Avoid physical or mental exhaustion.

- To avoid stirring up dust, do not sweep the house; it is preferable to mop or vacuum floors.

Smoking Promotes Pulmonary Tuberculosis (TB)

Up until the 19th Century, tobacco smoking was prescribed to TB patients. Up until a few decades ago, the cause and effect link between tobacco and TB was not accepted.

Currently, epidemiology has confirmed through a number of studies that a smoking habit is a significant risk factor for contracting TB. This was confirmed by the International Union Against Tuberculosis and Pulmonary Diseases, headquartered in Paris (France).[a]

Both tobacco use and TB are on the rise in developing countries such as Africa, Latin America and Asia. Smoking cessation programs are also beneficial for prevention of pulmonary TB.

a. Tobacco and tuberculosis: a qualitative systematic review and meta-analysis. Slama K, Chiang CY, Enarson DA, Hassmiller K, Fanning A, Gupta P, Ray C. Int J Tuberc Lung Dis. 2007 Oct;11(10):1049-61. Review. PMID: 17945060

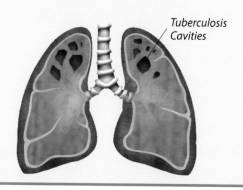

Tuberculosis Cavities

STOP SMOKING NATURALLY

The habit of smoking continues to be the leading cause of pulmonary disease throughout the world. If nobody smoked, there would be far fewer cases of bronchitis and cancer. But smoking cessation is possible –and using only natural methods.

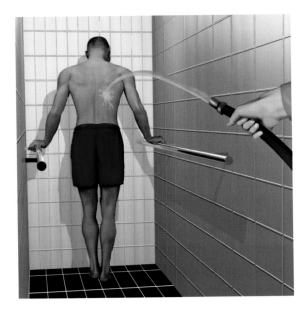

HYDROTHERAPY

Water is a great ally to free a smoker from the nicotine in the body and strengthen the willpower to stop using tobacco.

Water on the Inside (drinking)

Drink at least eight glasses of water a day for no less than 5 consecutive days, preferably before eating and up until 8 pm.

Drinking more water increases urine volume and elimination of toxic substances, including nicotine. The sooner nicotine is eliminated from the body, especially from the brain's neurons, the sooner the desire to smoke will disappear.

Water on the Outside

- **Sprayed onto the back**: This tones the nervous system and strengthens the will to stop smoking.
- **Baths in lukewarm water**: These sedate and relax, reducing the desire to smoke.

- **Rubdowns with cold water** in the morning: These activate blood circulation and stimulate the nervous system, making it unnecessary to turn to coffee (which in itself increases the desire to smoke).

A bath mitt soaked in cold water is great for morning stimulation rubdowns.

PHYSICAL THERAPY

Exercise, especially respiratory-type, helps eliminate many of the poisons deposited in the body by tobacco smoke –primarily carbon monoxide and tar.

- **Deep Breathing**: Do at least two or three sessions of 10 consecutive breaths per day. While filling the lungs with air, push the belly out so that air gets deep inside each lung.
- **A Brisk Walk**: Once per day, at least.
- **Sweating**: If possible, do some type of physical activity to the point of breaking a sweat, at least four times per week.

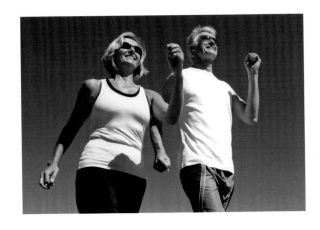

DIET THERAPY

An appropriate diet helps eliminate the desire to smoke, neutralizes the negative health effects of tobacco, and helps prevent weight gain.

- **Eat less in the evening** and more in the morning.
- Reduce or eliminate **meat** consumption, which triggers the desire to smoke and promotes development of cancer.
- Reduce or eliminate **highly fatty or spicy foods,** as these stimulate the desire to smoke.
- Avoid all **alcoholic beverages,** as alcohol weakens willpower and increases the desire to smoke.
- **Increase intake of:**
  – Fresh vegetable salads.
  – Fresh fruit, especially oranges and kiwis, for their high vitamin C content.
  – Garlic, radishes and cabbage.
  – Whole grains.
  – Nuts, such as walnuts and almonds.
  – Seeds, such as pumpkin, sunflower or sesame seeds.
  – Carrot juice, for its high content of beta-carotene, which is an antioxidant and protects the lungs.

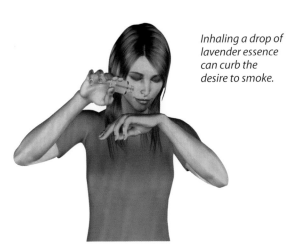

Inhaling a drop of lavender essence can curb the desire to smoke.

PHYTOTHERAPY

Medicinal herbs are very helpful for smoking cessation due to their safe and mild effects. Some examples are:

- **Calming Herbal Teas:** Such as passion flower (*Passiflora incarnata*), valerian (*Valeriana officinalis*), lemon balm (*Melissa officinalis*) and/or sweet orange flower (*Citrus sinensis*).
- **Pectoral Herbal Teas:** Green anise (*Pimpinela anisum*), peppermint (*Mentha piperita*), common mallow (*Malva silvestris*), licorice (*Glycyrrhiza glabra*) and/or coltsfoot (*Tussilago farfara*).
- **Inhalation of Essential Lavender Oil** (*Lavandula angustifolia*): Produces an effect of peace and wellbeing, and is very recommendable when the urge to smoke is high.

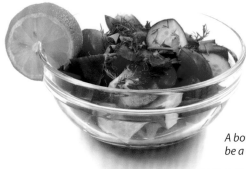

A bowl of raw salad with seeds should be a daily staple in the diet of an ex-smoker.

Tobacco's Three Major Poisons

Thousands of toxic substances have been identified in tobacco smoke, but there are three that should be eliminated in order to overcome addiction and improve health.

Poison	Effects	How to Get Rid of it
Nicotine	• Addiction (the need to keep smoking). • Narrowing of the arteries: Strokes, atherosclerosis, thrombosis.	Drink plenty of water (at least 8 glasses per day over 5 days).
Carbon Monoxide	• Sedation, mild numbing. • Lower oxygenation of the body's cells, especially neurons. • High doses can be deadly.	Deep breathing of fresh air.
Tar	• Irritation of the mouth, throat and bronchial passages. • Over a long period, mutations and cancer.	Once tar infiltrates the tissues in the mouth and respiratory organs, it takes many years to eliminate it.

Heart

The engine of life.

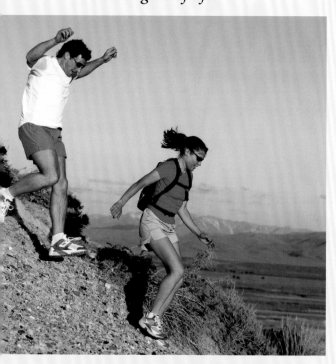

Clear arteries provide greater energy for the body and allow better physical and mental performance.

*T*he heart's never-ending, rhythmic beat stays with humans throughout their entire lives, beginning long before birth. Starting on day 23 of intrauterine life, the heart begins to beat; so by the moment of birth, it has already beaten more than 40 million times.

The heart is much more than a muscle: It is truly a super-muscle made of a special type of contracting fibers that can work continuously and with hardly any rest over an entire lifetime. This ability differentiates the heart from the rest of the body's muscles, which need to rest after exercise.

In order to beat without resting throughout life, the heart requires a constant blood supply for itself. This blood comes by way of the coronary arteries, which are the first branches exiting the body's greatest pipeline: the aorta. When coronary artery blood flow is decreased or interrupted, the heart protests with sharp, pressure-like pain –the main symptom of a heart attack.

Caring for the heart involves, more than anything, keeping coronary arteries clear to ensure blood can flow through them and supply the blood that the heart demands in order to perform its work.

To develop a healthy body, it is essential to know how to take care of the heart.

Facts and Figures About the Heart

0.5 sec	Time the heart rests between beats.
5%	Percentage of blood flow supplied by the heart for its own needs.
70 ml (2.37 fl oz)	Blood volume pumped through each ventricle (left and right, with each beat).
2 500 000	Liters pumped by the heart in a year.
37 000 000	Number of times the heart beats in a year.

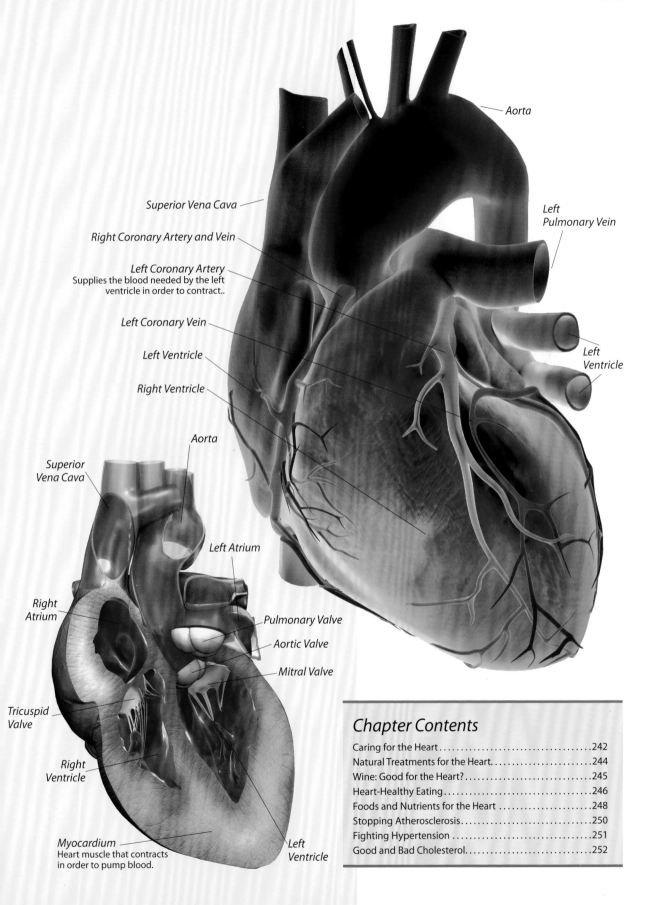

Aorta

Superior Vena Cava

Left
Pulmonary Vein

Right Coronary Artery and Vein

Left Coronary Artery
Supplies the blood needed by the left
ventricle in order to contract..

Left Coronary Vein

Left
Ventricle

Left Ventricle

Right Ventricle

Aorta

Superior
Vena Cava

Left Atrium

Right
Atrium

Pulmonary Valve

Aortic Valve

Mitral Valve

Tricuspid
Valve

Right
Ventricle

Myocardium
Heart muscle that contracts
in order to pump blood.

Left
Ventricle

Chapter Contents

Caring for the Heart

Modern medicine is capable of saving 90% of patients who arrive at the emergency room with myocardial infarction, but it cannot prevent it from happening: This depends on personal habits.

Do Not Smoke

Tobacco narrows arteries and decreases blood flow to the myocardium (heart muscle). Any amount of cigarettes is harmful to the heart.
See "Stop Smoking Naturally" in the chapter on Lungs.

Control Blood Pressure

All adults should measure their blood pressure at least once per year. A reading greater than 140/90 mm of mercury requires corrective measures and possibly treatment, excessive pressure levels damage the heart (see "Fighting Hypertension").

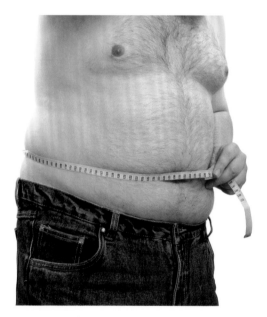

Waist size must be controlled in order to care for the heart. Over 102 cm (40 in) in men, or 88 cm (35 in) in women, is indicative of a high cardiovascular risk.

Exercise

Keeping the heart in good condition requires at least 30 minutes of vigorous exercise per day, or 40 minutes, 3 times per week. Vigorous exercise is exercise that causes perspiration.

With physical activity, the branches of the coronary arteries open up and the heart muscle receives better blood flow.

Heart-Healthy Eating

Low in saturated fats, low-salt, low-sugar and no meat, as shown in "Heart-Healthy Eating".

Fresh fruits and vegetables, nuts, whole grains and olive oil are especially beneficial for the heart.

The most heart-healthy exercise is walking at a vigorous pace, like an old saying: "We all have two doctors: the left leg and the right leg".

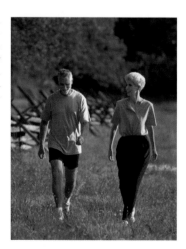

Watch the Abdomen

Waist size is an indicator of total body fat. The higher the number of fat cells, the greater the risk of type 2 diabetes and cholesterol deposits in the arteries.

If the waist measures over 102 cm (about 40 inches) in men, or 88 cm (about 35 inches) in women, a weight control program should be started.

CAREFUL WITH COFFEE

Although some statistical studies have not found a clear relationship between coffee intake and coronary disease, experiments have shown that mainly due to its

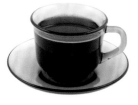

caffeine content, coffee has the following negative effects on cardiovascular health:

- It increases blood pressure slightly.
- It increases blood adrenaline levels.
- It promotes hardening of the arteries and makes dilation more difficult.
- It increases cholesterol levels and homocysteine in the blood.

Coffee intake triggers coronary events (angina and infarction) in sensitive people and also increases the seriousness of the cardiac infarction.[a]

At the University of Toronto (Canada), it was found that people under 59 years of age who are carriers of the gene called "CYP1A2*1F", that is responsible for the slow metabolization of caffeine, have a 67% greater risk of suffering a myocardial infarction, as compared to carriers of the gene "CYP1A2*1A", which provides for the quick metabolization of caffeine.[b]

This means certain people have a greater hereditary predisposition to eliminate caffeine slowly, and therefore coffee is more harmful for them. Because not everyone is able to find out if they are a carrier of the slow caffeine metabolization gene, it is safest to reduce or eliminate coffee intake.

a. Acute and long-term cardiovascular effects of coffee: implications for coronary heart disease. Riksen NP, Rongen GA, Smits P. Pharmacol Ther. 2009 Feb;121(2):185-91. PMID: 19049813
b. Coffee, CYP1A2 genotype, and risk of myocardial infarction. Cornelis MC, El-Sohemy A, Kabagambe EK, Campos H. JAMA. 2006 Mar 8;295(10):1135-41. PMID: 16522833

Reasons You Must See a Doctor

- Pressure-like chest pain. If accompanied by nausea, cold sweats, or palpitations, it could be a heart attack.
- Changes in the heart's beating patterns.
- Dizziness or fainting with no apparent cause.
- Blood pressure of 140/90 mm Hg or higher.

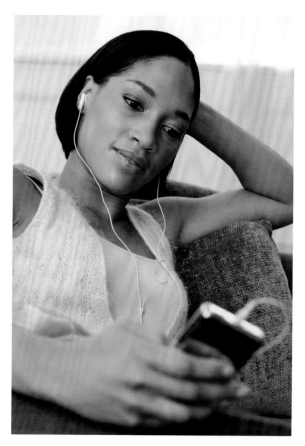

LISTEN TO MUSIC

An extensive study of 1,461 participants, many of whom had suffered an infarction,[a] found that listening to music has a favorable effect on the heart:

- It decreases blood pressure and heart rate, which eases the heart's work.
- It reduces anxiety and pain in heart patients.

Not just any type of music is beneficial for the heart, but rather the kind with these three characteristics:

- A pleasant melody.
- Little rhythm.
- A lot of harmony.

Ideally, the music listening sessions should last half an hour and be directed by a music therapy professional. The World Federation of Music Therapy[b] offers courses, training and certification for the therapeutic use of music.

a. Music for stress and anxiety reduction in coronary heart disease patients. Bradt J, Dileo C. Cochrane Database Syst Rev. 2009 Apr 15;(2):CD006577. PMID: 19370642
b. http://www.wfmt.info

Natural Treatments for the Heart

The heart is sensitive to heat and cold applied from the outside.

Cold Compress over the Heart

A cold compress applied over the heart relieves anxiety and stops tachycardia. It also achieves good results in arrhythmia.

Water Temperature: About 4 ˚C (39 ˚F).

Duration: 5-10 minutes.

Afterward: Cover the chest completely and rest for a few minutes.

Frequency: One to three times per day.

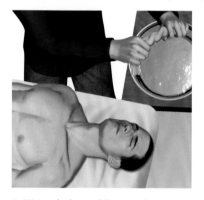

1. Wet a cloth in cold water, drain.

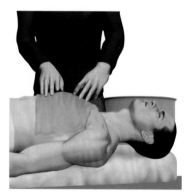

2. Place the cloth over the chest, in the heart area.

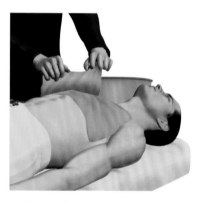

3. Cover with a wool or flannel blanket so the compress warms up as it pulls heat away from the heart.

Hot Compress over the Heart

A hot compress over the heart promotes vasodilation (widening) of the coronary arteries. It is recommended in cases of angina as a complementary treatment.

Water Temperature: About 42 ˚C (108 ˚F).

Duration: 5-10 minutes.

Afterward: Cover the chest completely and rest for a few minutes.

Frequency: One to three times per day.

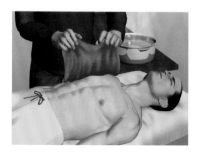

To keep the compress over the heart warm, soak the cloth in hot water again when the temperature decreases.

Hot Bath for the Arms

Due to a reflex mechanism, heat on the arms has a vasodilation effect on the heart and chest arteries.

Indications
• Hypertension.
• Angina.
• Heart Failure.

Water Temperature: 36-40 ˚C (97-104 ˚F). Hot water can continue to be added until it reaches 44 ˚C (111 ˚F).

Duration: 10-15 minutes.

Afterward: Dry the arms well, put on warm clothing and rest for a few minutes.

Frequency: One to two times per day.

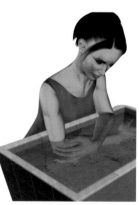

Place both arms into the bath at the same time.

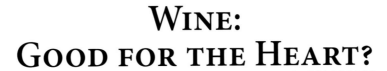

WINE:
GOOD FOR THE HEART?

It is not clear, as some have said, whether wine consumption improves cardiovascular health or prevents heart attacks.

After a few decades of statistical enthusiasm over the reported health effects of moderate consumption of wine and alcoholic beverages, from which the industry has financially benefitted in recent years more realistic studies have shown the many undesirable effects of wine and alcohol on health. The following can be understood from these recent studies:

• The positive evaluation of wine and alcoholic beverages on overall health is primarily a response to cultural and economic factors (the legend of wine) more than to contrasting scientific data.

• Epidemiological studies linking moderate alcohol consumption to lower mortality rates have greater systematic errors in data collection, according to work done by the University of California (San Francisco, United States)[a]; therefore, they do not serve to support the reported healthy effects of alcohol.

• Low alcohol consumption (less than 30 g per day, which is equivalent to two 150 ml glasses of wine, two glasses of beer or a glass of liquor) has the following undesirable effects:
– It increases the risk of breast, liver, mouth, throat and esophageal cancer, among others, according to a study of over a million women by the United States National Cancer Institute[b].
– It promotes hypertension.
– It causes predisposition to heavier drinking, along with its corresponding effects.

• No alcoholic beverage, including wine, can be considered a therapeutic remedy.

• Nobody who is abstaining from alcohol should be encouraged to drink in order to improve cardiovascular health, as recommended by the WHO. In fact, all drinkers should be encouraged to reduce alcohol consumption.

In light of recent scientific studies, the recommendation of Solomon the Wise is still valid "Do not look upon the wine when it is red…".

a. Moderate alcohol use and reduced mortality risk: systematic error in prospective studies and new hypotheses. Fillmore KM, Stockwell T, Chikritzhs T, Bostrom A, Kerr W. Ann Epidemiol. 2007 May;17(5 Suppl):S16-23. Review. PMID: 17478320

b. Moderate alcohol intake and cancer incidence in women. Allen NE, Beral V, Casabonne D, Kan SW, Reeves GK, Brown A, Green J; Million Women Study Collaborators. J Natl Cancer Inst. 2009 Mar 4;101(5):296-305. Epub 2009 Feb 24. PMID: 19244173

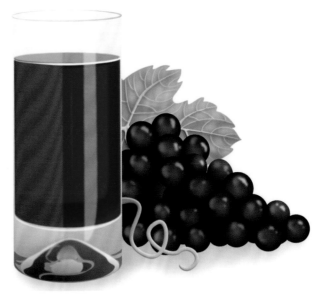

Grape Juice Is Much Better Than Wine
Grapes, especially its skin and seed, are the true source of resveratrol and other heart-protecting substances. What little good wine can have is the same as what grape juice leaves behind.

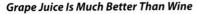

HEART-HEALTHY EATING

Five simple recommendations that can save many hearts.

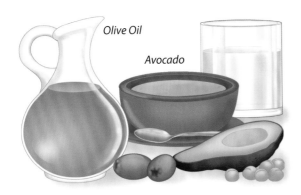

Olive Oil

Avocado

1. EAT FEWER FATS AND BETTER-QUALITY FATS

The diet needs to supply a certain amount of fat, which should not exceed 30% of the total calories consumed. For a 2,000 calorie diet, this means 67 grams of fat (a little more than 4 tablespoons of oil).

The typical Western diet is high in fat, up to 45% of total calorie intake, being primarily saturated fats from meat and milk. This fat is also accompanied by cholesterol, and promotes the production of more cholesterol in the body.

An excess of fat and cholesterol becomes deposited on the walls of the coronary arteries feeding the heart, reducing the amount of blood it receives and weakening it. When the blockage of a coronary artery is significant, the result is a heart attack.

Goals
- Reduce the total amount of fat consumed.
- Reduce or eliminate "trans" fats that are present in hydrogenated vegetable oils, some margarines and fried foods.
- Replace saturated fats (present primarily in meat, sausage, whole milk, cheese and butter) with unsaturated vegetable oils.

Alternatives
- Use unsaturated vegetable oils, such as olive oil and oil from seeds.
- Use tofu (soy cheese), guacamole and vegetable pâtés.
- Use vegetable drinks (milks) such as soy and oatmeal.

2. USE LESS SALT

Due to its sodium content, excessive salt in the diet hardens arterial walls and promotes hypertension, which overburdens the heart.

Goals
- Reduce or eliminate consumption of processed, canned and high-salt foods.
- Reduce salt intake to less than 6 grams per day.

Alternatives
- Use small amounts of unrefined sea salt (contains magnesium and other minerals that neutralize the effect of sodium).
- Use herbal salts, which are lower in sodium and have a high proportion of potassium, which neutralizes the negative effects of sodium.
- Use lemon, garlic and aromatic herbs to season foods.

Moses Warned Against Animal Fats

A few decades ago, science discovered that animal fat is not healthy.

But in the book of Leviticus, written over 3,000 years ago, Moses warned, "You shall not eat any fat, of ox or sheep or goat" (Lev. 7:23, NKJV). Pork is not mentioned here because pork meat and pork fat are not considered suitable for human consumption.

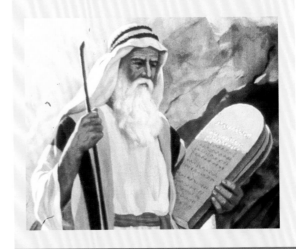

3. Eat Less Sugar

An excess of sugar in the diet is converted to fat and increases blood triglyceride levels (a type of fat), all of which promotes blockage of coronary arteries feeding the heart muscle.

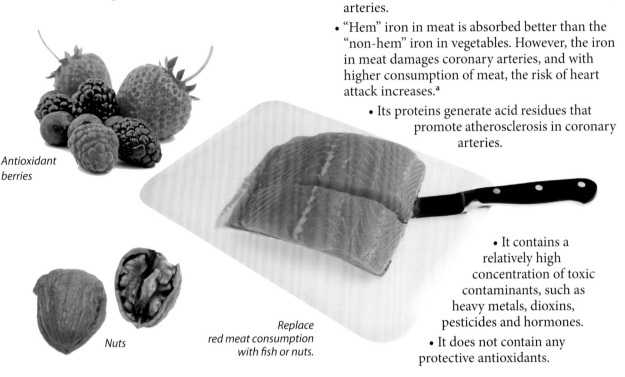

Antioxidant berries

Nuts

Replace red meat consumption with fish or nuts.

Refined or white sugar, whether chemically sucrose (common sugar), fructose, or glucose, does not contain the vitamins, minerals, fiber, or antioxidants needed by the heart, as compared to the naturally occurring sugar in fruit.

Goal
• Reduce or eliminate consumption of sweets, pastries, cakes and candies made with refined sugar and flour.

Alternatives
• When wanting to use sugar, use dried fruits such as raisins, prunes, apricots, dates or figs. These fruits sweeten, but in addition to sugar they provide:
  – Fiber, which regulates sugar absorption, preventing sudden increases in blood glucose levels that affect pancreatic function.
  – Artery-protecting antioxidants.
  – Vitamins and minerals.
• As sweeteners, use molasses (cane syrup), brown sugar (solidified cane juice) or maple syrup, which supply iron and other heart-healthy vitamins and minerals.

4. Eat Less Meat

Meat, especially red meats (beef, lamb or pork), is harmful for the heart due to the following reasons:
• It contains saturated fat and cholesterol that clog arteries.
• "Hem" iron in meat is absorbed better than the "non-hem" iron in vegetables. However, the iron in meat damages coronary arteries, and with higher consumption of meat, the risk of heart attack increases.[a]
• Its proteins generate acid residues that promote atherosclerosis in coronary arteries.
• It contains a relatively high concentration of toxic contaminants, such as heavy metals, dioxins, pesticides and hormones.
• It does not contain any protective antioxidants.

Goal
• Reduce or eliminate consumption of red meat, replacing it with fish at first, then vegetable "meats".

Alternative
• Use soy-based "vegetable meat" and other legumes, walnuts, and grains.

5. Increase Antioxidant Intake

Antioxidants protect arterial walls from the buildup of cholesterol and saturated fats. With healthy, clear arteries, the heart works much better.

Fruits (especially woodland berries), bright-colored vegetables, seeds and nuts, and whole grains are good sources of protective antioxidants.

---

a. Dietary iron intake and risk of coronary disease among men. Ascherio A, Willett WC, Rimm EB, Giovannucci EL, Stampfer MJ. Circulation. 1994 Mar;89(3):969-74. PMID: 8124837

FOOD AND NUTRIENTS FOR THE HEART

*Nutritional supplements have beneficial effects for the heart,
but do not replace the need to eat a healthy diet.*

WHOLE GRAINS

Eating whole grains improves artery condition and prevents atherosclerosis, as shown by a study of 1178 people done by Winston-Salem University in North Carolina (United States)[a].

A whole grain is complete just as nature provides it. Due to this, it has two parts that are very rich in cardio-protective nutrients, which are not present in refined flour:

• The germ, rich in polyunsaturated fatty acids and vitamin E.
• The bran, which has a high concentration of fiber, vitamins, minerals and antioxidant phytonutrients.

SOY

The Nutrition Committee of the American Heart Association has published a report after reviewing 22 studies on the effects of soy protein and isoflavones.[b] In contrast to the proteins in cow's milk, those in soy reduce LDL (bad) cholesterol by 3%, although it has not been shown to have a significant effect on HDL (good) cholesterol or on triglycerides.

This study concluded that soy products are good for cardiovascular health due to their elevated proportion of polyunsaturated fats, fiber, vitamins and minerals, and for their low saturated fat content.

OTHER HEART FRIENDLY FOODS

Flaxseed, garlic, walnuts, grapes, broccoli, and bananas are the healthiest foods for the heart.

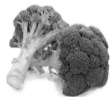

Broccoli

---

a. Whole-grain intake and carotid artery atherosclerosis in a multiethnic cohort: the Insulin Resistance Atherosclerosis Study. Mellen PB, Liese AD, Tooze JA, Vitolins MZ, Wagenknecht LE, Herrington DM. Am J Clin Nutr. 2007 Jun;85(6):1495-502. PMID: 17556684

b. Soy protein, isoflavones, and cardiovascular health: an American Heart Association Science Advisory for professionals from the Nutrition Committee. Sacks FM, Lichtenstein A, Van Horn L, Harris W, Kris-Etherton P, Winston M; American Heart Association Nutrition Committee. Circulation. 2006 Feb 21;113(7):1034-44. Epub 2006 Jan 17. PMID: 16418439

Heart Health Includes the Stomach

Up until a few decades ago, science had not discovered the close connection between food and cardiovascular health.

We now know how much our diet affects the condition of the heart and arteries.

Coronary artery blockage due to cholesterol deposits can be prevented with a diet rich in antioxidant fruit and seeds.

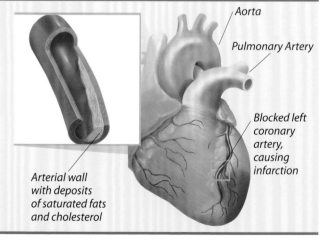

Aorta

Pulmonary Artery

Blocked left coronary artery, causing infarction

Arterial wall with deposits of saturated fats and cholesterol

Vitamin E

Vitamin E is an antioxidant from fats. It prevents the oxidation of LDL cholesterol, which is the first step in formation of atheromatous plaque in arteries.

Best Natural Sources: Sunflower seeds, almonds, wheat germ, virgin olive oil.

Precautions: It has been shown that even natural vitamin E supplements containing only alpha-tocopherol (one of its chemical forms) can have contradictory effects and do not reduce mortality from heart diseases.[a]

In order for vitamin E supplements to be truly effective in preventing heart diseases, they must meet the following criteria:

- Naturally-occurring, non-synthetic. The naturally-occurring chemicals can be differentiated from others because they are dextrorotary and begin with the letter "d", for example d-alpha-tocopherol. The synthetic forms start with "dl", for example, dl-alpha-tocopherol.
- Contain a mixture of different natural forms of vitamin E, in addition to the d-alpha-tocopherol, such as other tocopherols and tocotrienols.
- Do not use high doses (more than 400 IU per day), as they can have a counterproductive effect.
- Take vitamin E supplements along with vitamin C (250-500 mg of vitamin C with each dose of vitamin E).

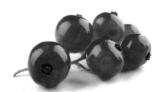

Red currants, a good natural source of vitamin C and antioxidants.

Other Nutrients for the Heart

Vitamin C

Vitamin C maintains the pliability of arteries, primarily the coronary arteries. It is a powerful antioxidant that recycles vitamin E.

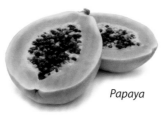

Papaya

Best Natural Sources: Acerolla, guava, currants, kiwi, citrus fruits. Meat, fish, milk, and eggs do not contain vitamin C.

Folic Acid and Vitamins B_6 and B_{12}

These reduce the level of homocysteine, which is an amino acid in the blood produced from meat proteins. A high level of homocysteine (more than 10 micromoles per liter) increases the risk of heart diseases and potentially Alzheimer's disease.

Best Natural Sources: Wheat germ, vegetables and seeds are good sources of folic acid and vitamin B_6. Vitamin B_{12} is not found in reliable levels in vegetables, although the bacteria in the colon and mouth can synthesize it.

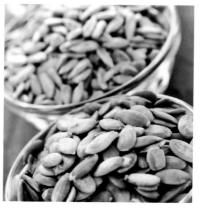

Pumpkin and sunflower seeds.

Lycopene

Lycopene is a bright red antioxidant vegetable pigment. A study done by Harvard University with 28,345 women showed that an increased level of lycopene in the blood is associated with at least a 50% decrease in the risk of cardiovascular diseases.[a]

Best Natural Sources: Tomato (tomato sauce has a high lycopene concentration), watermelon and papaya.

Magnesium

The greater the magnesium intake, the lower the risk of coronary disease and heart attack.

Best Natural Sources: Pumpkin and sesame seeds, almonds, legumes and whole-grain cereals. Meat and dairy are poor sources of magnesium.

a. Vitamin E in the primary prevention of cardiovascular disease and cancer: the Women's Health Study: a randomized controlled trial. Lee IM, Cook NR, Gaziano JM, Gordon D, Ridker PM, Manson JE, Hennekens CH, Buring JE. JAMA. 2005 Jul 6;294(1):56-65. PMID: 15998891

a. Plasma lycopene, other carotenoids, and retinol and the risk of cardiovascular disease in women. Sesso HD, Buring JE, Norkus EP, Gaziano JM. Am J Clin Nutr. 2004 Jan;79(1):47-53. PMID: 14684396

STOPPING ATHEROSCLEROSIS

Over the years, all of the body's arteries, especially the coronary arteries of the heart, become harder and narrower. Stopping this process, and even reversing it, is possible –and well worth the effort.

AVOID RISK FACTORS

All of the risk factors promoting arterial damage can be modified or controlled, except one: heredity.

- **Heredity**: There is an inherited predisposition for atherosclerosis. It is good to keep family history in mind when determining individual risk.
- **Cholesterol**: When levels are high, or not enough antioxidants are taken in, the arterial walls become damaged and allow the buildup of saturated fats.
- **Tobacco**: This is not only harmful for the smoker, but also for those exposed to second-hand smoke. If there are smokers in the family, the risk of heart disease increases by 20% –even among non-smokers.
- **Hypertension**: Damages arterial walls.
- **Stress**: Causes release of hormones, such as adrenaline, which narrows arterial walls.
- **Diet high in saturated fats, salt, sugar, and meat** (see "Heart-Healthy Eating").
- **Excess weight** and a sedentary lifestyle.
- **Excess of "hem" iron** (found in meats). This acts like a pro-oxidant and builds up in the body, being difficult to eliminate. In high levels, "hem" iron causes arterial damage.

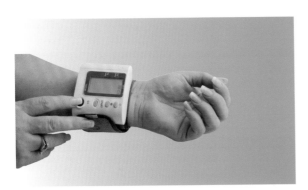

Progression of Arterial Damage

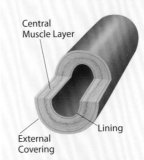

1. Normal Artery

Central Muscle Layer

Lining

External Covering

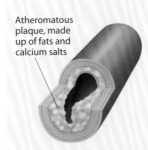

Early damage caused by oxidized LDL cholesterol

2. Early Damage to Arterial Lining

LDL cholesterol oxidizes due to a lack of antioxidants, then attacks and tears the lining that comes in contact with blood.

Atheromatous plaque, made up of fats and calcium salts

3. Fat Deposits and Formation of Atheromatous Plaque

Saturated fats and calcium first build up in the damaged area, narrowing the arterial lumen and making it difficult for blood to pass through it.

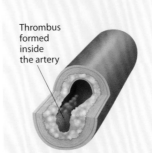

Thrombus formed inside the artery

4. Thrombosis and Complete Blockage

The slowed blood flow forms a clot or thrombus, blocking the arterial lumen almost completely. The result is a heart attack.

FIGHTING HYPERTENSION

Measurement of blood pressure alone rarely normalizes blood pressure readings if it is not accompanied by changes in diet and lifestyle, such as those suggested on this page.

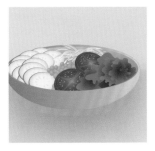

Stop using tobacco, alcohol, and coffee.

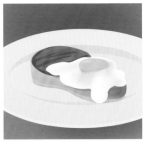

Eat fewer animal proteins (meat, eggs, cheese, etc.).

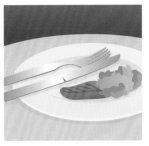

Reduce total calorie intake (simply eat less and stay a little hungry after finishing a meal).

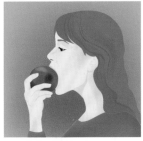

Take in enough natural antioxidants (at least 5 pieces or portions of fruit or vegetables per day).

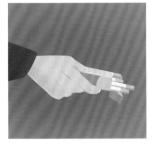

Make more than half of the diet raw foods (sprouted grains, fruits, vegetables, seeds, nuts), including at least one fresh vegetable salad per day.

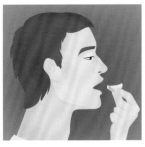

Eat 2 or 3 cloves of raw garlic per day, or have extracts or odorless pearls.

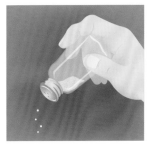

Reduce or eliminate added salt in foods.

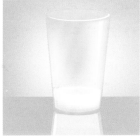

Reduce intake of whole milk, cured cheese, butter, and dairy products in general.

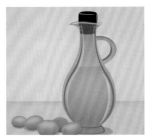

Use virgin olive oil as the main source of fat.

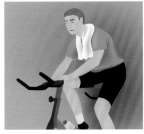

Exercise to the point of copious sweating or spend time in a sauna regularly.

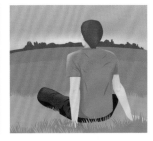

Relax under the sun, preferably within view of a country landscape or close to the sea.

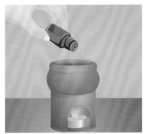

Inhale relaxing essential oils, such as lavender or citrus blossom.

GOOD AND BAD CHOLESTEROL

The importance of cholesterol cannot be stressed enough:
It is at least as dangerous for the heart and arteries to have little
antioxidants in the blood, as it is to have high cholesterol.

CHOLESTEROL: NOT SO BAD

- Cholesterol is a necessary component of blood, which is essential to life and a required building block for:
  – All the body's cell membranes.
  – The synthesis of sex hormones in the ovaries and testicles, and corticosteroid hormones in the adrenal glands.

- Twenty-five percent of the cholesterol circulating in the blood comes from food. The rest is synthesized by the liver, at a rate of about 1,000 mg per day.

- Having excessively low cholesterol promotes depression and lethargy.

- Cholesterol is only harmful for the arteries when it is high and the blood does not have enough protective antioxidants, such as vitamin E, vitamin C, beta-carotene, flavonoids and other vegetable pigments.

- Dyslipidemias are lipid metabolism disorders. In these cases, an increase in cholesterol or triglyceride levels is conditioned by hereditary factors, and not so much by diet.

- Cholesterol reduction does not necessarily reduce the risk of cardiovascular disease. The best results are obtained when, in addition to cholesterol reduction, natural antioxidant intake is increased.

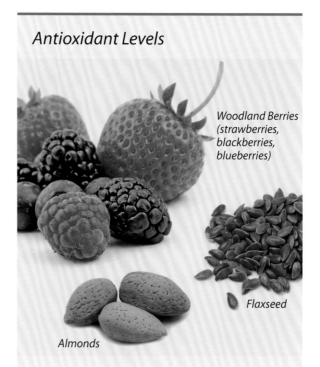

Antioxidant Levels

Woodland Berries (strawberries, blackberries, blueberries)

Flaxseed

Almonds

There is no overall test to measure the level of antioxidants in the blood, like there is for measuring cholesterol levels.
In order to ensure a high level of protective antioxidants in the blood, increase intake of:
- Nuts and seeds (rich in vitamin E).
- Bright-colored fruits, such as oranges, red grapes or woodland berries (rich in vitamin C, carotenoids and flavonoids).

Cholesterol: Blood Levels

According to the American Heart Association (www.americanheart.org)

Type of Cholesterol	Desired Level	Risk Level
HDL (good) cholesterol	60 mg/dL	Under 40 mg/dL in men, or under 50 mg/dL in women.
LDL (bad) cholesterol	Under 130 mg/dL	Over 160 mg/dL
Total Cholesterol	Under 200 mg/dL	Over 240 mg/dL

FOODS AND SUPPLEMENTS FOR CHOLESTEROL CONTROL

- **Regular Physical Activity**: This is the best way to raise HDL (good) cholesterol.
- **Garlic**: Fresh and as extracts, it reduces LDL cholesterol, dilates arteries and prevents buildup of platelets and thrombus (clot) formation.
- **Red grape juice**, including skin and seeds.
- **Walnuts**: In addition to being antioxidant, they reduce cholesterol and protect the arteries.
- **Flaxseed**: This reduces cholesterol and protects the arteries.
- **Sesame Seeds**: They reduce LDL (bad) cholesterol and increase HDL (good) cholesterol.
- **Artichokes**: Raw, cooked or as extracts, they reduce cholesterol production in the liver and increase production and release of bile (choleretic and cholagogue effects), which is also beneficial for cholesterol reduction.
- *Plantago ovata* **Seeds**: Very rich in mucilages and other types of soluble fiber that have a filling and laxative effect. They also stop absorption of cholesterol and glucose in the bowels.
- **Soy Lecithin**: Controls metabolism of fats.
- **Coenzyme Q10**: Natural antioxidant that improves heart performance.

The French Paradox

The so-called French paradox is that the French eat a large amount of saturated fats with cholesterol (butter, cheese, meat, pâtés, etc.), yet have lower cholesterol and less cardiovascular diseases than would be expected.

In a potentially anticipated and/or self-interested manner, the better health condition of the French was attributed to their wine intake, without taking into account the decisive influence of these other heart-healthy habits of the French population:

- High intake of vegetables (for example, vegetable broths) and salads.
- High fruit intake.
- Prevalence of olive oil.
- Generally small portions, with a limited number of calories per dish.

It is very likely that these characteristics of French cuisine, more than wine, are really responsible for the paradox.

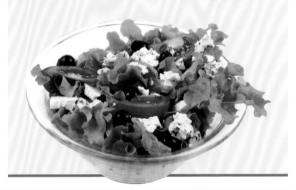

Cholesterol Is Not the Only Important Factor

High Cholesterol	High Antioxidants	**Risk of Cardiovascular Disease**
High Cholesterol	High Antioxidants	Low A high level of antioxidants protects against cholesterol oxidation and arterial damage.
	Low Antioxidants	High When there are no antioxidants, cholesterol oxidizes and damages arteries.
Normal or Low Cholesterol	High Antioxidants	Very Low
	Low Antioxidants	Medium A heart attack can happen with normal cholesterol if there are not enough antioxidants.

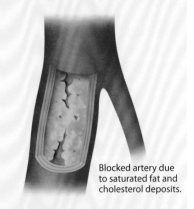

Blocked artery due to saturated fat and cholesterol deposits.

Cholesterol is required, although not enough by itself, to cause damage to arterial walls. If not enough antioxidants are consumed, cholesterol oxidizes, making it harmful.

Back

An extraordinary combination of stability and flexibility.

T he back is centered around the spine, the body's axis. The spine itself is a true marvel of structural design. The physiological curves formed by the spine make it better able to withstand weight than if it were completely straight; the hundreds of muscles and ligaments in the back act in conjunction to achieve stability and flexibility; and as a whole it is evidence of careful planning to achieve the goal of an upright posture.

This all leads to the conclusion that the human back is not the result of a progressive transformation away from the horizontal posture of mammals, but instead of intelligent design from the beginning. Thanks to this, the back defies the force of gravity and withstands mechanical stressors that come with an upright posture; and unlike any animal, it allows us to raise our heads to look into heaven.

Work, sports and the activities of daily living often place too many demands on the back: staying in or forcing uncomfortable positions, as well as turning, twisting, stretching or flexing movements. Add to this inadequate or lacking resting periods, and it is understandable that four out of every ten people suffer back pain at some point in their lives.

Learning to care for the back should be part of the school of life.

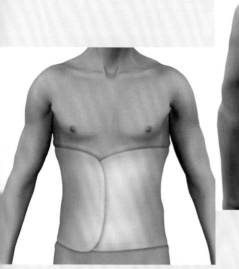

Wearing a lumbar support brace is an effective way to relieve and prevent back pain.

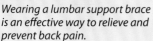

Facts and Figures About the Back

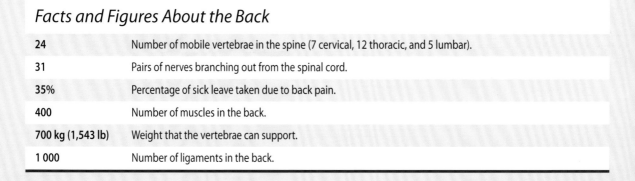

24	Number of mobile vertebrae in the spine (7 cervical, 12 thoracic, and 5 lumbar).
31	Pairs of nerves branching out from the spinal cord.
35%	Percentage of sick leave taken due to back pain.
400	Number of muscles in the back.
700 kg (1,543 lb)	Weight that the vertebrae can support.
1 000	Number of ligaments in the back.

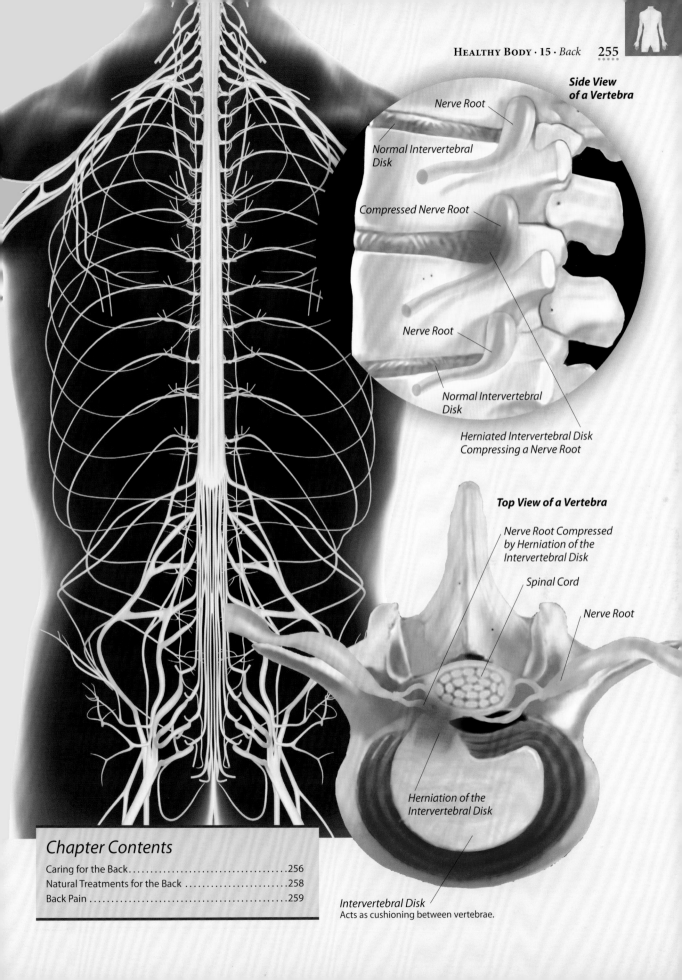

Side View of a Vertebra

Nerve Root

Normal Intervertebral Disk

Compressed Nerve Root

Nerve Root

Normal Intervertebral Disk

Herniated Intervertebral Disk Compressing a Nerve Root

Top View of a Vertebra

Nerve Root Compressed by Herniation of the Intervertebral Disk

Spinal Cord

Nerve Root

Herniation of the Intervertebral Disk

Intervertebral Disk
Acts as cushioning between vertebrae.

Chapter Contents

CARING FOR THE BACK

Back care should start in childhood by acquiring good posture habits.

DO NOT STRAIN THE BACK

- Avoid spending too much time in the same position, whether standing, sitting or laying down.
- Avoid spending too much time doing the same activity that requires back straining.
- Incorporate resting periods into the activity in order to do relaxation and stretching exercises.
- Never lift more than 25 kilos (55 lb) of weight.

AVOID SOFT SEATS

Sofas, armchairs, and soft seats in general promote over-curvature of the back. Hard seats are preferable because they allow the posture to remain more upright.

WEAR PROPER FOOTWEAR

Proper foot support protects the back. Conversely, shoes with extremely high heels (over 5 cm) or completely flat shoes overburden the back and cause a predisposition to back pain.

Soles capable of absorbing the impact of walking –running shoes, for example– protect the spine and help prevent back pain.

AVOID OBESITY

Every extra pound or kilogram accumulated on the body, especially the abdomen, adds work for the back. Losing weight relieves many types of back pain.

AVOID CONSTIPATION

Increased abdominal pressure caused by constipation promotes herniation of intervertebral disks, one of the most significant causes of lumbar pain and sciatica.

SWIM

Swimming is the best exercise for simultaneously strengthening and relaxing back muscles. Simply moving the arms and trunk in the water relieves many types of back pain.

GET ENOUGH REST

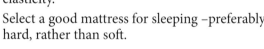

Lack of enough rest can trigger episodes of back pain.

- Make time to rest 7-8 hours per day. During sleep, muscles relax and spinal joints regain their elasticity.
- Select a good mattress for sleeping –preferably hard, rather than soft.

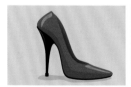

Bad

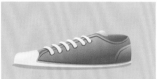

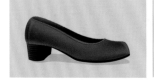

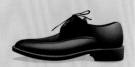

Good (2-5 cm or 0.8-2 in heels)

Reasons You Must See a Doctor

- Back pain radiating to the back of the thighs.
- Back pain accompanied by tingling or loss of strength in the legs.

MAINTAIN CORRECT POSTURE

Posture is a habit becomes automatic with repetition.

Caring for the back requires correction of bad posture habits acquired in daily life or at work that, because they seem more comfortable, change the biomechanics of the back. Bad posture habits tend to be more serious when they are acquired at a younger age.

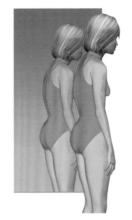
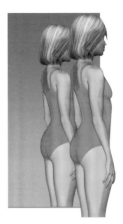

Looking in the mirror helps to perceive and correct postural defects that often go unnoticed.

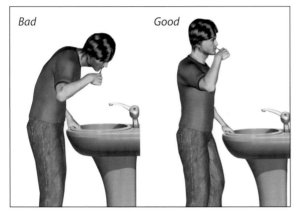

During Grooming

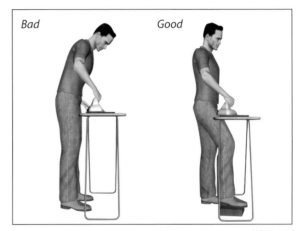

During Household Chores

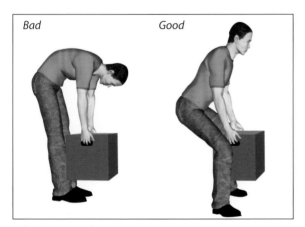

Lifting Heavy Objects

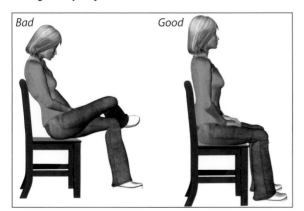

Sitting

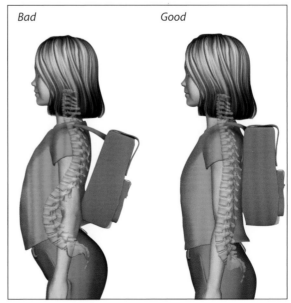

Carrying a Backpack

NATURAL TREATMENTS FOR THE BACK

Due to its large surface area, the back is very sensitive to physical stimuli, such as heat or pressure.

HEAT

Heat is the simplest and most effective remedy for back pain. By relaxing the back's powerful muscles, heat relieves stress on the vertebrae and decreases nerve root pressure. In this way, heat relieves back pain effectively and safely.

Heat can be applied several ways:
- Heating pad.
- Hot water bottle or bag: Always protect the skin with a cloth to prevent burns.
- Back compresses: See how to apply in "Natural Treatments for the Brain".

SPRAYED WATER

Spraying hot water onto the back combines the heat effect with the effect of water pressure. The result is deep relaxation and toning at the same time.

Spas have treatment chambers made especially for spraying streams of hot, pressurized water onto the back. This can be done at home in the bathtub by switching to a showerhead that allows water to be sprayed in a stream.

POULTICES

Poultices combine the effect of the product applied with that of heat (these are usually applied hot).

Mud or clay poultices relieve inflammation and pain in back muscles and joints; they should be left in place for 15-30 minutes.

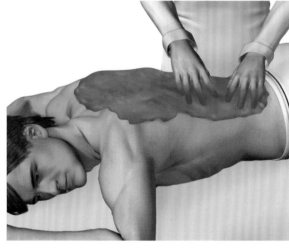

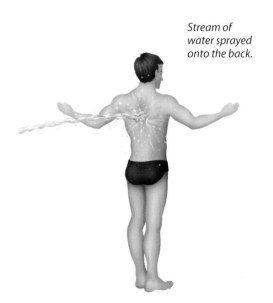

Stream of water sprayed onto the back.

Clay poultice on the back and shoulder. To increase the calming effect, hot clay is best.

SAUNA

Because of its purifying effect –toxins are eliminated with sweating– combined with the action of heat and moisture, saunas relive many types of back pain.

Saunas usually last 15-30 minutes and can be done daily or every other day.

BACK PAIN

Back pain is not the price paid for the ability to walk,
but rather a warning sign to watch posture and avoid stress.

In 90% of all cases, there is no organic change or deformity that can explain back pain. In these cases, pain is due to functional causes related to bad posture or excessive strain, and tends to disappear after two or three weeks of rest and simple treatments.

Common Causes

- Lower limb asymmetries (one leg longer than the other).
- Spinal deformities (scoliosis, kyphosis, lordosis).
- Intervertebral disk degeneration (herniated intervertebral disk).
- Osteoporosis.
- Osteoarthritis (wear and tear of the bones that worsens with age).
- Traumas.
- Rheumatic inflammations, such as arthritis or fibromyalgia.
- Vertebral infections, such as tuberculosis or brucellosis.
- Tumors.

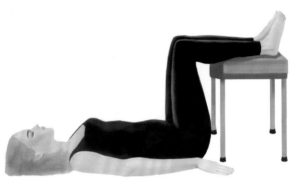

The Most Comfortable Position
Laying on a hard surface with the legs up, with an optional cushion under the lumbar area, is the position preferred by most who suffer back pain.

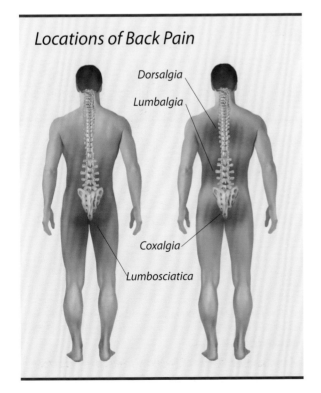

Locations of Back Pain

Dorsalgia

Lumbalgia

Coxalgia

Lumbosciatica

AVAILABLE TREATMENTS

When medication and physical therapy are unable to eliminate back pain, there are denervation procedures (sectioning pain-transmitting nerve fibers) and surgery.

Anti-inflammatory and Analgesic Medications

These are useful in acute cases, but their medium- and long-term effects are quite unsatisfactory. In addition, they have side effects, mainly for the stomach and the liver, and their continued use produces tolerance (need to increase the dose in order to obtain the same effect).

Physical Therapy

Physical therapies applied by qualified professionals (massage, hydrotherapy, electrotherapy, etc.) achieve the best results for back pain treatment.

In addition, physical therapy attempts to rehabilitate the posture and biomechanical imbalances that cause back pain.

Belly

An indicator of lifestyle, and of cardiovascular risk.

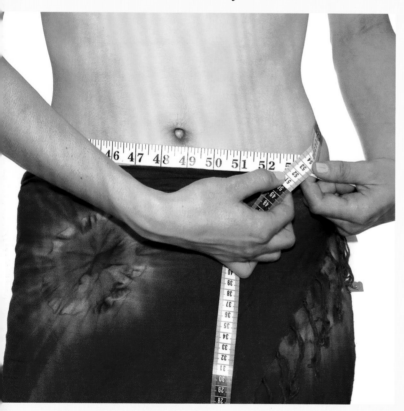

There is a direct relationship between abdominal circumference and the risk of having a heart attack.

Belly refers to the anterior wall of the abdominal cavity, from the lower part of the ribs in the chest to the coxal bones of the pelvis.

Fat accumulation on the belly and inside the abdominal cavity gives rise to what is known as central obesity. This type of obesity is closely related to cardiovascular disease. Abdominal size is therefore very important to health, as it is a reliable indicator of the risk of:

- Heart disease.
- Hypertension.
- Metabolic syndrome.
- Insulin resistance and type 2 diabetes.

Even more important than waist size is its proportion as compared to hip size, which is called "Waist to hip ratio".

The navel, located in the middle of the belly, is the scar left by the umbilical cord detaching after birth. The blood vessels that provided everything needed for fetal development passed through this cord. The navel reminds us that we were in our mothers' womb for nine months.

Caring for the belly is as easy as living a healthy, active life.

Facts and Figures About the Belly

12 mm Hg	Normal intra-abdominal pressure.
88 cm (about 35 in)	Maximum recommended waist measurement for women.
102 cm (about 40 in)	Maximum recommended waist measurement for men.

Waist-to-Hip Ratio

This is calculated by dividing waist circumference by hip circumference.

	Normal	Moderate Risk	High Risk
Men	Less than 0.95	0.96-1	Over 1
Women	Less than 0.8	0.81-0.85	Over 0.85

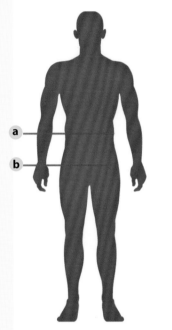
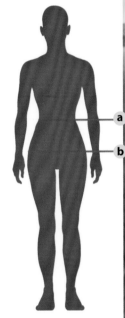

(a) Waist measurement at the navel.
This is measured at navel level.
In men, it should be under 102 cm (about 40 inches).
In women, it should be under 88 cm (about 35 inches).

(b) Hip size.
This is measured at the hips' widest point.

(1) Alba Line
(2) Abdominal Rectus Muscle
(3) Abdominal External Oblique Muscle
(the internal and transverse obliques are located below this)
(4) Abdominal Internal Oblique Muscle
(5) Inguinal Ligament

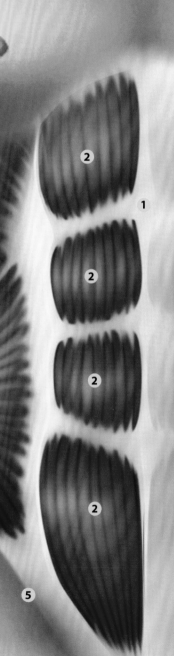

Chapter Contents

CARING FOR THE BELLY

Caring for the belly includes preventing muscle distension and fat accumulation, which are promoted by a sedentary lifestyle.

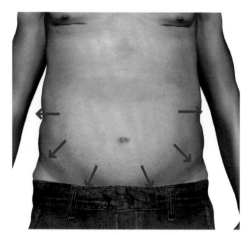

ABDOMINAL EXERCISES

Abdominal exercises are the most effective for strengthening muscle structure, but any other exercise or sport also works.

Goals
- To prevent abdominal distension, promoted by intra-abdominal pressure and a sedentary lifestyle.
- To stop fat accumulation in the belly.

Frequency
- Do 3-6 sessions per week.
- Each session should include at least three sets, with a short resting period between each.
- Each set should include at least 10 repetitions of each exercise.

Precautions
- Follow the advice on this page to prevent muscle injury.
- The best results are obtained with consistency and repetition, which are much preferred over an intense but sporadic effort.
- Do not do any exercise that causes pain or increases existing pain.

CONTROL WAIST SIZE

The abdomen is a pressurized cavity. The organs located in the abdomen tend to continually press against the abdominal wall, or belly.

Fat also tends to accumulate in the belly. All of this causes waist size to increase over the years. It has been shown that the greater the waist size, the higher the risk of cardiovascular diseases and type 2 diabetes (see previous unit).

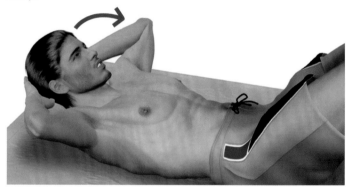

Trunk Flexion
Lay in a supine decubitus (face up) position on a hard but cushioned surface.
Look up, keeping chin away from chest.
Place hands behind the head.
Slowly lift the abdomen and head until they reach a 30-degree angle from the floor, or up to 45 degrees once trained. Breathe out with every flexion.

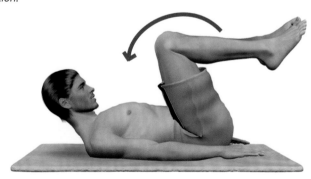

Leg Flexion
Lay in a supine decubitus (face up) position on a hard but cushioned surface.
Stretch out arms and place the palms of the hands on the floor.
Lift the knees toward the shoulders.
Lift the head, as if trying to see the navel.

DEVELOPING A FLAT BELLY

A bulging belly indicates the need to adopt healthy habits,
both in the diet as well as in posture and physical exercise.

REDUCE CALORIE INTAKE

Taking in fewer calories reduces abdominal fat. Those to be sure to reduce include:

- White sugar added to meals.
- Cakes, pastries, ice cream and other refined products –that is, those lacking in vegetable fiber.
- Animal fats (fatty meats, sausage, butter, cheese).
- Fried foods.

KEEP AN UPRIGHT POSTURE

An upright posture –shoulders back and the back straight– tenses abdominal muscles and contributes to a flat belly.

PREVENT CONSTIPATION

Fecal and gas retention in the bowels makes the belly puff out. Eating enough vegetable fiber (whole grains, fruits and vegetables –preferably raw), and doing physical activity contribute to prevention of constipation.

AVOID EXCESSIVE INTESTINAL GASSES

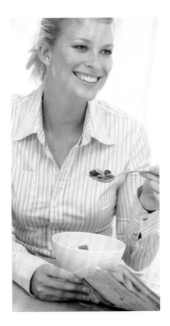

- Infusions or extracts made from anise (*Pimpinella anisum*) or fennel (*Foeniculum vulgare*).
- Chewing slowly.
- Charcoal taken before meals (a teaspoon dissolved in water).

PREVENT FLUID RETENTION

Both fluid and fat build up in the belly. An anti-natural diet, the effect certain female hormones, or poor kidney, heart, or liver function increase fluid retention, especially in the abdomen. To get rid of fluids:

- Reduce or eliminate salt intake.
- Take diuretic herbs (as infusions or extracts) such as horsetail (*Equisetum arvense*) or white birch (*Betula alba*).

REDUCE STRESS LEVELS

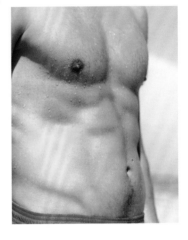

It has been shown that chronic or regular stress promotes fat accumulation in the belly, due to the action of the hormone, cortisol; the level of this hormone increases in stressful situations.[a] Stress also tends to make people consume more food and exercise less, all of which contributes to fat accumulation in the belly.

REDUCE OR ELIMINATE ALCOHOL CONSUMPTION

Even in moderate or small amounts, alcohol increases cortisol levels, promoting fat accumulation in the belly.

---

a. Chronic stress and obesity in adolescents: Scientific evidence and methodological issues for epidemiological research. De Vriendt T, Moreno LA, De Henauw S. Nutr Metab Cardiovasc Dis. 2009 Apr 9. [Epub ahead of print] PMID: 19362453

Liver

*A silent laboratory
inside the abdomen.*

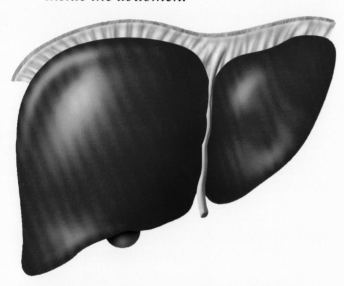

The liver is the body's great purification factory. A healthy diet promotes its detoxification function and reducing or eliminating alcohol consumption and intake of other toxins that overwork it, are the best help for its numerous functions.

*T*he liver is the largest organ in the body, and quite possibly the one that performs the most functions. Some of the most significant of these are:

- Filtration of the blood that it receives through the portal vein coming from the intestine.

- Production of bile, the digestive juice required for digesting fats and absorbing vitamins A, D, E and K.

- Elimination of medications and toxins from the blood, including alcohol and many other drugs. The liver performs this detoxification function by way of thousands of chemical reactions with which it neutralizes and deactivates foreign substances circulating in the blood. Were it not for the liver, alcohol consumed would stay in the blood for days and days, perpetuating its toxic effects. But the liver is subjected to overburdening and damage each time it has to eliminate alcohol or other toxins from the blood.

- Storage of glucose from foods, and release of glucose when energy is needed for muscle activity or other bodily functions. In the absence of glucose, the liver can obtain it from the amino acids in proteins and the fatty acids produced by fats.

The liver works a great deal, although in silence, and requires special care.

Facts and Figures About the Liver

1.5 liters (3.17 US pt)	Volume of blood that passes through the liver every minute.
2 liters (4.23 US pt)	Volume of bile produced by the liver in a day.
20%	Percentage of Western women over 40 who have gallstones.
90%	Percentage of alcohol consumed that is eliminated by the liver. The rest is eliminated in urine and breath.

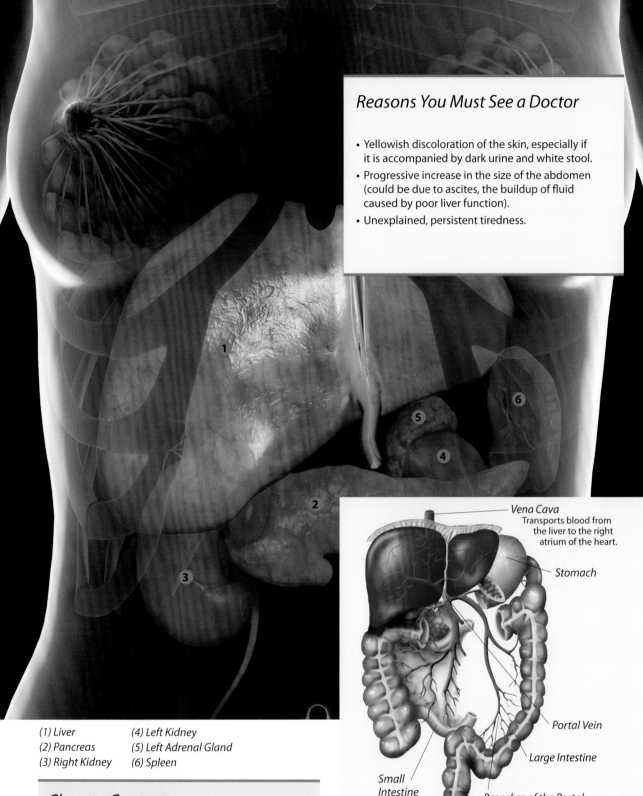

Reasons You Must See a Doctor

- Yellowish discoloration of the skin, especially if it is accompanied by dark urine and white stool.
- Progressive increase in the size of the abdomen (could be due to ascites, the buildup of fluid caused by poor liver function).
- Unexplained, persistent tiredness.

(1) Liver
(2) Pancreas
(3) Right Kidney
(4) Left Kidney
(5) Left Adrenal Gland
(6) Spleen

Vena Cava
Transports blood from the liver to the right atrium of the heart.

Stomach

Portal Vein

Large Intestine

Branches of the Portal Vein System

Small Intestine

Portal Vein System
The portal vein is the large vein in the abdomen that transports nutrient-rich –and toxin-filled– blood from the bowel to the liver.
The liver absorbs nutrients and eliminates toxins received from the bowel by way of the portal vein.

Chapter Contents

CARING FOR THE LIVER

*An orderly life and healthy diet are
the best care the delicate liver could receive.*

PHYSICAL REST

When the liver is overburdened or debilitated due to some disorder, it needs to rest. Physical rest is needed because one of the liver's functions is to provide chemical energy to muscles. By letting the muscles rest, the liver also rests, promoting its recovery.

- All types of vigorous or prolonged exercise should be avoided during the chronic phase of hepatitis, and with liver diseases in general.
- Bed rest is recommended during the acute phase of hepatitis.

A SENSIBLE DIET

In order to take good care of the liver, the most ideal diet is light and nutritious, requiring it to work very little, and with the following characteristics:
- The most natural and least processed possible.
- Without extra artificial additives.
- Low in fat.
- Moderate protein content.
- Rich in complex carbohydrates (whole grains, legumes, tubers).
- Low in salt.

REDUCE OR ELIMINATE ALCOHOL

In addition to viral hepatitis, alcohol consumption is the primary cause of liver disorders such as cirrhosis.

Ethyl alcohol is a foreign substance to the body that greatly alters the function of neurons and poisons the entire body. After being consumed, alcohol must be eliminated from the blood as quickly as possible. Only 10% of consumed alcohol is eliminated through the breath and the urine produced in the kidneys. The only organ capable of freeing the body completely from the toxic alcohol is the liver.

In order to neutralize and destroy alcohol molecules, the liver must perform an important metabolic task through the enzyme, alcohol dehydrogenase. The liver is capable of eliminating the alcohol toxin, but upon doing so, it becomes overburdened and could become ill.

CAREFUL WITH CHEMICALS AND MEDICATIONS

When the liver is affected by some disorder, revealed sometimes only by an increase in blood transminase levels, extra precautions must be taken in order to protect against chemicals and medications that overburden the liver.

- Avoid contact with chemicals, especially pesticides, solvents and sprays.
- Avoid any type of drug, including the caffeine in coffee.
- Do not take any medication, with or without a prescription, without first consulting a physician. Many medications can overburden a weakened liver and worsen latent liver failure.

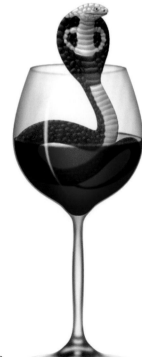

Do not look on the wine when it is red, when it sparkles in the cup, when it swirls around smoothly; at the last it bites like a serpent and stings like a viper.
Solomon the Wise
(Proverbs 23:31-32, NKJV)

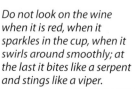

ALCOHOL:
NATURAL DETOXIFICATION

*The recommendations in this unit are a true detoxifying cure for alcohol.
They also serve to regenerate the liver.*

LIVER PROTECTORS AND REGENERATORS

Radish

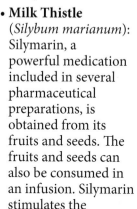

- **Radishes** (*Raphanus sativus*): Eaten fresh in a salad or as a juice, these increase bile production, detoxifying and decongesting the liver. Radishes contain a sulphurated glycoside that through enzymatic hydrolysis coverts to raphanol, a stimulant for the regeneration of hepatocytes (liver cells).

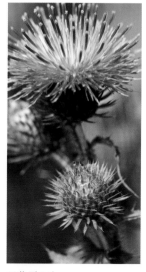

- **Milk Thistle** (*Silybum marianum*): Silymarin, a powerful medication included in several pharmaceutical preparations, is obtained from its fruits and seeds. The fruits and seeds can also be consumed in an infusion. Silymarin stimulates the regeneration of liver cells damaged by toxins such as ethyl alcohol.

Milk Thistle

ANTI-ALCOHOL SUPPLEMENTS

These facilitate the liver's detoxification work:
- Vitamins B_1, B_2, B_6, B_{12}.
- Folic acid.
- Vitamin E.
- Magnesium and zinc.
- Brewer's yeast, wheat germ, flaxseed and soy lecithin.

ANTI-ALCOHOL DIET

These foods help the liver detoxify itself from alcohol and reduce the urge to drink:
- High quantities of fruits and vegetables.
- A salad every day.
- One or two glasses of fruit juice every day.
- Foods rich in vegetable proteins, such as legumes, nuts and soy products.
- Whole grains.
- Alkalinizing, cleansing broth (see Ch. 20).

INHALATION OF AROMATIC ESSENCES

Inhalation of aromatic essences sedates and balances the nervous system, helping to control the urge to drink. The following essences are particularly effective:
- Lavender (*Lavandula angustifolia*).
- Lemon Balm (*Melissa officinalis*).
- Citrus Blossom (Bitter orange, *Citrus aurantium*).

COLD RUBDOWNS

Rubdowns are done progressively with a glove or cloth soaked in cold water, rubbing the arms and legs first, and then the chest and abdomen. Due to the effects, they help overcome alcohol dependency and drug addiction.
- They improve blood circulation.
- They increase resistance to cold, which prevents having to turn to alcohol.
- They tone the nervous system, increasing will power.
- They produce optimism and increase life energy.

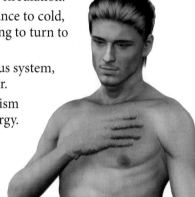

Natural Treatments for the Liver

All forms of heat contribute to the liver's recovery.

Heat on the Liver Area

Heat has a toning effect on liver function, promoting the release of bile and relaxing bile duct spasms that cause biliary colic.

Heat can be applied several ways:

- **Sunlight on the Liver**: This is a highly recommendable way to apply heat onto the liver. Exposing the abdomen to the sun for 15-20 minutes, preferably during the middle of the day, and during a period where it heats up quite a bit. This can be done through a window. Protect the chest and head from the sun.
- **Compresses on the Liver**: These are applied the same way as chest compresses, only on the liver area. Compresses are kept in place for 15 minutes, soaking the cloth in hot water when it cools down. See "Natural Treatments for the Lungs".
- **Hot Clay Poultices on the Liver**: This can be kept on for one or two hours per day.
- **Derivative Compress on the Liver**: The goal of this compress is to attract blood from the inside of the abdomen to the abdominal wall. A cloth soaked in cold water and drained is placed over the liver, then covered with a blanket until noticing a pleasant heat. This can be kept in place the entire night.

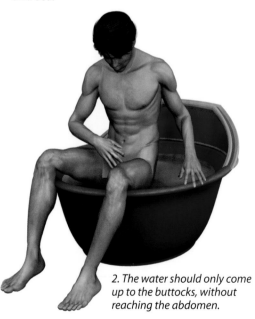

1. Sit on a stool placed inside a tub designed especially for sitz baths, or inside a large container. With a large enough container, this can also be done on a bed.

2. The water should only come up to the buttocks, without reaching the abdomen.

3. Using a bath mitt, sponge, towel or rough cloth soaked in bath water, rub the entire lower abdomen, from the navel to the genitals.

"Vital Bath"

The "vital bath" is a variant of the sitz bath, but for the lower abdomen, and can be done sitting or on a bed. It was popularized by Dr. Adrian Vander in Europe in the mid-20th Century; he enthusiastically recommended it as a general revitalizer for the body.

Beneficial Effects

The "vital bath" stimulates abdominal skin, triggering a reflex that stimulates circulation through the internal organs, primarily the liver.

- It stimulates all of the liver's functions, especially bile production and detoxification.
- It activates blood circulation throughout the entire body, increases defenses, stimulates hunger and invigorates the entire body.

Water Temperature: The water should be lukewarm or cool (4-16 °C, or 30-61 °F). The effect is more intense with colder water and vigorous rubbing.

Duration: 15-20 minutes.

Afterward: Dry the skin, cover the entire body with a blanket and rest for a few minutes.

Frequency: One to three times per day, preferably after meals.

Ideal Daily Schedule for Liver Patients

This is a suggested schedule. Better progress will be made when more days are spent this way in the life of a person with hepatitis or chronic liver disease.

8:00 A.M. GET UP
- Drink two glasses of water.
- Take 10 breaths.

BREAKFAST
- A bowl of muesli with vegetable milk (soy, oat, rice or almond).
- Add a tablespoon of one or several of the following nutritional supplements to the muesli: Wheat germ, brewer's yeast, lecithin, crushed flaxseed sprouts.
- A kiwi or an orange, along with another piece of fruit.
- A medicinal herb tea.

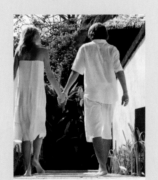

MORNING ACTIVITIES
- Reading, meditation and/or prayer.
- A leisurely walk.
- A glass of fruit juice.
- Sunlight, compresses or hot clay poultices on the liver.

LUNCH
- Fresh salad made of a variety of vegetables, including onion and radishes. Slices of fresh baby artichoke can be added. Dress with olive oil, lemon and very little salt.
- Potatoes, yucca or yam with vegetables; or legume puree with potatoes.
- A handful of nuts (walnuts, almonds, hazelnuts, pine nuts or others).

AFTERNOON ACTIVITIES
- Nap.
- Half a glass of carrot juice. A few tablespoons of spinach, radish or other vegetable juice can be added.
- Core bath.

SUPPER
- Vegetable broth or puree.
- Tofu.
- An apple or other piece of fruit.
- A medicinal herbal tea.

BEFORE BEDTIME
- Reading, meditation and/or prayer.
- Place a derivative compress on the liver.

10:00 P.M. BEDTIME

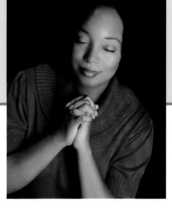

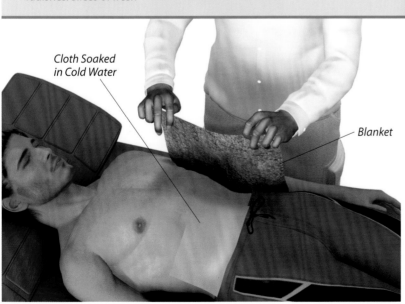

Cloth Soaked in Cold Water

Blanket

Derivative Compress on the Liver
Reduces inflammation and tones the liver.
The cloth placed over the skin should be soaked in cold water. Then, cover with a blanket to hold in body heat.

VIRAL HEPATITIS B AND C

PREVENTION

The viruses of these types of hepatitis are transmitted through the blood, unlike the hepatitis A viruses, which are transmitted by foods –mainly oysters and other raw shellfish.

Any procedure that puts a person in contact with somebody else's blood can transmit the hepatitis B or C viruses.

Despite any lack of symptoms, people who have the hepatitis B or C virus in their blood should act responsibly to avoid transmission to others. These simple guidelines are very useful in preventing transmission of hepatitis.

The hepatitis B and C viruses are not transmitted through coughing, sneezing, sharing cutlery or glassware, or by casual interpersonal contact.

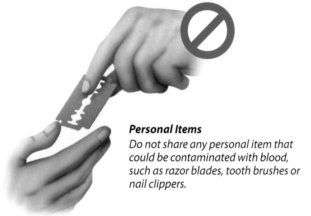

Syringes and Needles
Do not reuse or share syringes or needles.

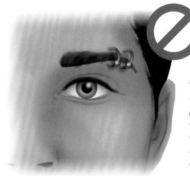

Tattoos and Piercings
Do not get tattoos or piercings, as they pose an unnecessary risk of contracting hepatitis, local infection and anatomic injury.

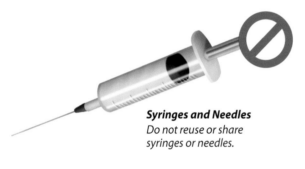

Personal Items
Do not share any personal item that could be contaminated with blood, such as razor blades, tooth brushes or nail clippers.

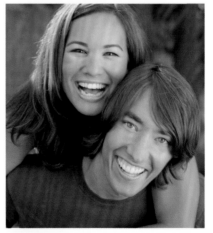

Sexual Contact
Do not have sex with anybody other than a steady partner. If this guideline is ignored, use a condom.

Transfusions and Surgical Procedures
Do not have transfusions, surgical procedures or dental treatments at unrecognized hospitals or clinics where there is no guarantee that all preventive measures will be taken.

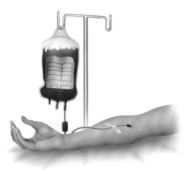

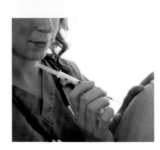

Hepatitis B Vaccine
Recommended for healthcare personnel who are at risk of contacting hepatitis B, and for newborns of mothers who are infected with or carry hepatitis B. It is also recommended for people who have hepatitis C.

VIRAL HEPATITIS B AND C

QUESTIONS AND ANSWERS

*Stopping the progression of viral hepatitis B and C
to chronic hepatitis and liver cirrhosis is the primary goal.*

If a blood test detects hepatitis C antibodies, is chronic hepatitis unavoidable?

Hepatitis C antibodies indicate that at some point there was contact with the virus in one of the ways it is transmitted. This contact has been able to cause acute hepatitis C, which usually runs its course without being diagnosed.

The fact that a person has been infected with the hepatitis C virus does not necessarily mean that the virus is still present and will cause chronic hepatitis that will eventually result in liver cirrhosis. Between 25-50% of people who have been contaminated with this virus never develop chronic hepatitis, and the virus disappears from the blood after a few months.

A healthy lifestyle contributes to eliminating the hepatitis virus without it causing chronic hepatitis and cirrhosis.

Should everyone who has chronic hepatitis B or C be treated with interferon?

The decision to treat chronic hepatitis with interferon is not easy to make. A liver disease specialist should make the decision in every individual case with the following in mind:

1. The patient's condition.

2. Blood and other diagnostic tests, including liver biopsy.

3. Factors of a prognosis predicting a positive response to interferon treatment.

The response to interferon treatment is positive in 40-60% of cases. Its administration causes side effects. Therefore, it should not automatically be applied in all cases of chronic hepatitis.

In any case, whether chronic hepatitis is treated with interferon or not, the patient should follow a strict lifestyle to protect the liver.

Can the hepatitis C virus survive outside the body and still transmit the infection?

The hepatitis C virus can survive up to 4 days in a drop or splatter of blood. In order to clean contaminated surfaces, it is recommended to dilute bleach in water (one part bleach in 10 parts water), as chlorine is very effective against the hepatitis virus.

Are blood transfusions completely safe nowadays?

All donated blood must undergo screening for the hepatitis B and C viruses, among others. The advanced testing techniques used allow post-transfusion risk of hepatitis to be nearly eliminated.

However, there is a small chance that a person could become infected with the hepatitis C virus after a blood or blood product transfusion, which the United States Centers for Disease Control and Prevention calculates is less than one case for every two million transfused units.[a]

What should a pregnant woman do if she is a carrier of the hepatitis B virus?

The newborn must be vaccinated against hepatitis B at birth, as well as receive a dose of anti-hepatitis B immunoglobulin.

Can hepatitis B or C be passed between people who live in the same house?

The hepatitis B or C virus is only transmitted by contact with the blood of an infected person.

---

a http://www.cdc.gov/ncidod/diseases/hepatitis/c/faq. htm; http://www.cdc.gov/spanish/enfermedades/Hepatitis/ HepatitisCpreguntasfrecuentes.htm

CARING FOR THE GALLBLADDER

*The gallbladder is a bile storage site where calculi or stones often form,
causing dangerous complications.*

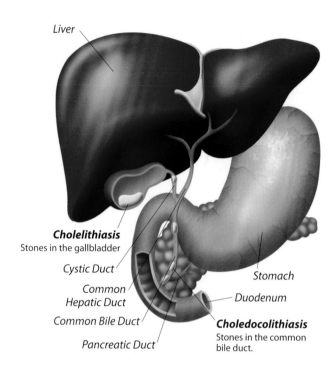

Liver

Cholelithiasis
Stones in the gallbladder

Cystic Duct

Common
Hepatic Duct

Common Bile Duct

Pancreatic Duct

Stomach

Duodenum

Choledocolithiasis
Stones in the common
bile duct.

GALLSTONES

Bile is made up of bile salts, cholesterol, lecithin and water. When it becomes thick, "bile clay" and bile calculi or stones form inside the gallbladder, in a process known as cholelithiasis.

Symptoms

Gallstones go unnoticed in half of all cases, causing no discomfort. However, they can cause complications which are sometimes serious, such as:
- **Biliary Colic**: Pain on the liver side that radiates to the back, with nausea and vomiting.
- **Cholecystitis**: Inflammation of the gallbladder requiring urgent surgical intervention.
- **Choledocolithiasis**: Passage of a stone from the gallbladder to the common bile duct, causing jaundice and fever.

Risk Factors

The possibility of stones forming in the gallbladder increases with the following risk factors:
- Women over 40 years of age with two or more children.
- Increase in blood cholesterol levels.
- Diet high in saturated or hydrogenated fats.
- Use of oral contraceptives (the pill).
- Drastic weight loss diets, attempting to lose weight quickly.

Treatment

It is very difficult –and risky– to try to dissolve gallstones to promote natural elimination. The gallstones or small fragments can become dislodged when trying to dissolve them, and then pass into the common bile duct, causing a serious complication with fever, jaundice and pancreatitis.

The only safe solution for gallstone treatment is cholecystectomy, which is the surgical removal of the gallbladder with its stones still inside.

CARING FOR THE GALLBLADDER

The goal of caring for the gallbladder is to facilitate its functioning as a bile deposit site and prevent stone formation on its inside, by way of the following recommendations:

- Reduce fat intake, especially saturated fats (mainly animal origin) and hydrogenated or "trans" fats (such as in bakery goods, margarines, and fried foods).

- Increase intake of plant fiber, which retains part of the bile acids and cholesterol in the bowels, preventing them from being reabsorbed and producing more bile.

- Drink teas or extracts from choleretic plants (those that improve bile flow, making it more fluid) and cholagogues (which facilitate emptying of bile), such as:
  – Boldo (*Peumus boldus*).
  – Globe Artichoke (*Cynara scolymus*).
  – Dandelion (*Taraxacum officinalis*).
  – Fumitory (*Fumaria officinalis*).

CARING FOR THE PANCREAS

*The pancreas is a silent, hidden organ inside the abdomen,
whose good function depends on the quality of the diet.*

CARING FOR THE ENDOCRINE PANCREAS

The primary threat to the good function of the endocrine pancreas is a sudden increase in blood glucose levels caused by foods with a high glycemic index, with large amounts of refined sugars (sweets, candies, pastries, cakes with flour and white sugar, etc.).

These foods and products force the Langerhans cells in the endocrine pancreas to secrete insulin urgently in order to reduce blood sugar levels. The constant stimulus caused by a diet high in sweets eventually overburdens the pancreas, affecting insulin secretion and promoting the onset of type 2 diabetes.

Diet for Prevention of Type 2 Diabetes
• Choose foods with a low glycemic index, which causes a slow and moderate increase of blood glucose levels.
• Reduce intake of refined sugars.
• Increase intake of vegetable fiber, which slows the starch digestion and regulates sugars absorption. The more fiber a food contains, the more slowly it is digested and the less of an increase it causes in glucose levels.

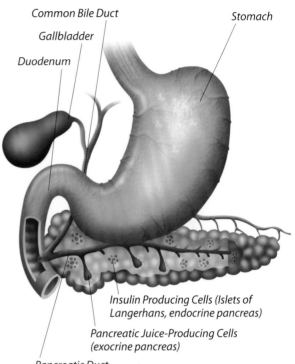

Common Bile Duct
Gallbladder
Duodenum
Stomach
Insulin Producing Cells (Islets of Langerhans, endocrine pancreas)
Pancreatic Juice-Producing Cells (exocrine pancreas)
Pancreatic Duct
Transports pancreatic juice to the duodenum.

Pancreas: A Dual-Function Organ
The pancreas is an organ with two types of highly specialized cells: Those of the exocrine pancreas, which produce pancreatic juices for digestion, and those of the endocrine pancreas, which are in charge of producing insulin.

CARING FOR THE EXOCRINE PANCREAS
• Reduce or eliminate consumption of alcoholic beverages, a common cause of pancreatitis.
• Reduce intake of high-fat foods and products, such as fried foods, sauces and meat dishes.
• Increase intake of fiber-rich, whole-grain foods, and reduce refined products that are high in white flour and sugar. This benefits both the exocrine pancreas, which produces pancreatic juices for digestion, as well as the insulin-producing cells.
• Increase consumption of papaya and pineapple, two fruits that are rich in digestive enzymes that aid digestion and ease the work of the pancreas.
• Early recognition of symptoms of a poorly functioning pancreas:
  – Flatulence, heavy digestion.
  – Poorly digested stool that is sticky, foamy and contains excessive fat (steatorrhea).
  – Pain around the abdomen, following the path taken by a belt.
• Diagnose gallstones and treat them with surgery.

Stomach

*Food storage
area and
digestive juice
factory.*

*T*he primary function of the stomach is
to mix consumed food with gastric juices,
thereby beginning the complex process of
digestion.

The inside of the stomach has the peculiarity
of being able to reflect mood. Anger makes
it turn red; fear, pale; excitement, it begins
to contract; stress, it starts to secrete juices.
All of this is due to the fact that there is a
direct connection between the brain and the
stomach, by way of the autonomic nervous
system. Any anxiety or emotion affects
stomach function.

Because the stomach can break down and
digest proteins, it is worthwhile to question
why it does not digest itself, being that it is
primarily made up of proteins. This does
not occur in normal conditions, thanks to
the stomach's true mucus barrier that wraps
around it like a film and protects its inside
from the acidy juices. When this mucus
barrier is breached, stomach juices attack the
stomach's own wall, causing gastritis (irritation
of the mucosa) and stomach ulcer (erosion
and substance loss in the mucosa).

The stomach needs special care in order to
preserve the protective mucus barrier. This
care includes regular meals, respecting the
stomach's needed rest periods.

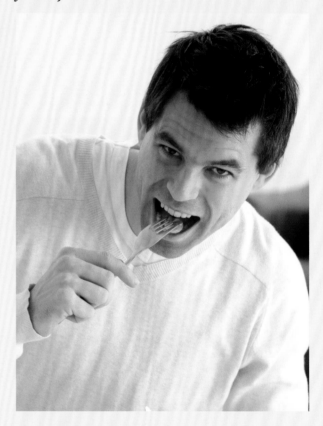

*Good stomach function is reflected in the facial expression,
and reflects favorably on the whole body.*

Facts and Figures About the Stomach

2 liters (4.23 US pt)	Stomach capacity.
2.5	pH of gastric juice (very acid).
3 days	Time it takes to completely renew the mucus layer that lines the stomach.
3 liters (6.34 US pt)	Volume of gastric juices secreted throughout the day.

Esophagus

Fundus

Stomach Body

The Stomach's Mucus Barrier

The mucus barrier protects the stomach wall against the chemical attack of hydrochloric acid and pepsin. These two substances are the primary ingredients in gastric juices, secreted by the stomach to digest foods, mainly proteins.

Thanks to its impermeability, the mucus barrier prevents the stomach wall to be self-digested by the gastric juices.

The mucus barrier is made up of a layer of viscous mucus and cylindrical-shaped mucosal cells that line the stomach.

The primary cause of gastritis and ulcers is some breach in the mucus barrier due to stress, infectious agents or stomach irritants.

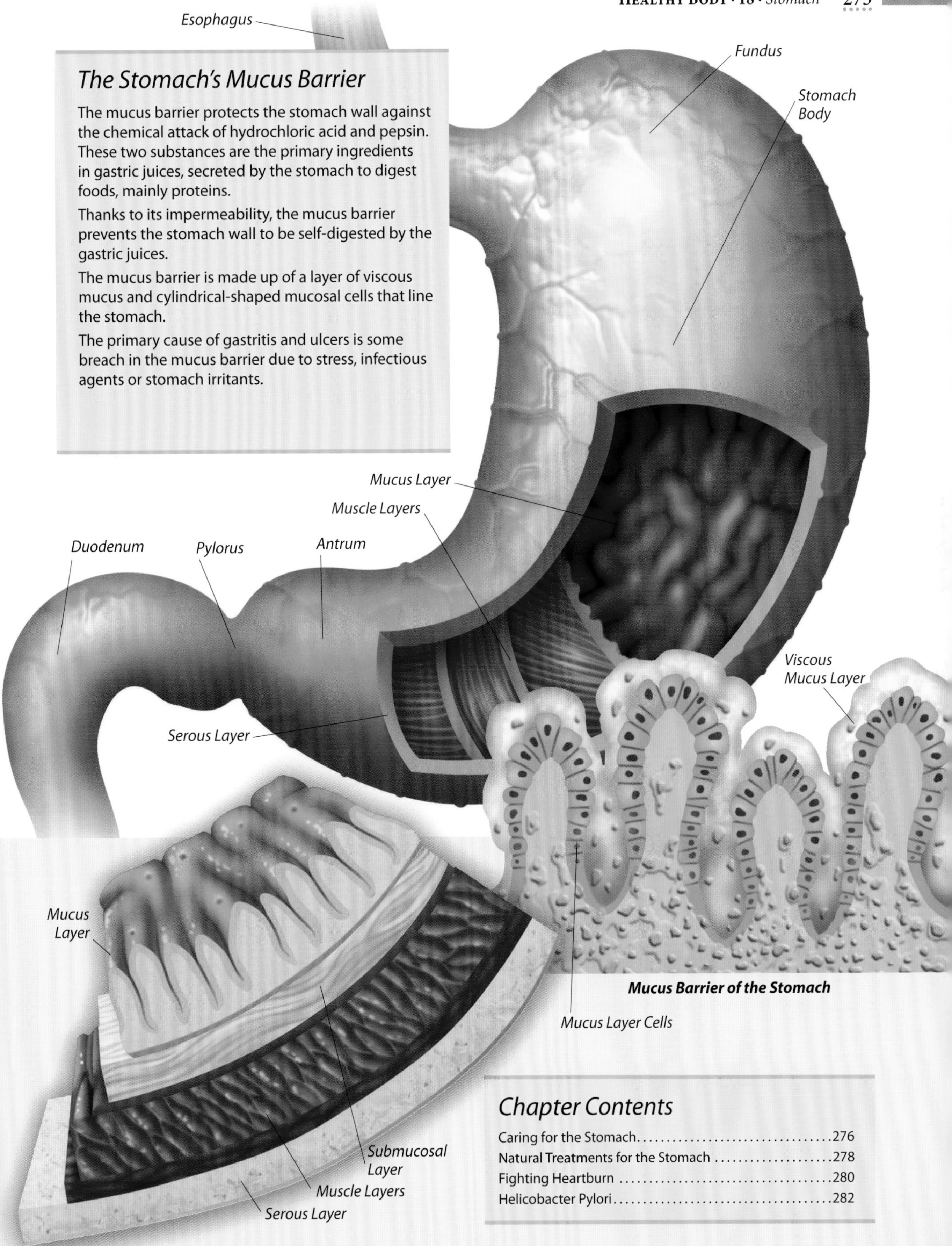

Mucus Layer

Muscle Layers

Duodenum

Pylorus

Antrum

Serous Layer

Viscous Mucus Layer

Mucus Layer

Mucus Barrier of the Stomach

Mucus Layer Cells

Submucosal Layer

Muscle Layers

Serous Layer

Chapter Contents

CARING FOR THE STOMACH

*The stomach works every day, and is often overburdened
by an excess of food. Allowing it to rest is the primary way to care for it.*

WATCH MEDICATIONS

Nearly all medications affect the stomach. However, some are especially aggressive, as they breach the mucus barrier that protects the stomach.
• Anti-inflammatories.
• Aspirin.
• Corticosteroids.
• Iron salts.

AVOID STOMACH IRRITANTS

Stomach irritants are products that increase acid secretion and weaken the mucus barrier. Although there is broad individual variability, the following products are the most irritating for the stomach, and the primary causes of indigestion:
• Coffee.
• Alcoholic beverages.
• Carbonated beverages.
• Spicy condiments.
• Pickled products.
• Fried foods.
• Fatty foods.

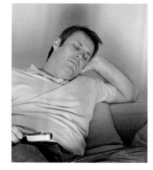

If you are stressed, it is best to rest, relax and even sleep, rather than eat.

STAY A LITTLE HUNGRY

When the stomach is filled with food, it sends an electrical signal to the brain informing it that it has reached the level of satiety. So, eating stops.

If the stomach becomes used to taking in large volumes of food with every meal, it takes longer to send the signal of satiety to the brain. In this way, more and more tends to be eaten, and the stomach ends up overburdened; obesity is the inevitable result.

It is recommended to eat only up to three quarters of what one could potentially eat. This improves digestion and prevents the feeling of heaviness after eating, and puts an end to excess weight.

WATCH EXTREME TEMPERATURES

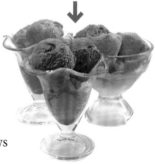

Avoid foods or drinks that are extremely hot or cold, as in both cases a certain level of inflammation is caused in the mucosa. Cold slows digestion.

Ideally, the stomach should receive food and beverages at a lukewarm temperature.

EAT ON A REGULAR SCHEDULE

The entire digestion process is subjected to biological rhythms. Listening to the internal clock's calls for food consumption –trying to eat at the same time every day– facilitates the stomach's work.

It is just as important to avoid snacking between meals, in order to allow the stomach to rest at least a few hours between one meal and the next.

Drink Solid Foods and Eat Liquids

This old hygiene adage emphasizes the importance of chewing and insalivating solid foods well, until they become almost liquid. In this way, the stomach's work is made easier.

On the other hand, liquids such as juice and broths should stay in the mouth for a while, as they also need to be insalivated for good digestion.

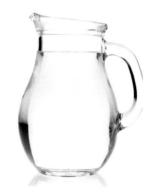

DO NOT DRINK LIQUID DURING MEALS

Drinking liquids with meals dilutes digestive juices, slowing digestion and potentially causing a heavy feeling in the stomach, belching or flatulence.

It is best to drink liquids, preferably plain water, 5-15 minutes before a meal.

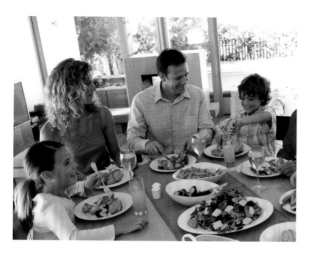

CALM, PLEASANT MEALTIMES

The stomach works better when these simple suggestions are followed:

• Take small bites and chew slowly. This way, foods arrive at the stomach more insalivated and broken down, making the stomach's work easier.

• Do not eat while doing other activities, such as walking or driving.

• Avoid arguments and anxiety while eating. Make mealtimes pleasant and calm.

• Slow down the hustle and bustle of life, setting aside more time for eating and sleeping.

AVOID MIXING TOO MANY FOODS

A meal with too many different foods or products, especially when they are high in fat and protein, overload the stomach and slow digestion. The simpler the meal is, the more healthful it will be.

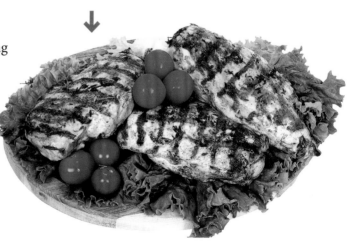

TAKE A LEISURELY WALK AFTER MEALS

A leisurely walk helps the stomach digest well, more than a nap. At a gentle pace, digestive secretions are activated and foods are better absorbed.

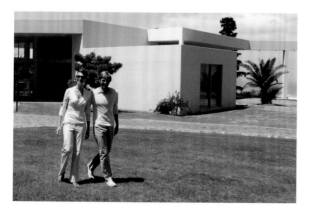

Reasons You Must See a Doctor

• Persistent stomach pain accompanied by cold sweats and general malaise: This could be a heart attack.

• Vomiting blood (usually black in color).

• Black stool (could be due to blood coming from the stomach or bowels).

NATURAL TREATMENTS FOR THE STOMACH

The stomach tends to respond well to fasting, heat and medicinal herbs.

STOMACH RUBDOWN

Rubbing the stomach increases blood flow to the digestive organs, increases appetite and tones the stomach in cases of indigestion or slow digestion.

How to Do

Use a bath mitt or cloth soaked in cold water. Rub vigorously until abdominal skin becomes a healthy reddish color.

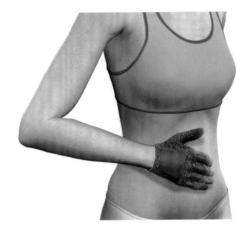

FASTING

Simple fasting is the most effective remedy for indigestion and heaviness in the stomach. By allowing the stomach to rest, regeneration of the mucosal cells is promoted and good function is restored.

Duration

Keep in mind that all of the stomach's mucosal cells renew every 3 days, so fasting a day or two at most allows sufficient rest for good digestive function.

How to Do

During a fasting period, water, teas, purifying vegetable broth or diluted fruit juices are allowed.

FRUIT CURE

The fruit cure also provides rest and relief for overloaded stomachs. Any fresh fruit is good for the stomach, although there are some that are especially recommended.

The fruit cure is really an alternative to fasting, recommended especially for those who cannot tolerate fasting, or who want the curative effect of some fruit in particular.

These are some of the most recommended fruits for the fruit cure:
- Papaya and pineapple: For the stomach.
- Apples: For the stomach and bowels.
- Pears: For the stomach and the kidneys.
- Grapes: For the heart and the liver.
- Figs: For the bowels and the blood.
- Cherries and strawberries: For the joints.
- Bananas: For hypertension.
- Mango: For the skin.

Duration

Fruit cures usually take 3 days, but they can be continued up to a week or more in special cases.

How to Do

Depending on the type of fruit, one to three kilos (2.2 to 6.6 lb) can be eaten per day, in 4 or 5 sittings.

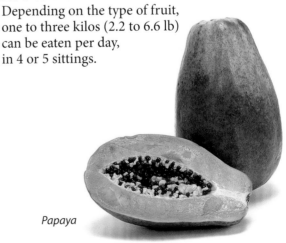

Papaya

MEDICINAL HERBS

The stomach responds quite well to digestive medicinal herbs, whether as teas or phytotherapy preparations. The best plants are mentioned for each group.

- **Protective Herbs**: These contain soothing mucilages that create a protective layer inside the stomach.
  - Common plantain (*Plantago major*).
  - Mallow (*Malva silvestris*)
- **Healing Herbs**: These contain flavonoids with anti-inflammatory action. They increase secretion of protective mucus in the stomach and promote healing of the mucosa that has been eroded by an ulcer or gastritis.
  - Yarrow (*Achillea millefolium*)
  - Comfrey (*Symphytum officinale*).
  - Dragon's blood (*Croton lechleri*): Tree in the Amazon with sap that is healing and hemostatic (stops bleeding). It is taken as 4-6 drops in a little water or juice before meals.
- **Stomach Toning Herbs**: These increase the production of gastric juices, increase appetite and promote digestion when it is heavy or slow. They tend to be bitter-tasting.
  - Peppermint (*Mentha piperita*).
  - Gentian (*Gentiana lutea*).
  - Chamomile (*Matricaria chamomilla*).
  - Yarrow (*Achillea millefolium*)
- **Hot Infusion for the Stomach**: This is an example of a general-use infusion for relieving indigestion and promoting regeneration of the stomach's mucus barrier. Place a teaspoon of each of these plants in half a liter of near-boiling water, and let stand for a few minutes while it cools. Drink up to two or three cups per day.
  - Anise (*Pimpinella anisum*).
  - Passion Flower (*Passiflora incarnata*).
  - Licorice (*Glycyrrhiza glabra*).
  - Yarrow (*Achillea millefolium*).

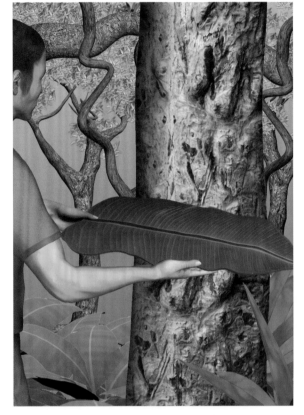

Dragon's blood is the sap of a tree in the Amazon that is very effective in treating stomach disorders.

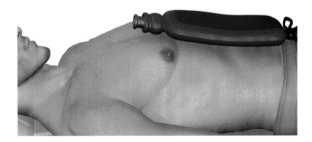

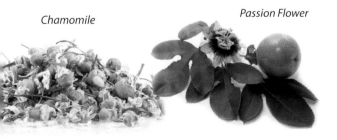

Chamomile

Passion Flower

HOT WATER BOTTLE ON THE STOMACH

Stomach pains, especially when associated with anxiety, are relieved by applying a source of mild heat, such as a hot water bottle. Heat relaxes stomach spasms and helps fight vomiting.

FIGHTING HEARTBURN

Permanently beating heartburn requires much more than just taking an antacid. Lifestyle changes are required and, in some cases, surgery is needed to correct the reflux-causing hiatal hernia.

Having acid in the stomach is normal; and if the mucus barrier in this organ is intact, the acid does not cause any symptoms. However, the esophagus is very sensitive to this acid. When there is reflux, stomach juices ascend into the esophagus, causing a burning sensation and even pain.

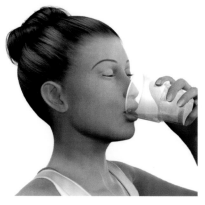

Drinking a glass of water is the best way to relieve heartburn.

WATER

Water dilutes gastric juices and has better results than milk or other drinks. Drinking water also increases the production of the protective mucus in the stomach mucosa.

FOODS THAT RELIEVE HEARTBURN

- Raw or cooked carrots.
- Raw or roasted apples.
- Papaya and pineapple, for their rich content of digestive enzymes and fiber.
- Raw cabbage juice (two tablespoons).
- Raw potato juice (two tablespoons).

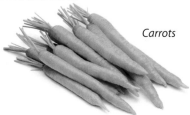

Carrots

CHEMICAL ANTACIDS

- Baking Soda: This provides immediate relief for heartburn, but is not recommended because it is absorbed into the blood and overburdens the kidneys and heart.
- Aluminum and Magnesium-Based Antacids: These are better-tolerated, but produce a rebound effect and can eventually decrease calcium absorption.
- H_2 receptor antagonists (omeprazole and others): Well-tolerated, although their continued use has side effects that stem from a lack of acid in the stomach.

FOODS OR PRODUCTS TO BE REDUCED OR ELIMINATED

- Fried foods, fatty foods, spices, fast food (tends to have a high fat content).
- Alcoholic beverages, coffee and tobacco.
- Milk: Contrary to what used to be believed, drinking milk is not a good heartburn remedy. Milk only has a temporary neutralizing effect, but produces a rebound effect with increased acid secretion in the stomach.
- Carbonated beverages, such as sodas and beer. Carbon dioxide (CO_2), the gas that forms the bubbles, stimulates acid secretion in the stomach.
- Certain medications, especially anti-inflammatories such as ibuprofen and aspirin.

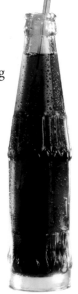

REDUCE PRESSURE ON THE STOMACH

- Avoid tight-fitting clothing or belts.
- Keep an upright posture.
- Do not go to bed or lie down immediately after eating. Have a small evening meal, or none at all.
- Sleep on the left side. Sleeping on the right side promotes reflux toward the esophagus.
- Avoid constipation: Increased pressure caused by stool retention in the abdomen promotes acid reflux from the stomach.
- Lose weight, reducing especially abdominal fat (see "Developing a Flat Belly" in Chapter 16).

SLEEP AT AN INCLINE

Raise the head of the bed to keep the head and chest somewhat elevated as compared to the abdomen. This reduces nighttime acid reflux into the esophagus.

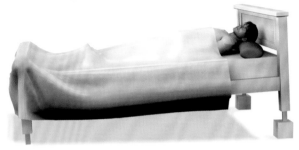

Raise the Head of the Bed to Sleep at an Incline
Put a few blocks of wood or bricks under the legs at the head of the bed, raising it 10-15 cm (4-6 inches).

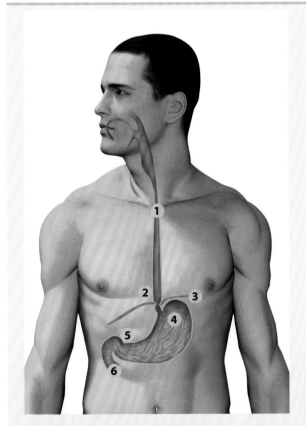

Normal Esophagus and Stomach
(1) Esophagus
(2) Lower Esophageal Sphincter
(3) Diaphragm
(4) Stomach
(5) Pylorus
(6) Duodenum

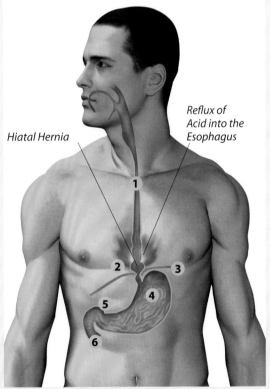

Hiatal Hernia

Reflux of Acid into the Esophagus

Hiatal Hernia
A hiatal hernia is the most common cause of reflux and heartburn. In reality, the acid is not felt in the stomach, but rather in the esophagus when the acid moves upward.

HELICOBACTER PYLORI

There are natural remedies that contribute to the eradication of this bacteria, the discovery of which has revolutionized the traditional treatment of gastritis and stomach ulcers.

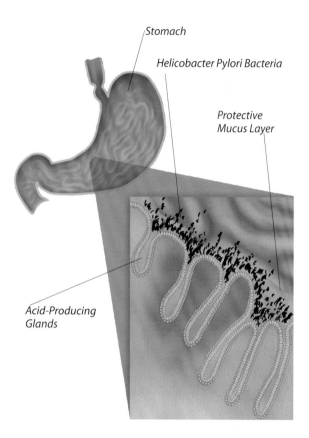

Stomach

Helicobacter Pylori Bacteria

Protective Mucus Layer

Acid-Producing Glands

THE HELICOBACTER PYLORI BACTERIUM

A few decades ago, it was thought that no bacteria could live in the stomach's acidic environment. However, in 1982, two Australian scientists discovered that the bacterium called Helicobacter pylori is able to survive the acid of gastric juice, as well as cause the following diseases:

- **Gastritis**: The Helicobacter causes inflammation of the mucosa and affects the mechanisms that protect against the acid.
- **Stomach or Duodenal Ulcer**: In 90% of ulcers, there is an infection by Helicobacter pylori in the stomach mucosa.
- **Stomach Cancer**, both adenocarcinoma and lymphomas. The Helicobacter bacterium is not carcinogenic itself, but rather acts as a cancer promoter.

TRANSMISSION OF THE INFECTION

About three quarters of the world's population has Helicobacter pylori bacteria in their stomach. However, the mere presence of this bacteria is not enough to cause damage to the stomach or cause a stomach ulcer or cancer. Other aggressive factors are required, such as an unbalanced diet, stress, coffee, alcohol, tobacco or certain medications (mainly aspirin, anti-inflammatories or corticosteroids).

Infection with Helicobacter pylori can pass from person to person, and is more common when the following circumstances are present:

- Poor overall hygiene.
- Diet low in vegetable antioxidants.
- Advanced age.

ERADICATION

Conventional treatment for the eradication of Helicobacter from the stomach includes antagonists and several antibiotics combined. This treatment tends to be effective, but there are resistant cases in which the bacteria persists in the stomach.

All foods or plants mentioned hereafter have been shown to be effective *in vitro* (and some *in vivo*) against Helicobacter, and are useful to complement conventional treatment for eradication of the bacteria.

- **Honey**: The antibacterial effect of honey has also been shown against Helicobacter pylori. This has been confirmed by research done with Manuka honey,[a] a typical product of New Zealand. A teaspoon of honey (5-10 g) half an hour before a meal can contribute to the eradication of Helicobacter.

---

a. Susceptibility of Helicobacter pylori to the antibacterial activity of manuka honey. al Somal N, Coley KE, Molan PC, Hancock BM. J R Soc Med. 1994 Jan;87(1):9-12. PMID: 8308841

- **Broccoli** (*Brassica oleracea*): According to a study by the Tokyo University of Science (Japan)[b], eating 70 g of broccoli florets for two months can reduce the bacterial colonization of Helicobacter pylori by 50%, in addition to soothing gastritis. Both broccoli and cabbage, as well as other plants in the crucifer family, are effective against Helicobacter due to their high content of sulfurane, an antioxidant and anticarcinogenic substance.

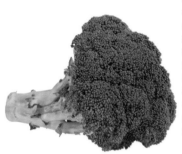

Broccoli or cabbage complement the antibiotic and antagonist-based eradication treatment such as omeprazole, obtaining better results; they can be consumed raw or as juices, as well as steamed

- **Garlic** (*Allium sativum*): At the University of Castilla - La Mancha (Ciudad Real, Spain), garlic extract rich in allacin and thiosulfinate has been shown to be an effective inhibitor of the growth of Helicobacter pylori *in vitro*.[c] Garlic oil is also effective.[d]

- **Cranberry** (*Vaccinium macrocarpon*): The antibacterial effect of these berries on the germs that cause urinary tract infections has been studied extensively. But studies done by Tokai University School of Medicine (Japan) have shown that due to their polyphenol content, cranberries are also active against Helicobacter pylori, inhibiting their growth.[e] This berry can be consumed fresh (a handful two or three times per day) or as juice (two or three glasses per day).

- **Antioxidant Berries** (woodland fruits): The combination of cranberries with other berries rich in anthocyanins with high antioxidant power such as blueberries, sauco berries, raspberries and strawberries, has also been shown to be active *in vitro* against Helicobacter.[f]

- **Propolis**: A natural antibiotic made by bees for their own needs from the resin and sap of various trees. Studies by the University of Messina (Italy) show that propolis is very effective *in vitro* as a Helicobacter growth inhibitor,[g] due to which it is recommended to complement to eradication treatment.

- **Chili Peppers** (*Capsicum frutescens*): Various studies *in vitro* show that the alkaloid capsaicin, responsible for the spicy effect of chili peppers, is capable of inhibiting the growth of Helicobacter pylori bacteria.[h] Despite this possible beneficial effect, the incidence of stomach cancer is elevated in countries such as Mexico, where consumption of chili peppers is high. A study by the National Institute of Public Health in Cuernavaca (Morelos, Mexico) found that the greater the consumption of chili peppers, the higher the risk of stomach cancer.[i] Therefore, consumption of chili peppers as a way to fight Helicobacter pylori is not recommended.

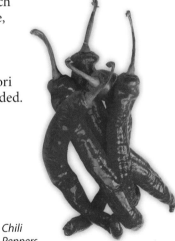

Chili Peppers

b. Dietary sulforaphane-rich broccoli sprouts reduce colonization and attenuate gastritis in Helicobacter pylori-infected mice and humans. Yanaka A, Fahey JW, Fukumoto A, Nakayama M, Inoue S, Zhang S, Tauchi M, Suzuki H, Hyodo I, Yamamoto M. Cancer Prev Res (Phila Pa). 2009 Apr;2(4):353-60. PMID: 19349290

c. Allyl-thiosulfinates, the bacteriostatic compounds of garlic against Helicobacter pylori. Cañizares P, Gracia I, Gómez LA, Martín de Argila C, Boixeda D, García A, de Rafael L. Biotechnol Prog. 2004 Jan-Feb;20(1):397-401. PMID: 14763870

d. The effect of simulated gastric environments on the anti-Helicobacter activity of garlic oil. O'Gara EA, Maslin DJ, Nevill AM, Hill DJ. J Appl Microbiol. 2008 May;104(5):1324-31. Epub 2007 Nov 20. PMID: 18028365

e. Growth inhibitory action of cranberry on Helicobacter pylori. Matsushima M, Suzuki T, Masui A, Kasai K, Kouchi T, Takagi A, Shirai T, Mine T. J Gastroenterol Hepatol. 2008 Dec;23 Suppl 2:S175-80. PMID: 19120894

f. Berry anthocyanins as novel antioxidants in human health and disease prevention. Zafra-Stone S, Yasmin T, Bagchi M, Chatterjee A, Vinson JA, Bagchi D. Mol Nutr Food Res. 2007 Jun;51(6):675-83. Review. PMID: 17533652

g. Antibacterial effect of plant extracts against Helicobacter pylori. Nostro A, Cellini L, Di Bartolomeo S, Di Campli E, Grande R, Cannatelli MA, Marzio L, Alonzo V. Phytother Res. 2005 Mar;19(3):198-202. PMID: 15934015

h. Capsaicin as an inhibitor of the growth of the gastric pathogen Helicobacter pylori. Jones NL, Shabib S, Sherman PM. FEMS Microbiol Lett. 1997 Jan 15;146(2):223-7. PMID: 9011042

i. Capsaicin consumption, Helicobacter pylori positivity and gastric cancer in Mexico. López-Carrillo L, López-Cervantes M, Robles-Díaz G, Ramírez-Espitia A, Mohar-Betancourt A, Meneses-García A, López-Vidal Y, Blair A. Int J Cancer. 2003 Aug 20;106(2):277-82. PMID: 12800206

Bowels

Thanks to them, food from the outside world becomes a part of us.

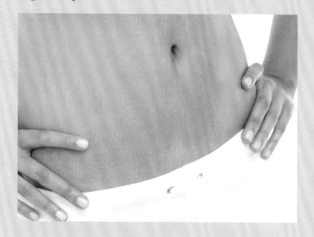

If the small intestine were smooth, its surface area would measure about 0.56 square meters (6 square feet). However, thanks to numerous intestinal villi, the surface capable of absorbing nutrients increases to 8.4 m² (90.4 square feet).

*T*he small intestine is the connection between the food coming from the outside world and the environment of the inside world. This section of the bowels works as a complex chemical processing system, designed to break down food and prepare it to enter the bloodstream and become part of us. If food were to enter the bloodstream directly without first being processed in the bowels, it would cause a severe allergic reaction and turn out to be a deadly poison.

The large intestine (cecum, colon, sigmoid colon and rectum) was long considered simply a transportation organ, designed to get rid of what is left after digestion.

Today, however, we know that the large intestine houses a complex world of beneficial bacteria required for digesting food, producing vitamins and contributing to the good functioning of the immune system. Our wellbeing depends on the enormous number of bacteria contained in our large intestine. It is estimated that we have nearly as many beneficial bacteria in the large intestine as we have in cells in the entire body (about 70 trillion, that is, millions of millions, or 70^{12}).

The bowels are much more than just a passageway; they hold part of the outside world (food and bacteria) within a person.

Facts and Figures About the Bowels

1 liter (2.11 US Pints)	Volume of gas typically produced each day inside the bowels (methane and hydrogen, primarily).
8 meters (26.2 ft)	Average length of the digestive tract, from the stomach to the anus.
8.4 m² (90.4 sq ft)	Total absorption area of the small intestine.
50	Number of different bacteria living within the large intestine, making up the bacterial flora.
200 to 300 g (7 to 10.6 oz)	Weight of stool with a diet rich in vegetable fiber (50-100 g in a meat diet).
10^{11} (one hundred billion)	Number of bacteria in one gram of normal stool.

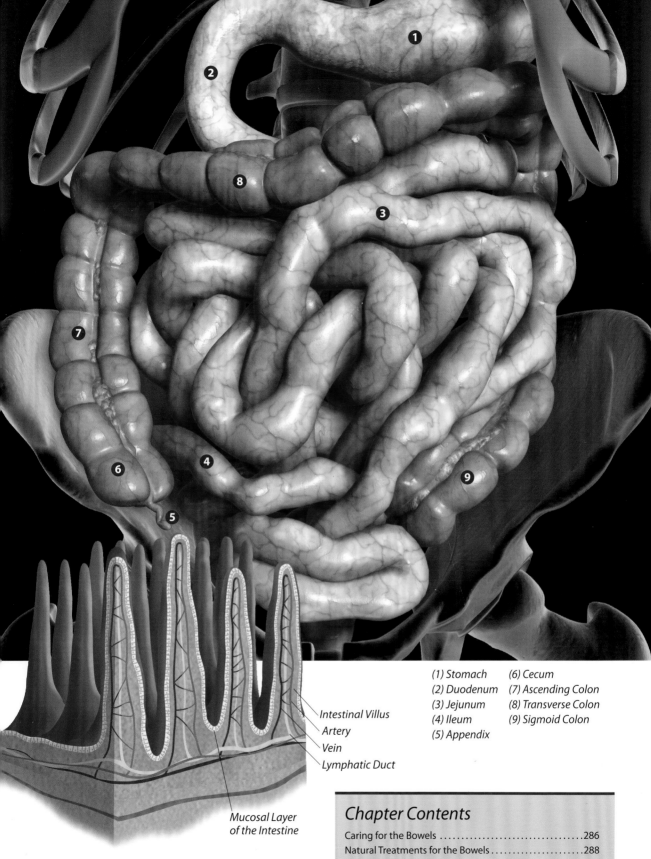

Intestinal Villus
Artery
Vein
Lymphatic Duct

Mucosal Layer
of the Intestine

(1) Stomach	(6) Cecum
(2) Duodenum	(7) Ascending Colon
(3) Jejunum	(8) Transverse Colon
(4) Ileum	(9) Sigmoid Colon
(5) Appendix	

Intestinal Villi
Microscopic projections coming out of the mucosa lining the small intestine and where nutrients are absorbed from foods and taken to blood or lymph (fatty acids).

Chapter Contents

Caring for the Bowels

The best way to care for the bowels is to consume enough fiber.
It is estimated that one quarter of digestive diseases are
due to not eating enough fiber.

Drink Water

The bowels require water. When mildly dehydrated, the body first resorts to the water in stool, extracting nearly all of its water and drying it out. When stool becomes dry, the bowels must work hard to move and eliminate it.

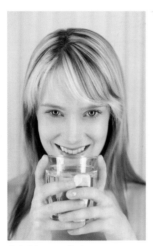
Drinking too little water promotes constipation.

Avoid Bowel Stressors

There are certain substances in foods that require more work for the bowel to digest, causing biochemical stress. With intestinal disorders, the following bowel "stressors" should be avoided:

- Refined products that are high in sugar and white flour and low in fiber, such as cakes and pastries.
- Animal fats and processed fats (hydrogenated).
- Lactose, especially in those who are unable to tolerate this milk sugar.
- Gluten, especially in celiacs, as well as in people who are sensitive to this wheat protein.
- Meat.

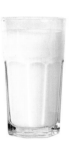
Due to its lactose content, cow's milk is one of the primary bowel stressors.

Consume Probiotics

Probiotics are living organisms –usually bacteria– that live in the human bowels and make up the bacterial flora.

An unbalanced diet, antibiotics or other reasons cause the number of beneficial bacteria in the bowels to decrease, affecting the composition of bacterial flora, and leading to the appearance of pathogenic germs such as certain fungi (like *Candida albicans*). The most common species of probiotics are:

- *Lactobacillus acidophillus* and *Lactobacillus casei.*
- *Bifidobacterium parvus*, one of the beneficial bacteria in yogurt.
- *Lactobacillus plantarum 299v*: A bacterial species recently researched and marketed as a pharmaceutical preparation. This bacterium, which has remarkable probiotic properties, is unique in that it is very resistant to stomach acid and survives the journey to the large intestine where it balances bacterial flora. It has had good results in irritable bowel, flatulence and diarrhea.

Good sources of probiotics are sauerkraut, which is rich in *Lactobacillus*, and yogurt.

Prevent Excess Gas

- Chew slowly and eat smaller amounts.
- Do not combine more than 3 or 4 types of food in the same meal.
- Avoid cooked vegetables such as artichokes, leeks and cabbage. These same vegetables do not tend to cause flatulence if they are eaten raw.
- Remove skin from legumes by mashing them.
- Decrease or eliminate white bread.
- Decrease or eliminate sweets made with white sugar.
- Decrease or eliminate milk and dairy products.
- Do not drink anything during meals.
- Take probiotic and digestive enzyme supplements.
- Take activated vegetable charcoal (2-6 capsules before each meal, with water).
- Drink infusions or extracts of carminative medicinal herbs (which eliminate gas) such as fennel (*Foeniculum vulgare*), anise (*Pimpinella anisum*) and caraway (*Carum carvi*).

Fiber Content of Food

The recommended daily amount of fiber is 25 g.

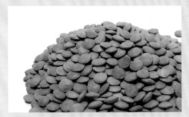

A bowl of lentils: 15 g

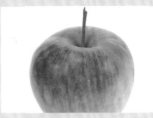

An apple: 8 g

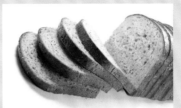

100 g of whole wheat bread: 6.9 g

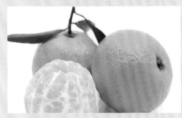

An orange: 6 g

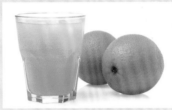

UA glass of orange juice: 0.5 g

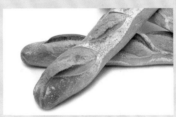

100 g of white bread: 2.3 g

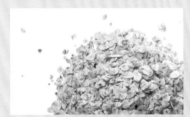

A tablespoon of whole oats: 1 g

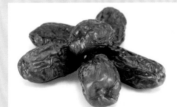

A date: 1 g

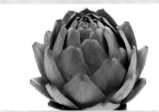

An artichoke: 5 g

CONSUME ENOUGH FIBER

The human intestine can break down, digest and absorb any food ingredient except vegetable fiber. Fiber is eliminated with stool exactly the way it entered through the mouth, only larger –due to its ability to retain water.

About 25 g of vegetable fiber is required for stool to be sufficiently large and for proper bowel function. Of the two types of fiber –insoluble (bran) and soluble (mucilage and pectin)– the latter is most recommended.

The Benefits of Fiber

- Promotes the feeling of fullness, thereby preventing obesity.
- Keeps stool soft and voluminous, facilitating its journey through the bowels.
- Regulates glucose entering the blood, preventing surges in blood glucose and thereby reducing insulin needs.
- Reduces reabsorption of biliary acids, making the liver utilize more cholesterol for bile production and reducing its level in the blood.
- Stimulates growth of bacterial flora in the bowels (beneficial intestinal bacteria), causing more vitamins to be produced.
- Prevents the following diseases: Diverticulosis and diverticulitis, inflammatory bowl disease, gallstones, hemorrhoids and colon cancer.

Reasons You Must See a Doctor

- Blood in the stool.
- Abdominal cramping after eating, especially if accompanied by diarrhea.
- Constipation that does not improve with ordinary diet changes.
- Pain with bowel movements.

NATURAL TREATMENTS FOR THE BOWELS

When applied on the abdomen, the bowels are sensitive to pressure and temperature stimuli.

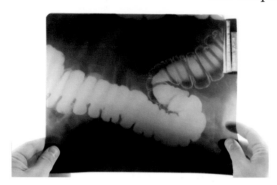

BOWEL MASSAGE

Lie on a hard surface and relax.

Using the 3 middle fingers of both hands, massage the surface of the midsection making a semicircular movement, from right to left.

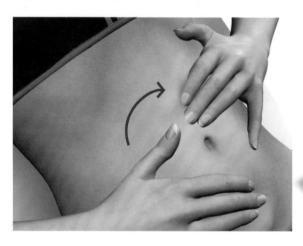

SITZ BATH

A warm sitz bath tones abdominal muscles and promotes bowel movements. It also helps heal anal fissures.

Water Temperature: Warm (20-30 ˚C, or 68-86 ˚F)

Duration: 5-10 minutes.

Afterward: Rub skin vigorously to dry, then get dressed.

Frequency: One to three times per day, preferably before meals.

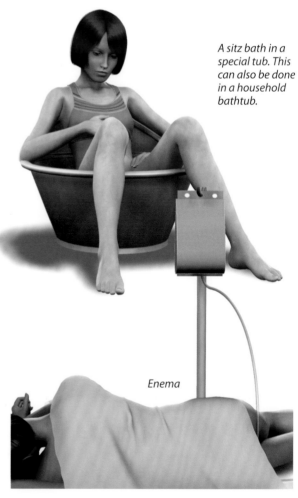

A sitz bath in a special tub. This can also be done in a household bathtub.

ENEMAS

Along with a fiber-rich diet, introducing aqueous liquids into the anus with a tube softens stool and makes it easier to pass, helping keep the bowels clear.

Enemas are usually done with half a liter of warm water. Optionally, add a teaspoon of salt or other laxative or soothing medicinal herb infusion.

Enema

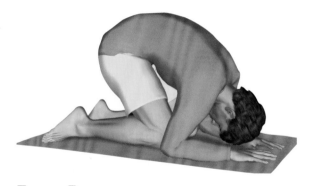

MIDSECTION WRAP

A midsection wrap relaxes and reduces inflammation of the abdominal organs. When applied cold, it produces a derivative effect, that is, it redirects blood from the internal organs to the abdominal wall. This decongests and reduces inflammation in the bowels in cases of enteritis or colitis from a variety of causes.

The steam formed by applying the wrap dilates skin pores and promotes elimination of toxins through the skin.

Water Temperature: Water should be cool or cold (4-16 °C, or 30-61 °F). The colder the water, the more intense the effect.

Duration: One to three hours. It can be left on overnight.

Afterward: Rub skin vigorously to dry, then get dressed.

Frequency: Once per day, on an empty stomach.

FETAL POSITION

Kneel on the floor, sitting back on legs, then curving the body down and forward. This position relaxes abdominal muscles and stimulates bowel movements.

Midsection Wrap

Wet, drained cotton cloth

Cool or cold water

Wool cloth for preserving heat

Digestion, Absorption and Elimination

Proper bowel function requires the complete digestion of foods, proper absorption of their nutrients and satisfactory elimination of the waste products as stool.

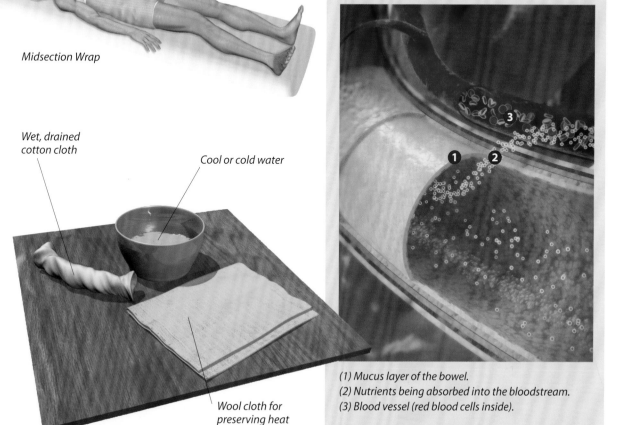

(1) Mucus layer of the bowel.
(2) Nutrients being absorbed into the bloodstream.
(3) Blood vessel (red blood cells inside).

FIGHTING CONSTIPATION

*Sufficient fiber and water intake prevents constipation
as well as up to one quarter of all digestive diseases.*

EXERCISE

A sedentary lifestyle promotes constipation. Movement is needed for toning abdominal muscles. Taking a brisk walk is a good bowel movement stimulator.

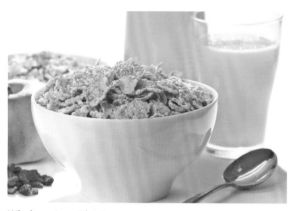

Whole grains with juice

CONSUME MORE FIBER

In order to consume more fiber, it is enough to eat more fruit, vegetables and whole grains every day. However, soluble fiber from plants in the *Psyllyum*. family can also be taken. This soluble fiber is preferred over the insoluble fiber in bran, which can irritate the bowels.

DRINK ENOUGH FLUIDS

Without enough water intake, the body absorbs water from stool, making it dry and harder to eliminate.

USE NATURAL TREATMENTS FOR THE BOWELS

Bowel massage, enemas and sitz baths are effective remedies against constipation and have no undesirable effects.

REDUCE MEAT INTAKE

Meat does not supply any fiber. Additionally, it promotes the development of the "enemy" bacteria responsible for decay (unlike vegetable fiber, which promotes the development of beneficial bacteria).

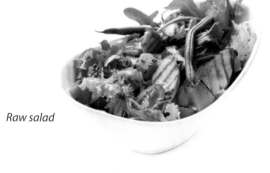

Raw salad

WATCH BOWEL MOVEMENTS

Follow "Steps for Healthy Bowel Movements" (separate unit).

TRAVEL

Traveling or leaving the usual environment tends to slow bowel movements. Help prevent constipation while traveling by drinking water, increasing fruit and fiber intake and setting aside time for bowel movements.

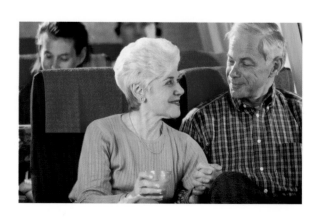

EAT MORE FRESH FRUIT

All fresh fruits are excellent natural laxatives due to their water and fiber content. Even apples help fight constipation (apples are a bowel regulator: they prevent constipation and stop diarrhea).

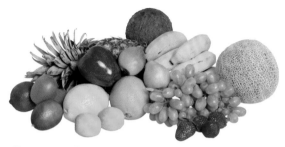

GENTLE LAXATIVES

- Magnesium Salts: Magnesium is a hydrophilic (water-attracting) mineral that pulls water into the bowels, softening stool.
- Aloe Vera: The juice or gel of this plant is a natural softener for digestive tract mucosa. Take a few tablespoonfuls with water before bedtime to help with the next morning's bowel movement.
- Infusion of cascara sagrada (*Rhamnus purshiana*) or senna (*Cassia angustifolia*) with mallow leaves (*Malva sylvestris*).

Characteristics of Good Bowel Movements

WHEN?
- Ideally, bowel movements should occur in the morning before leaving the house.

HOW OFTEN?
- At least once per day.

HOW?
- Stool should come out without great effort.
- Bowel movements should not cause pain, but rather relief after stool is eliminated.

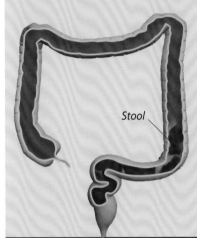

Stool

With enough fiber and water, stool acquires the necessary size and consistency for a good bowel movement.

Size Does Matter

British surgeon Denis Burkitt (1911-1993) did extensive research on the beneficial effect of vegetable fiber for the bowels and overall health. During his stay in Uganda (Africa) as a missionary doctor, he observed that the stool weight of Africans following their traditional diet was much heavier than that of Westerners.

From his research, Dr. Burkitt confirmed that the smaller the stool, due to a diet poor in fiber, the greater the risk of diverticulitis and colon cancer, appendicitis, hemorrhoids, gallstones and even gastroduodenal ulcers.

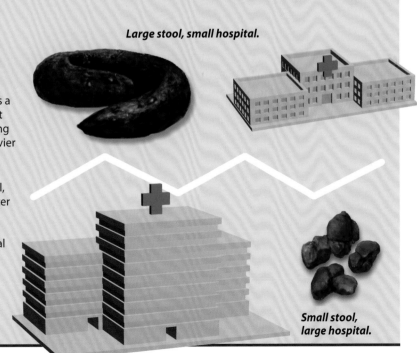

Large stool, small hospital.

Small stool, large hospital.

COLON CANCER PREVENTION

*Although some cases of colon cancer are hereditary,
the majority can be prevented by following these recommendations.*

DECREASE OR ELIMINATE MEAT INTAKE

Both red meat (pork, veal and lamb) and white meat (chicken and turkey) promote colon cancer. This is due not only to their lack of the fiber needed by the colon, but also to the carcinogenic substances formed at high temperatures with cooking or grilling.

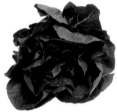

Leafy vegetables: good sources of anti-cancer folates.

DECREASE OR ELIMINATE ALCOHOL INTAKE

Alcohol has been found to particularly promote colon cancer in people who consume few folates or folic acid. This vitamin is found primarily in leafy vegetables, seeds and legumes.

DECREASE FAT INTAKE

There is a direct link between the total amount of fat in the diet, especially animal fat, and the risk of colon cancer.

Recently, it has been shown that trans-fatty acids, which are formed by industrial hydrogenation of vegetable oils to obtain solid fats or by frying foods, promote colon cancer. Certain margarines, sauces and pastries are the main sources of trans-fatty acids.

A study by the University of North Carolina (United States) has shown that trans-fatty acids promote the development of adenomatous polyps in the colon, which are considered pre-cancerous lesions.[a]

INCREASE FIBER INTAKE

The protective effect of fiber against colon cancer has now been well established, despite some research that had called it into question. Fiber retains water and increases the size of stool, speeding up elimination. This reduces the time that colon mucosa remains in contact with carcinogenic substances that may be in stool.

AVOID OBESITY

Overweight people have an excess of blood insulin, a hormone that promotes cell growth in the mucosal cells of the colon.

EXERCISE MORE

Exercise has been shown to have a protective effect against colon cancer, possibly because exercise decreases blood insulin levels.

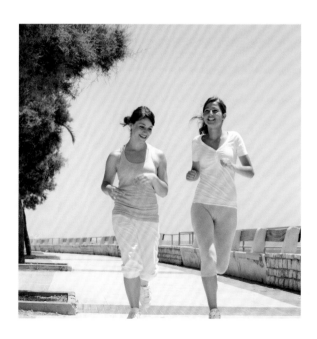

---

a. Consumption of trans-fatty acid and its association with colorectal adenomas. Vinikoor LC, Schroeder JC, Millikan RC, Satia JA, Martin CF, Ibrahim J, Galanko JA, Sandler RS. Am J Epidemiol. 2008 Aug 1;168(3):289-97. Epub 2008 Jun 27. PMID: 18587137

Travel Time through the Digestive Tract

While traveling through the large intestine, the water in stool passes into the bloodstream, and stool becomes solid.

Little water is extracted if stool travels through the large intestine quickly, resulting in **diarrhea**. If it travels through very slowly, a great deal of water is extracted from it, resulting in the dry stool typical to **constipation**.

The stool traveling slowly through the large intestine or colon allows prolonged contact between stool and the intestinal mucosa. The consequences of this slow travel are:

- Internal self-intoxication, due to the absorption of toxic substances formed in stool as a result of decay. Self-intoxication causes predisposition to headaches as well as chronic and degenerative diseases.
- Increased risk of colon cancer: If there are carcinogenic substances in stool from meat and meat products, its prolonged contact with intestinal mucosa promotes degeneration into cancer.
- *Predisposition to formation of diverticula in the colon, hemorrhoids and anal fissures, all due to increased pressure inside the bowels from dry, hard stool.*

HOW TO MEASURE DIGESTIVE TRAVEL TIMES

The most objective way to measure travel time from the mouth to the anus is to consume a certain amount of a marker product. The most recommended is vegetable charcoal, found in drugstores. Vegetable charcoal is not at all harmful, but rather very beneficial for the bowels due to its adsorption power (ability to retain toxins).

1. Take about 5 g of vegetable charcoal (about 2 teaspoons, or about 20 vegetable charcoal capsules) with a few sips of water.

2. Note the time and date of consumption.

3. Immediately start keeping an eye on stool.

4. When stool starts looking black, it is a sign that the charcoal has completely passed through the bowels. Count the number of hours between taking the marker charcoal and the first appearance of black stool.

5. If stool does not appear black, repeat the test with a larger amount of charcoal.

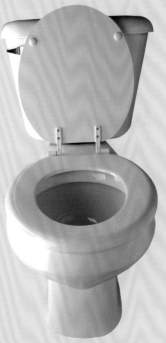

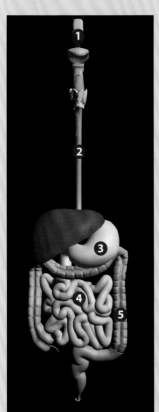

(1) Mouth
1 minute.

(2) Esophagus
A few seconds.

(3) Stomach
About 4 hours.

(4) Small Intestine
About 4 hours.

(5) Large Intestine
12-16 hours.
Fast passage: Diarrhea.
Slow passage: Constipation.

Travel Time from Mouth to Anus	Results
20-24 hours	Ideal.
Up to 30 hours	Acceptable.
48 hours (2 days)	Sluggish bowels.
72 hours (3 days) or more	Toxic bowels.

HEALTHY BOWEL MOVEMENTS

A satisfying bowel movement is the end-result of good digestion.
To achieve it, learning to have a bowel movement is almost
as important as learning to eat.

Having a bowel movement is a physiological act that is reflexive and repetitive –almost ceremonious. This ideal time for a bowel movement is in the morning after getting up. In order for this to happen, get up ten or fifteen minutes early, if necessary.

Whether in the morning or any other time, however, the important thing is to educate the bowels, setting aside a set time each day for bowel movements. The following four steps are recommended for proper bowel movements.

1. DRINK A GLASS OF WATER

Upon waking, drink a glass or two of room-temperature water. This cleanses the stomach of the mucus that builds up overnight and stimulates the bowel movement reflex.

2. PREPARE FOR A BOWEL MOVEMENT

Get in a position that allows for a bowel movement and relax, waiting as long as necessary for the bowel movement to occur. Squatting is the normal position for a bowel movement. This has been done all throughout the ages and across cultures. In the 19th Century, however, pedestal toilets became popular, allowing bowel movements to occur in a seated position.

Having a bowel movement in a seated position seems more comfortable. However, it promotes many disorders because it forces the abdomen and thorax to strain more to force out stool.

Advantages of Squatting for Bowel Movements

- Fewer anal fissures. If there is already a fissure, bowel movements are less painful and healing is faster.
- Fewer hemorrhoids. If they are already present, swelling and pain are reduced.
- Less diverticulosis (formation of small pouches in the walls of the large intestine).

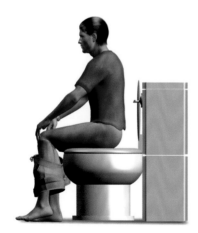

**Seated Position
(customary in Western societies)**
This seems to be more comfortable, but requires more straining, which overburdens abdominal and thoracic organs.

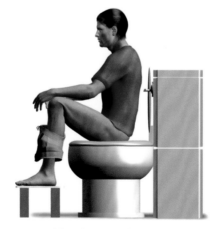

Footstool for Elevating the Legs
This allows for a more physiological position for bowel movements, even while seated. Although not as beneficial as the "squatting" position, this intermediate solution helps prevent anal fissures, hemorrhoids, diverticula and hernias.

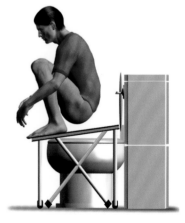

Squatting Position
Heels should touch the buttocks and thighs should touch the belly.
Perineal muscles distend and abdominal muscles push out the bowel content better.
There are also other toilet models that are even with the floor surface, thus allowing bowel movements in the squatting position

- Fewer abdominal hernias, including inguinal hernias.
- Less need to increase pressure in abdomen and thorax with the straining of a bowel movement. This increased pressure, called "Valsalva's maneuver", reduces blood flow to the brain and coronary arteries, promoting fainting, strokes and other cardiovascular events.

3. CHECK STOOL

Stool should be visually checked immediately for anything unusual that could signal a disorder or disease.

Characteristics of normal stool

- **Weight**: Over 200 g is recommended (indicating presence of enough vegetable fiber).
- **Density**: Same or less than water, such that it floats. Dense stool that sinks in water contains little fiber and is indicative of a diet poor in vegetable fiber.
- **Consistency**: Enough to preserve a cylindrical shape.
- **Color**: Brown.
- **Other Characteristics**: Not foamy, no blood, mucus or undigested food.

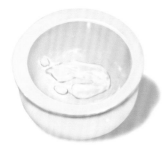

Whitish Stool (Acholic)
Can be due to a bile drainage problem.

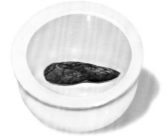

Bloody Stool (Rectal Bleeding)
Contains red blood, generally due to anal fissures, hemorrhoids, intestinal polyps, diverticulitis or colon cancer.

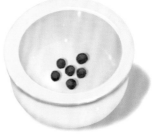

Dry Stool
Also called pellet stools. Associated with constipation, colon diverticulosis or irritable bowel.

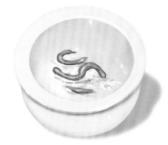

Ribbon-Like Stool
Associated with irritable colon with bowel spasm.

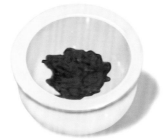

Black, tarry stool (melena)
Due to presence of blood coming from the stomach or small intestine.

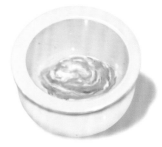

Forthy stool (steatorrhea)
Contains undigested fats due to a deficiency in pancreatic enzymes.

4. CLEANSE THE ANUS

Along with having bowel movements in a seated position, the use of bath tissue for anal hygiene is another habit of modern Western society.

The cellulose in bath tissue scratches and irritates the delicate skin and mucosa of the anus. It also does not achieve complete cleansing.

On the other hand, water completely removes stool, which is hydrosoluble, without causing skin irritation.

The most sanitary and healthy method for cleansing the anus after a bowel movement is simply washing it with water.

Device for cleansing the anus with water after a bowel movement, eliminating the need for bath tissue. Water from a showerhead or a bidet works the same way.

Kidneys and Bladder

The body's filtration and waste elimination system.

*A*long with the liver, the kidneys are the body's great purifiers, due to their ability to eliminate waste products and neutralize toxins. Kidneys are able to eliminate potentially deadly poisons, such as urea. When the kidneys are not working, the buildup of urea in the blood can result in death after just a few days.

The kidneys work around the clock to maintain a constant water ratio in the body and avoid pooling or dehydration. They have three main functions:

• Excretory Function: Consists of filtering the blood to eliminate water-soluble toxic metabolic waste through urine.

• Regulatory Function: Kidneys control the level of potassium, sodium and of other minerals in the blood. This chemical regulation by the kidneys must be extremely precise, because a tiny variation in the concentration of certain minerals is incompatible with life. Therefore, for example, an increase in potassium levels causes muscle weakness and even paralysis; a decrease results in cardiac arrest.

• Hormonal Function: The kidneys produce several very important hormones for balance in the body, including renin (regulates balance of body fluids and blood pressure) and erythropoietin (stimulates production of red blood cells in bone marrow)

The bladder regulates urine elimination. Along with the kidneys, it makes up part of a precise waste filtration and elimination system that requires care.

Facts and Figures About the Kidneys and Bladder

30 cm (11.8 in)	Length of each ureter, from the kidney to the bladder.
950	Liters of blood that pass through each kidney in 24 hours.
142 g (5 oz)	Weight of each kidney.
1 000 000	Number of blood filtration units in each kidney, which are called nephrons.

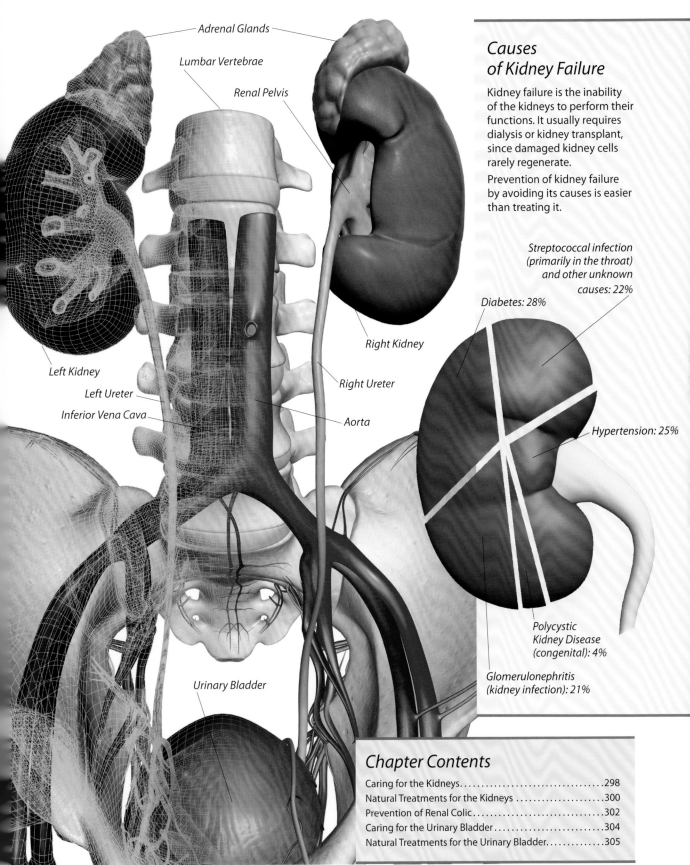

Adrenal Glands

Lumbar Vertebrae

Renal Pelvis

Right Kidney

Left Kidney

Left Ureter

Inferior Vena Cava

Right Ureter

Aorta

Urinary Bladder

Causes of Kidney Failure

Kidney failure is the inability of the kidneys to perform their functions. It usually requires dialysis or kidney transplant, since damaged kidney cells rarely regenerate.

Prevention of kidney failure by avoiding its causes is easier than treating it.

Streptococcal infection (primarily in the throat) and other unknown causes: 22%

Diabetes: 28%

Hypertension: 25%

Polycystic Kidney Disease (congenital): 4%

Glomerulonephritis (kidney infection): 21%

Chapter Contents

Caring for the Kidneys

Drinks, food, glucose levels, blood pressure, and certain infections are the factors that most influence kidney health.

Drink Water

Kidneys need water in order to eliminate waste products. The less water there is in the body, the more chemical work they must perform to concentrate all of the toxins to be eliminated.

Water is needed in the morning before eating and before meals. To prevent having to get up to urinate at night, avoid drinking water three or four hours before going to bed. This recommendation is especially important for older men who may have an enlarged prostate.

If there is already renal failure, the kidneys are unable to concentrate the waste products in the urine. In this case, water intake must be under medical supervision in order to prevent edema in the body.

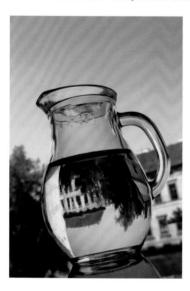

Sweat

Sweating eliminates waste products from the bloodstream, taking some of the work away from the kidneys. Each sweat gland acts like a tiny kidney, eliminating toxins and cleansing the blood. When sweating, the kidneys take a short break from their purification work.

The easiest way to sweat is through physical activity, which provides two benefits at the same time.

Ways to Promote Sweating

Be physically active

Take a sauna or steam bath

Drink a tea made from sudorific herbs

Diaphoretic (Sweat-Inducing) Herbs

- White willow (*Salix alba*): Preparation from its bark.
- Meadowsweet (*Filipendula ulmaria*): Infusion from its leaves and flowers.
- Blackcurrant (*Ribes nigrum*): Juice made from its fruit.
- Elderberry (*Sambucus nigra*): Infusion made from its flowers.
- Linden (*Tilia cordata*): Infusion made from its leaves and flowers.

EAT MORE FRUITS AND VEGETABLES

All juicy fruits and vegetables help the kidneys eliminate water and waste substances, primarily uric acid and urea. On the other hand, meat and meat products overburden the kidneys due to the type of proteins they contain.

When there is renal failure, the kidneys are unable to eliminate all of the potassium provided by fruits and vegetables; because they are very rich in potassium, fruit juice and vegetable broth intake must be restricted.

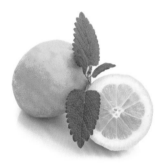

Lemon juice diluted in water alkalinizes urine and promotes elimination of acid residue from metabolism, such as uric acid.
In this way, lemons promote kidney function and prevent the formation of stones in the urine.

DECREASE OR ELIMINATE MEAT INTAKE

A study by Harvard University (United States) shows that a diet high in animal meat protein accelerates the deterioration of kidney function in women with mild kidney failure.[a]

Many people are unaware that they have mild-grade kidney failure and that a meat diet is causing them great harm.

---

a. The impact of protein intake on renal function decline in women with normal renal function or mild renal insufficiency. Knight EL, Stampfer MJ, Hankinson SE, Spiegelman D, Curhan GC. Ann Intern Med. 2003 Mar 18;138(6):460-7. PMID: 12639078

WATCH BLOOD SUGAR AND BLOOD PRESSURE

Diabetes and hypertension are the two main causes of kidney failure. If they are not properly controlled, both disorders tend to progress silently, causing progressive kidney damage.

CAREFUL WITH THROAT AND URINARY INFECTIONS

Tonsil or throat infections caused by streptococcal bacteria can damage kidneys irreversibly if they are not treated properly. Penicillin and other similar antibiotics are very effective in fighting these bacteria that could cause kidney damage, but they must be complemented by a healthy lifestyle (see "Caring for the Throat", Chapter 9).

If they spread up into the kidneys, recurring urinary tract infections can also cause permanent damage.

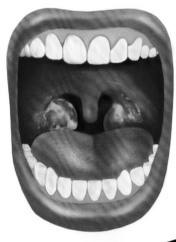

Tonsillitis with patches of pus caused by streptococcus, which is harmful for the kidneys.

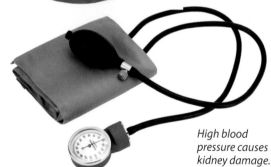

High blood pressure causes kidney damage.

Reasons You Must See a Doctor

- Blood in the urine.
- Frequent urination at night.
- Urine that is always clear and transparent, evening the morning or after sweating.
- Swollen eyelids or ankles.

NATURAL TREATMENTS FOR THE KIDNEYS

Local heat, fruit, and diuretic herbs are very beneficial for the kidneys.

HOT COMPRESS OVER THE KIDNEY AREA

Just like a hot sitz bath, a hot compress over the kidney area relaxes the urinary tract and relieves pain in cases of renal colic or urinary tract infection.

Water Temperature: About 42 ˚C (108 ˚F)
Duration: 10-15 minutes.
Afterward: Dry skin well and put on warm clothing.
Frequency: One to three times per day.

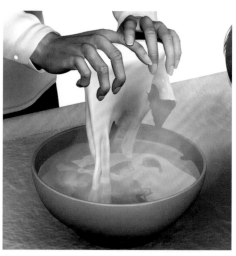

1. Wet a cloth in hot water, then drain.

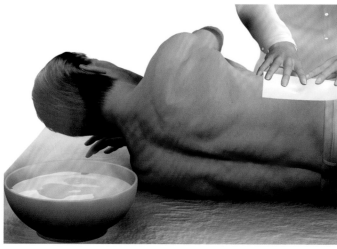

2. Place the cloth over the affected kidney.

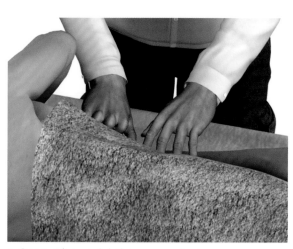

3. Cover with a wool cloth to preserve heat.

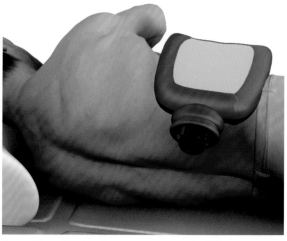

As an alternative to a hot compress over the kidney, a hot water bottle or bag achieves a similar effect.

HOT SITZ BATH

A hot sitz bath has a significant relaxing effect for a spasmodic urinary tract due to renal colic or an infection. Therefore, it is very good for relieving the pain of renal colic and urinary tract infections.

Water Temperature: Hot (36-42 ˚C (97-108 ˚F).

Duration: 10-15 minutes, adding hot water as needed to keep a steady temperature.

Afterward: Dry the skin well and put on warm clothing.

Frequency: One to three times per day, preferably before meals.

CLEANSING BROTH

Cleansing broth is made by cooking mineral-rich vegetables, such as onion and celery. It is usually made with 4 onions and a stalk of celery in a liter of water, boiled for about 10 or 15 minutes. Spinach and even nettle can be added.

The cleansing broth has the following effects:

• Helps eliminate waste products, such as uric acid.

• Promotes urine production in kidneys.

• Provides potassium, magnesium, calcium, iron and other minerals.

Caution: Due to its high potassium content, cleansing broth is not good to use once kidney failure has been diagnosed.

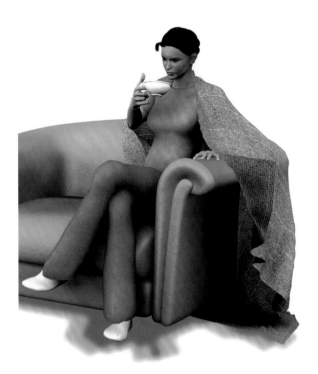

DIURETIC HERBS

Medicinal herbs that have a diuretic effect increase urine volume and promote the elimination function of the kidneys. These are the most effective and well-tolerated:

• **European White Birch** (*Betula alba*): Relieves kidney inflammation and stimulates elimination of water and waste products. It is used as a tea (20 g of leaves and/or buds per liter of water) or a preparation of root bark.

• **Horsetail** (*Equisetum arvense*): In addition to being diuretic, this herb provides silicon, a mineral needed by the tissues of the skin, nails and bones. It is taken as a preparation (about 30 g per liter of water).

• **Corn** (*Zea mays*): The corn stigmas, also called silk, relieve kidney inflammation and promote urine production. These are taken as an infusion (30 g per liter of water).

• **Meadowsweet** (*Filipendula ulmaria*): Depurative and antirheumatic taken as an infusion (about 30 g of flowers and leaves per liter of water).

FRUIT CURE

A fruit cure one to three days in length provides relieve for kidneys that are overburdened by animal proteins and salt.

The fruit cure is done by having only the selected fruit as food throughout the entire day, in whatever quantity is desired.

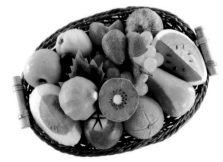

The most recommended fruits for the kidneys, due to their diuretic (urine volume increasing) and cleansing (waste product elimination promoting) effects are: Melons, watermelon, pears, grapes and cherries.

PREVENTION OF RENAL COLIC

One out of every ten adults will have a urinary stone at some time in life. Stones grow for months or years before causing any symptoms.

DRINK ENOUGH WATER

Drinking water decreases the concentration of the substances that form stones in urine. This decreases the risk of these substances causing a stone to form.

How much is enough? Water needs vary depending on the time of year and level of physical activity. But in general, in order to prevent kidney stones, enough water must be taken in so that urine is always clear. This usually means 1.5 or 2 liters per day.

The ideal types are distilled water, which contains absolutely no mineral salts (or any other toxins usually present in drinking water) or low-mineral water.

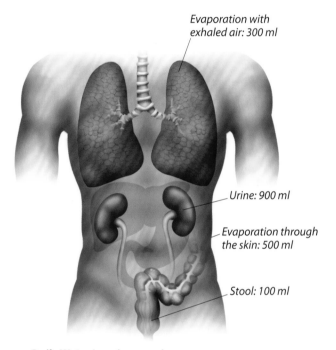

Evaporation with exhaled air: 300 ml

Urine: 900 ml

Evaporation through the skin: 500 ml

Stool: 100 ml

Daily Water Loss (average)
Every day, about 1 800 ml of water is lost. A typical diet provides about 400 ml, due to which at least another 1 400 ml should be taken in (about one and a half liters, or about 8 glasses)

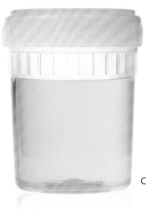

Water intake must be enough for the urine to be clear in color. The recommended amount is 1.5 to 2 liters per day.

Clear Urine

GET PHYSICAL ACTIVITY

With exercise, calcium is deposited in bones, where it is needed for strength. On the other hand, in sedentary people, blood and urine calcium levels increase, promoting stone formation.

REDUCE MILK AND CHEESE INTAKE

Cow's milk contains a high amount of calcium, which is needed for a calf's speedy development. Human babies do not need as much calcium as calves (which is the reason breast milk contains one third of the calcium that cow's milk contains). By consuming large amounts of milk and cheese, adults could be taking in too much calcium. Excessive calcium is eliminated with the urine, and is prime material for development of urinary stones.

DECREASE OR ELIMINATE MEAT

An excess of proteins in the diet, such as with a meat diet, increases the elimination of calcium with urine, predisposing a person to stone formation (and osteoporosis). Meat consumption also increases elimination of uric acid and phosphorus with urine, components that along with calcium make up the majority of urinary stones.

FOLLOW AN ANTI-STONE DIET

Those who have a tendency to develop urinary stones, especially those made up of calcium oxalate (the most common), can reduce the risk of developing new stones by nearly one-half by following a special diet, according to a study by the University of Bonn (Germany).[a] This diet consists of:

Increasing:
- Water (about 2.5 liters per day).
- Vegetable fiber, present in fruit, vegetables, whole grains, legumes.
- Potassium: High levels in fruit juices, tomatoes and vegetables in general.
- Vitamin B_6: Good sources are wheat germ, sesame seeds, bananas, avocado and legumes. Can also be taken in supplements.

Decreasing:
- Alcoholic beverages: Alcohol promotes the formation of urinary stones.
- Proteins in general, especially those of animal origin.
- Salt.
- Cholesterol.
- Vitamin C supplements: No more than 1 000 mg per day is recommended, since ascorbic acid is converted to oxalate, one of the components of stones. This limit only affects the vitamin C in supplements, not that which occurs naturally in fruit.

a. The efficacy of dietary intervention on urinary risk factors for stone formation in recurrent calcium oxalate stone patients. Siener R, Schade N, Nicolay C, von Unruh GE, Hesse A. J Urol. 2005 May;173(5):1601-5. PMID: 15821507

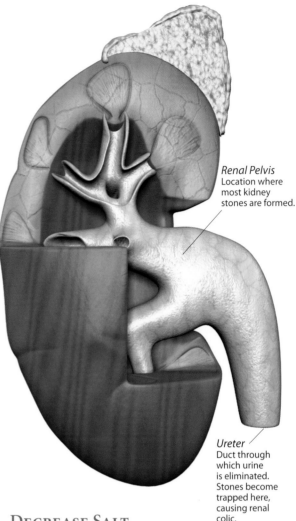

Renal Pelvis
Location where most kidney stones are formed.

Ureter
Duct through which urine is eliminated. Stones become trapped here, causing renal colic.

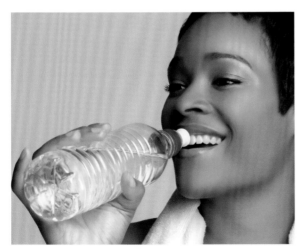

TAKE MAGNESIUM AND VITAMIN B_6

Magnesium and vitamin B_6 hinder the formation of stones in urine. Vitamin B_6 reduces elimination of oxalates, which are salts that make up stones.

DECREASE SALT AND CONDIMENTS

An excess of salt causes calcium loss with urine, which promotes stone formation. Many condiments, sauces, appetizers, sausages and luncheon meats contain high levels of salt.

Daily salt intake should not exceed 6 grams, equivalent to 2 400 mg of sodium.

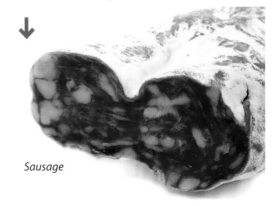

Sausage

CARING FOR THE URINARY BLADDER

*Cystitis and urinary incontinence
are the most common bladder disorders.*

PREVENTING CYSTITIS (BLADDER INFECTION)

The spread of bacteria through the urethra up into the urinary bladder is the most common cause of cystitis (bladder inflammation, presenting as burning with urination). Women are more susceptible to this type of infection due to the anatomical characteristics of the female urethra, which is shorter than that of a man.

These simple recommendations for women can prevent development of cystitis:

- Always cleanse genitals from front to back to avoid spreading bacteria from the anus to the urinary opening.
- Use pads if needed, rather than tampons, as these compress and irritate the urethra and promote genital and urinary infections.
- Wear cotton undergarments.
- Do not hold urine when feeling the urge to urinate.
- Avoid the use of force during sexual penetration, trying instead to keep movements gentle. If necessary, use a vaginal lubricant.
- Cleanse external genitalia before and after penetration, both in women and men. Simple cleansing with water is enough.
- Drink plenty of water during the day to avoid concentrated urine.
- Eat plenty of oranges, lemons and kiwis, as vitamin C protects against infection.
- Avoid antacids, as they can change urine pH and promote cystitis.
- If there are signs of infection, use the "Natural Treatments for the Urinary Bladder".
- In case of recurrent cystitis after sexual intercourse:
  - Use a male condom for penetration. When it is first removed from its packaging, it is sterile, which reduces the risk of infection in a woman.
  - Try to urinate after sexual intercourse with the goal of flushing out bacteria that might have ascended through the urethra.
  - In some cases, a single dose of nitrofurantoin or other urinary anti-infective medication can yield good results.

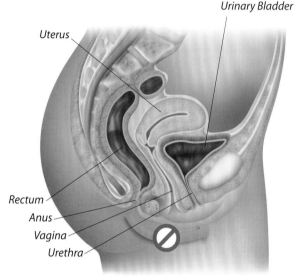

Cleansing from back to front brings germs from the anus that can spread to and travel up the urethra, causing cystitis.

STOP ADULT URINARY INCONTINENCE

Urinary incontinence is a lack of bladder control resulting in the involuntary loss of urine. The muscle weakness that comes later in life promotes incontinence. Although it is more common in women, it can also occur in men.

The following recommendations can stop the tendency to suffer urinary incontinence before it reaches the point of requiring protective padding, medication or surgery.

- Do pelvic floor muscle exercises (Kegel exercises): These muscles are exercised when trying to stop urine flow midstream. Contracting these muscles voluntarily for a few seconds several times per day (always with an empty bladder) improves urinary control.
- Bladder training: Schedule a specific time to urinate, such as every two or three hours.
- Walk half an hour to an hour per day.
- Avoid constipation.

NATURAL TREATMENTS FOR THE URINARY BLADDER

Cranberries and hydrotherapy are the most effective natural treatments for the bladder.

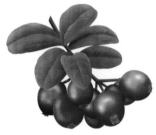

Cranberries

CRANBERRIES

Cranberries (*Vaccinium macrocarpon*) have been shown to be very effective for treatment and prevention of urinary tract infections. Bacteria that cause these infections, primarily the bacteria called *Escherichia coli*, have the ability to develop resistance quickly to traditional antibiotics. Cranberries, however, work differently than antibiotics by decreasing bacterial adhesion to urinary bladder walls, and do not produce resistance.

- **Recommended Daily Dose**: 1-2 glasses (200-400 ml) of diluted juice, or 3-6 tablespoons (45-90 ml) of concentrated juice.

- **Use During Pregnancy**: A study done with 400 pregnant women at the University of Toronto (Canada) has shown that drinking cranberry juice during pregnancy is safe, and a good alternative to the use of antibiotics.[a]

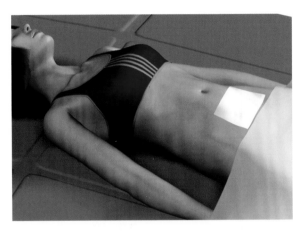

COMPRESS OVER THE PELVIC AREA

In cases of acute cystitis, a hot compress over the pelvic area relieves burning and discomfort with urination.

It is usually applied hot, but in cases of interstitial cystitis (a special type of chronic bladder inflammation) applying it cold has better results.

Water Temperature: About 42 °C (108 °F). Once it cools, soak it again in hot water.

Duration: 10-15 minutes.

Afterward: Dry skin well and put on warm clothing.

Frequency: One to three times per day.

STEAM BATH FOR THE BLADDER

A steam bath over the perineum and pelvic area reduces inflammation in the genital and urinary organs, and relives the burning of cystitis.

The simplest way to do the steam bath consists of filling a bidet with extremely hot water, sitting over it without allowing the water to touch the skin, and covering legs with a towel.

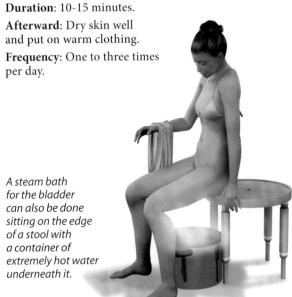

A steam bath for the bladder can also be done sitting on the edge of a stool with a container of extremely hot water underneath it.

a. Safety and efficacy of cranberry (vaccinium macrocarpon) during pregnancy and lactation. Dugoua JJ, Seely D, Perri D, Mills E, Koren G. Can J Clin Pharmacol. 2008 Winter;15(1):e80-6. Epub 2008 Jan 18. Review. PMID: 18204103

Male Genitalia

Reproductive cell factory and conduit for urine elimination.

The male genital organs are designed to produce reproductive cells and deposit them as close as possible to the female ovum. In addition, they are designed for the passage of urine.

The prostate is the gland in charge of producing seminal fluid in which sperm swim and where they obtain their energy and nutrients for their long journey through the uterus and Fallopian tubes.

Seminal fluid produced by the prostate contains mainly proteins, fatty acids and minerals. Its pH is alkaline, for partial neutralization of the acidic vaginal environment. Sperm could not survive in the acidic vagina without the seminal fluid produced by the prostate.

In addition to a healthy diet and lifestyle, local hygiene is essential to caring for the male genitalia. It cannot be overlooked that in the male genitalia is the location of the most common type of cancer in men –prostate cancer– which is related to meat and milk intake.

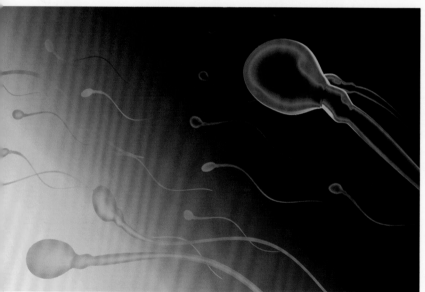

Sperm swimming in semen, trying to reach their target: The female ovum.

Facts and Figures About the Male Genitalia

35 ˚C (95 ˚F)	Temperature required for the testicles to produce sperm.
25 to 35	Age of highest production of the hormone testosterone in the testicle.
18 cm (7 in)	Distance a sperm cell can travel in an hour.
50 000 000	Number of sperm produced by a young man every day.

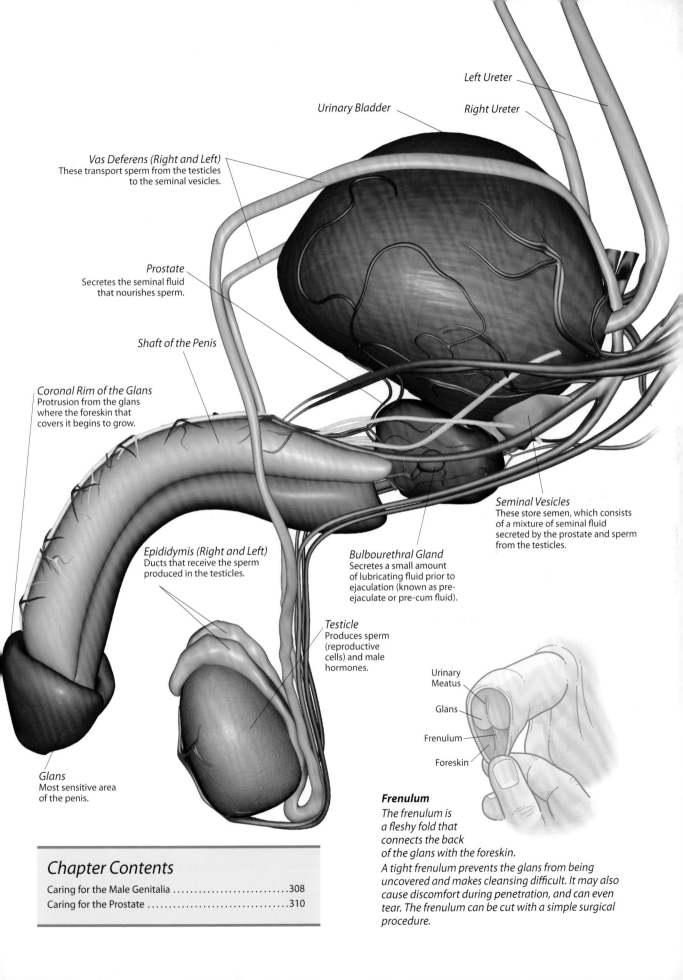

Left Ureter

Right Ureter

Urinary Bladder

Vas Deferens (Right and Left)
These transport sperm from the testicles
to the seminal vesicles.

Prostate
Secretes the seminal fluid
that nourishes sperm.

Shaft of the Penis

Coronal Rim of the Glans
Protrusion from the glans
where the foreskin that
covers it begins to grow.

Epididymis (Right and Left)
Ducts that receive the sperm
produced in the testicles.

Bulbourethral Gland
Secretes a small amount
of lubricating fluid prior to
ejaculation (known as pre-
ejaculate or pre-cum fluid).

Seminal Vesicles
These store semen, which consists
of a mixture of seminal fluid
secreted by the prostate and sperm
from the testicles.

Testicle
Produces sperm
(reproductive
cells) and male
hormones.

Glans
Most sensitive area
of the penis.

Urinary
Meatus

Glans

Frenulum

Foreskin

Frenulum
*The frenulum is
a fleshy fold that
connects the back
of the glans with the foreskin.
A tight frenulum prevents the glans from being
uncovered and makes cleansing difficult. It may also
cause discomfort during penetration, and can even
tear. The frenulum can be cut with a simple surgical
procedure.*

Chapter Contents

CARING FOR THE MALE GENITALIA

Daily cleansing of the penis is part of bodily hygiene habits.

PENILE HYGIENE

Sloughed-off cells and leftover urine accumulate in the space between the foreskin and the glans, forming a whitish substance called smegma. This occurs primarily in uncircumcised males.

Poor hygiene and the resulting accumulation of smegma under the foreskin in uncircumcised males promote infection of the glans by bacteria and fungi, known as balanitis. These infections are accompanied by bad odor, itching, pain and irritation of the penis.

The glans must be washed daily, especially if covered by foreskin –such as in uncircumcised males. In this case, the foreskin must be pulled back as far as possible without forcing it. Plain water is usually enough to eliminate smegma and prevent infection.

Signs of Poor Hygiene

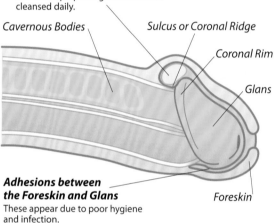

Smegma
Whitish substance that accumulates in the balanopreputial groove. Must be cleansed daily.

Cavernous Bodies

Sulcus or Coronal Ridge

Coronal Rim

Glans

Foreskin

Adhesions between the Foreskin and Glans
These appear due to poor hygiene and infection.

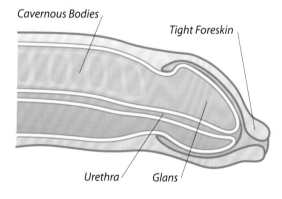

Cavernous Bodies

Tight Foreskin

Urethra   Glans

Phimosis

Tightness of the foreskin that prevents the glans from being uncovered.

In babies, a certain extent of phimosis is normal, and is usually corrected in the first few years. At 3 years of age, the foreskin can be retracted in 90% of boys.

Application of corticosteroid cream to the foreskin over several weeks may resolve phimosis without circumcision.

Caution: Do not force retraction of a baby's foreskin by pulling the skin back. This can cause tears and scarring that tighten the foreskin even further.

Reasons You Must See a Doctor

• Inability to retract foreskin to completely uncover the glans in an older child or adult.
• Discovery of a lump or hardness with palpation of the testicles, even if it is not painful.
• Paraphimosis.
• Blood in the semen.

Paraphimosis
Paraphimosis is an accident that happens to uncircumcised males when, after retracting the foreskin, it is unable to be returned to its original position. This is usually due to a tough or fibrous foreskin.

Paraphimosis requires urgent medical care, as it can cause serious penile complications due to lack of circulation to the foreskin and glans.

CIRCUMCISION

Male circumcision is one of the oldest-known surgical procedures. There is a great deal of controversy in the medical community regarding the need to routinely circumcise all boys. In addition to the religious implications of circumcision, there are medical arguments that are for and against it:

Advantages of Circumcision

- Better cleansing of the glans and the coronal ridge.
- **Prevents phimosis**, that is, the tightening of the foreskin, which causes predisposition to infections and discomfort with penetration.
- **Prevents Infection** of the glans (called balanitis) and reduces the risk of penile cancer in men and cervical cancer in his sexual partner.
- **Reduces the Risk of HIV Infection** (AIDS Virus). According to the World Health Organization (WHO), male circumcision reduces the chance that a male become infected with HIV during heterosexual sex by 60%.[a,b] However, it is worth mentioning that circumcision does not protect the woman against HIV, and only protects the man partially. It therefore cannot be considered a prevention method in itself.

a. http://www.who.int/hiv/topics/malecircumcision/en/index.html
b. http://data.unaids.org/pub/PressRelease/2007/070328_mc_recommendations_sp_es.pdf

Disadvantages of Circumcision

- **Unprotected Glans**: The glans is one of the most sensitive areas of the body. Those who defend the practice of circumcision only when needed argue that the glans needs the protection of the foreskin: "The foreskin is to the glans as the eyelid is to the eye".
- **Decreased Sensitivity**: Permanently exposing the delicate skin around the glans reduces sensitivity. However, it must be noted that this decrease does not affect sexual pleasure, which is produced in the brain by a combination of sensations, and not just by stimulation of the glans.
- **Surgical Complications**: Although rare, there can be complications after a circumcision, including bleeding, infection, hematoma and suture rejection.

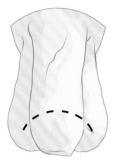

Uncircumcised Penis

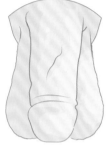

Circumcised Penis

The decision to perform a circumcision on a baby boy should be under medical advice. According to some groups, there are ethical considerations surrounding the rights of parents to opt for circumcision because of ritualistic reasons. In any case, if a circumcision is performed, the earlier it is done, the less discomfort for the boy.

DO NOT WEAR TIGHT PANTS

The fashion of tight pants forces the testicles to remain up against to the body, warming them up to the body's own temperature of 36.5 °C (97.7 °F). This decreases sperm production, because at 35 °C (95 °F) or greater, this physiological process is stopped (which is the reason the testicles are located outside the abdomen).

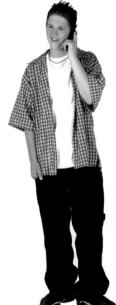

Wearing loose-fitting pants promotes male fertility.

TESTICULAR SELF-EXAMINATION

Just as women should periodically examine their breasts, men should also examine their testicles for abnormalities from time to time.

In its early stages, testicular cancer is not painful and does not cause any symptoms; therefore, the only way to detect it early is to palpate the testicles in search of any lumps.

A shower is recommended beforehand so that scrotal skin is soft and clean.

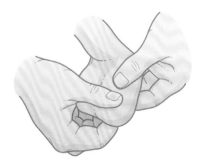

Gently palpate each testicle between the thumb and forefinger, looking for any lump or abnormality.

CARING FOR THE PROSTATE

*The main goals are prevention of prostate cancer and keeping the size
from enlarging enough to make urination difficult.*

ADVICE FOR EASIER URINATION

The most uncomfortable symptoms of age-related benign prostate hypertrophy are those related to urination: Difficulty urinating (dysuria) and frequency of urination (pollakiuria). The following advice helps urination and relieves the symptoms of a hypertrophied prostate.

- Maintain regular and safe sexual activity; ejaculation helps reduce prostate inflammation.
- Decrease or eliminate intake of caffeine, which is present in drinks such as coffee, tea, *yerba mate*, and certain soft drinks. Caffeine narrows the neck of the bladder, making it difficult for urine to pass through it.
- Decrease or eliminate alcoholic beverages, which have a similar effect to that of caffeine.
- Avoid hot spices, as they irritate the urinary tract and make urination difficult.
- Avoid nasal decongestants and antihistamines, which relax bladder muscles and make urination difficult.
- Avoid cold temperatures, as they promote urinary retention.
- Avoid straddling, such as with horseback and bicycle riding; it causes congestion of the prostate.
- Avoid constipation.
- Avoid stress, as it affects the urinary reflex.
- Take medicinal herb preparations for the prostate such as *Sabal serrulata* (Saw palmetto) and *Pygeum africanum*.

PROSTATE CANCER PREVENTION

Prostate cancer is the most common malignant tumor in non-smoking men. The many epidemiological studies performed suggest that prostate cancer can be prevented by the following four factors.[a]

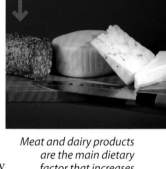

Meat and dairy products are the main dietary factor that increases the risk of metastatic prostate cancer.

- **Diet**: This is the most influential factor, both in prevention and advancement.
  – Risk Increasers[b]: Red meat and processed meat (such as bacon), milk, cheese, and dairy products in general.
  – Risk Reducers[c]: Tomato sauce, tomatoes, and watermelon, due to their high lycopene content; broccoli, cabbage, radishes, and other crucifer family plants; omega-3 fatty acids; vitamins D and E; and selenium.
- **Pesticides**: Occupational exposure to pesticides, such as in farmworkers, increases the risk of prostate cancer.
- **Vasectomy**: After much scientific controversy, a recent study by the "Fred Hutchinson Cancer Research Center" in Seattle (Washington, United States) has not found any link between vasectomy and the risk of prostate cancer.[d]

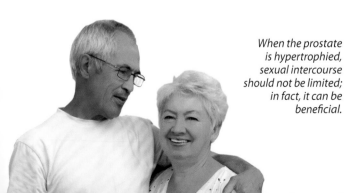

When the prostate is hypertrophied, sexual intercourse should not be limited; in fact, it can be beneficial.

a. Prostate cancer prevention: past, present, and future. Fleshner N, Zlotta AR. Cancer. 2007 Nov 1;110(9):1889-99. Review. PMID: 17893870
b. A prospective study on intake of animal products and risk of prostate cancer. Michaud DS, Augustsson K, Rimm EB, Stampfer MJ, Willet WC, Giovannucci E. Cancer Causes Control. 2001 Aug;12(6):557-67. PMID: 11519764
c. Role of diet in prostate cancer development and progression. Chan JM, Gann PH, Giovannucci EL. J Clin Oncol. 2005 Nov 10;23(32):8152-60. Review. PMID: 16278466
d. Vasectomy and the risk of prostate cancer. Holt SK, Salinas CA, Stanford JL. J Urol. 2008 Dec;180(6):2565-7; discussion 2567-8. Epub 2008 Oct 19. PMID: 18930503

Prostate Foods

- **Tomato**: Its natural red colorant, lycopene, is a powerful antioxidant that protects against prostate cancer.
- **Nuts**: These provide polyunsaturated fatty acids, vitamin E and zinc, which are all beneficial nutrients for the prostate.
- **Squash Seeds**: These reduce inflammation of the prostate and make urination easier.
- **Soy**: Thanks to the mild estrogenic action of the isoflavones that it contains, soy stops excessive enlargement of the prostate and protects against degeneration into cancer. Soybeans, soymilk or soy drinks, and tofu are the best natural sources of isoflavones.

Hot Stream of Water over the Pelvic Area

The hot stream of water from the shower over the pelvic area often helps to start urine flow and empty the bladder when urination is difficult.

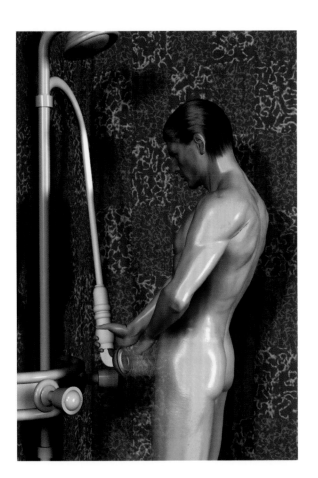

Vital Bath

The vital bath is a variant of the pelvic sitz bath. It reduces prostate inflammation and improves urination. See more details on use in "Natural Treatments for the Liver", in Chapter 17.

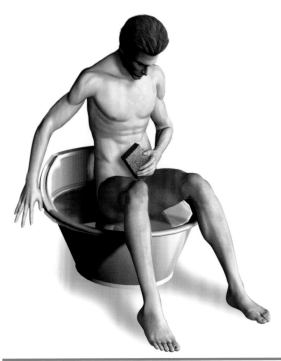

Tomato + Soy

A study by the "Wayne State University" in Detroit (Michigan, United States) showed that when taken together, the lycopene in tomatoes and the isoflavones in soy increase their preventive action against prostate cancer.[a]

According to this same study, in prostate cancer patients, taking 15 mg of lycopene with 40 mg of isoflavone extracts twice a day over 6 months reduces the level of PSA (a prostate cancer marker) and slows tumor progression.

- For 15 mg of natural lycopene, eat 600 g of tomatoes (about two large tomatoes).
- There are 40 mg of natural isoflavones in 150 g of tofu or 1.5 liters of soy drink.

a. Lycopene and soy isoflavones in the treatment of prostate cancer. Vaishampayan U, Hussain M, Banerjee M, Seren S, Sarkar FH, Fontana J, Forman JD, Cher ML, Powell I, Pontes JE, Kucuk O. Nutr Cancer. 2007;59(1):1-7. PMID: 17927495

Female Genitalia

The anatomical site for the miracle of life.

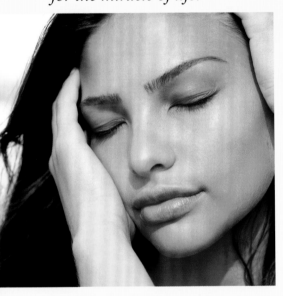

Caring for the female genitalia requires much more than local hygiene.
A healthy diet and lifestyle contribute significantly to the good function of these delicate organs.

The female genital organs are varied and complex, requiring a great deal of special care. The vulva and vagina are continually subjected to the threat of infection. Because their humidity and temperature levels are an ideal location for the development of many germs, the vulva and especially the vagina always need systems ready to protect against infection.

The most significant and effective system for preventing vaginal infections is keeping an acidic environment that inhibits bacterial development. This vaginal acidity is achieved thanks to the lactic acid produced by Doderlein's bacilli (*Lactobacillus acidophilus*), rod shaped bacteria normally found in the vagina. Any foreign product, such as soaps or contraceptive foams, or any local irritation, makes the vagina lose its acidity and promotes infection by bacteria such as *Gardnerella vaginalis*, or by fungi such as the *Candida* family, which manifests as abnormal vaginal discharge.

The most complex and amazing function in the known universe takes place inside the uterus: Gestation of a human being that begins with two microscopic reproductive cells. Human life begins in the female uterus, but for some women who do not undergo gynecological exams, it can also end there, as cervical cancer is one of the most common cancers next to breast cancer.

Facts and Figures About the Female Genitalia

4.5	Normal pH of the vagina (acidic).
5 ml (1 teaspoon)	Space inside a non-pregnant uterus, equivalent to a spoonful of coffee.
10 l (21 US pt)	Space inside a full-term pregnant uterus, two thousand times greater than a non-pregnant uterus.
400	Average number of menstrual cycles a woman has throughout her lifetime.
200 000	Number of ova present in each ovary at birth, of which about 200 become mature over a lifetime.

Fallopian Tubes

They carry the ovum from the ovary to the uterus. Fusion between sperm and ovum occurs in its distal third.

The tubes are often the location of infections, generally due to germs that come up from the vagina.

Ovaries

The ovaries take turns releasing an ovum, or reproductive cell, each menstrual cycle. During a woman's fertile life, the ovaries produce female hormones (estrogen and progesterone).

Uterus

Hollow muscular organ that is able to hold a developing fetus.

Vagina

The vagina normally cleans itself, making it unnecessary to clean inside it. The vaginal walls produce a fluid that transports dead cells and germs to the outside.

Urinary Bladder

Rectum

Uterus

Cervix

Urinary Bladder

Pubic Bone

Urethra

Vagina

Vulva

Chapter Contents

CARING FOR THE FEMALE GENITALIA

Hygiene, periodic gynecological exams, and responsible sexual behavior are the best ways to care for the female genitalia.

GENITAL HYGIENE

- **Cleansing**: Clean the genitals once per day with running water, moving fingers through the folds between the labia majora and labia minora. Avoid over-cleaning as it removes beneficial bacteria and protective substances from skin. In general, the genitals should be cleaned no more than once per day.
  - Clean the genital area from front to back to avoid spreading bacteria such as *Escherichia coli* and *Candida* fungi from the anal area to the vagina and urinary opening.
  - Avoid frequent douching, as it eliminates the normal protective vaginal flora.
  - During menstruation, clean external genitalia with water once or twice per day. Feminine cleansing cloths may also be used. If using tampons, change them at least three times per day.

- **Soap**: If using soap, it should be very mild and have a neutral or slightly acid pH (around 6.3). Unless it is needed, use soap only every two or three days rather than daily.

- **Other Intimate Products**: Avoid anything that alkalinizes vaginal pH, such as regular soaps and shampoos, certain intimate soaps and deodorants, diaphragms with spermicide, and contraceptive foams. The vagina needs to keep a slightly acid pH in order to prevent fungal and bacterial infections.

- **Careful with Tampons**: Regular use of tampons is not recommended, as it dries out the vaginal mucosa.
  - Tampons must be changed every six to eight hours.
  - Do not leave tampons in place overnight.
  - High-absorbency tampons promote the spread of streptococcus, staphylococcus, and other bacteria which can result in toxic shock.

- **Undergarments**: Prefer cotton garments, as they absorb moisture and keep the skin dry better than synthetic fabrics.
  - Avoid clothing that is too tight, as it blocks needed air circulation in the genital area.
  - Do not leave on a wet bathing suit.
  - Panty liners: Use only on the last days of the period, not daily, as they block natural perspiration. Watch out for those that have perfume and deodorants that irritate and change the vagina's natural acidity.

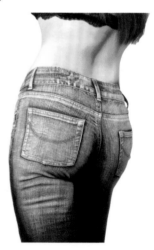

Moisture and lack of air circulation are the primary enemies of genital hygiene.

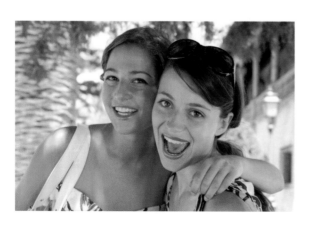

AVOID SEXUAL PROMISCUITY

It has been shown that the greater the number of sexual partners over a lifetime, especially before age 21, the higher the risk of cervical cancer.

The immaturity of the vaginal mucosa and the cervix in adolescents explains the greater risk of infection with the human papillomavirus (HPV) after having sexual intercourse.

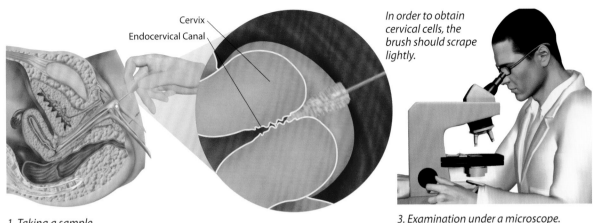

Cervix

Endocervical Canal

In order to obtain cervical cells, the brush should scrape lightly.

1. Taking a sample.

3. Examination under a microscope.

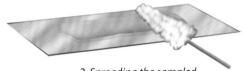

2. Spreading the sampled substance on a slide.

AVOID INTERCOURSE AT AN EARLY AGE

Starting to have sexual intercourse early not only promotes vaginal infection with the herpes virus, the human papillomavirus, and various bacteria, but it also increases the risk of invasive cervical cancer.

A study by the Institut Català d'Oncologia (Barcelona, Spain)[a] showed that women who had sexual intercourse for the first time between the ages of 17-21 have a 1.8 times greater risk of invasive cervical cancer as compared to those who began having intercourse after age 21. For those who started their sexual life at the age of 16 or earlier, the risk is 2.31 times greater. Another study by the University of Washington[b] has found similar results in women who began having sexual intercourse before the age of 21.

HAVE PAP EXAMS

- **What are they?** They consist of obtaining cervical cells by scraping them off and then examining them under the microscope. No anesthesia is required.

- **Why are they done?** They are done because they are the most effective test for prevention and early detection of cervical cancer, one of the most common types of cancer in women.

- **Who should have them done?** All women starting at the age of 21 or one year after having sexual intercourse for the first time.

- **How long must they be done?** Up until 70 years of age. They are no longer needed after a hysterectomy (surgical removal of the uterus).

- **How often must they be done?** Every two or three years, or every year if prior results were abnormal.

- **What if the results are positive?** A positive Pap exam can be due to inflammation of the cervix, or its infection with human papillomavirus (HPV), and does not necessarily imply that there is already some precancerous lesion. Colposcopy (cervical exam with a microscope) and biopsy help confirm the diagnosis.

a. Early age at first sexual intercourse and early pregnancy are risk factors for cervical cancer in developing countries. Louie KS, de Sanjose S, Diaz M, Castellsagué X, Herrero R, Meijer CJ, Shah K, Franceschi S, Muñoz N, Bosch FX; International Agency for Research on Cancer Multicenter Cervical Cancer Study Group. Br J Cancer. 2009 Apr 7;100(7):1191-7. Epub 2009 Mar 10. PMID: 19277042

b. Age of diagnosis of squamous cell cervical carcinoma and early sexual experience. Edelstein ZR, Madeleine MM, Hughes JP, Johnson LG, Schwartz SM, Galloway DA, Carter JJ, Koutsky LA. Cancer Epidemiol Biomarkers Prev. 2009 Apr;18(4):1070-6. Epub 2009 Mar 24. PMID: 19318437

Reasons You Must See a Doctor

- Abnormal vaginal bleeding at any age.
- Persistent pelvic pain.
- Abnormal vaginal discharge.

Natural Treatments for the Female Genitalia

Food, plants, baths, and massages contribute to feminine wellbeing.

Foods that Promote Hormonal Balance

- Squash seeds, sesame seeds, sunflower seeds, or flaxseed.
- Walnuts and almonds.
- Legumes, including soy.
- Soy drinks and tofu (soy "cheese").
- Raw or cooked carrots or carrot juice.

Hormone-Regulating Plants

- **Soy** (*Glycine max*): Isoflavones extracted from soybeans imitate some of the beneficial effects of the estrogen produced by the ovaries as well as partially compensate for the lack of it during menopause. The daily dose of isoflavones is 60-80 mg per day.

- **Red Clover** (*Trifolium pratense*): Contains isoflavones that increase the effect of soy isoflavones. Can also be taken as extracts.

- **Black Cohosh** (*Cimicifuga racemosa*): A bush native to the eastern North America. It fights the effects of decreased estrogen during menopause, such as hot flashes, melancholy, and anxiety. It is taken as 1-2 g of root powder or rhizome per day, or 20-40 mg of extract, 2 times per day. After 6 months of treatment, it should be stopped for a while.

- **Sage** (*Salvia officinalis*): Has a mild estrogenic action, thanks to which the hormonal system is balanced. Leaves are taken as an infusion.

Red Clover

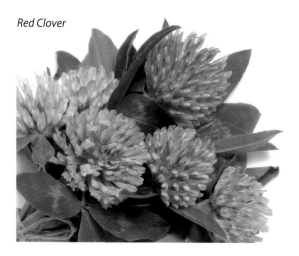

Sitz Bath

A sitz bath with warm or room temperature water is very useful for feminine hygiene, especially with a genital infection. In order to achieve an antiseptic and protective effect, one of the following products may be added to bathwater:

- Lemon Juice: 2-3 lemons per liter of water.
- Vinegar: 3-4 tablespoons (45-60 ml) per liter of water.
- Tea Tree Oil (*Melaleuca alternifolia*): 10 drops per liter of water.
- Pau d'Arco Preparation (*Tabebuia impetiginosa*): 60 g of bark for every liter of water, cooked for 5 minutes.

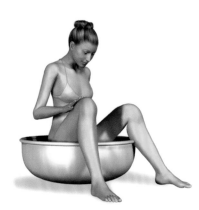

Essence Massage

Place 3-5 drops of essence of lemon balm or sage onto the pelvic area, without touching the genitals, and massage gently. Has a relaxing and sedative effect that is especially useful for painful menstrual periods.

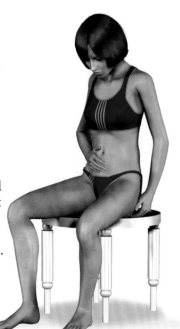

PROS AND CONS OF HPV VACCINATION

A PERSONAL DECISION

Infection with the human papillomavirus (HPV) is one of the most common sexually transmitted diseases and can cause cervical cancer.

REASONS TO VACCINATE

- The human papillomavirus (HPV) is very widespread and is passed between people through sexual contact. If an adolescent is considering the possibility of beginning a sexual life early, having intercourse without a condom, or changing sex partners often, she should be vaccinated.
- Adolescents and young women have a greater chance of becoming infected after unprotected intercourse than adult women. The risk increases greatly with smoking.
- There is no treatment for the infection by this virus. Once it has spread, the virus remains for many years until the immune system eliminates it.

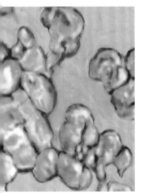

Genital wart caused by a type of HPV.

REASONS NOT TO VACCINATE

- Pap exams are very good at early detection of cervical cancer. If a woman undergoes this exam every two or three years, it is highly improbable that she will have cervical cancer throughout her life. In the case of a positive result due to dysplasia or some other precancerous cervical lesion, this exam detects it in time to treat the lesion. It has been estimated that it takes 10 years for a precancerous lesion to become cervical cancer.
- The likelihood of contracting an HPV infection is proportional to the number of sexual partners throughout life. In addition, it increases greatly when intercourse begins at a young age.
- The HPV vaccine only protects against certain types of the virus: More than 40 types of HPV virus are known, but the vaccine only protects against the 4 major types:
  - HPV type 16 and type 18, which cause 70% of cervical cancers.
  - Against two types of HPV which cause 90% of cases of genital warts.
- The HPV vaccine can create a sense of false security against high-risk sexual activities. It should be made clear that the vaccine does not protect against the genital herpes virus, AIDS-causing HIV, syphilis, gonorrhea, or other venereal diseases.
- The HPV vaccine is only effective in women who have never been exposed to HPV. This is the reason that it should be placed at 11 or 12 years of age. If an adolescent has already had sexual intercourse and has been exposed to some form of HPV, the vaccine does not protect them against this type of virus.
- Pregnancy or allergy to any component of the vaccine.
- For some families, the high cost of the vaccine.

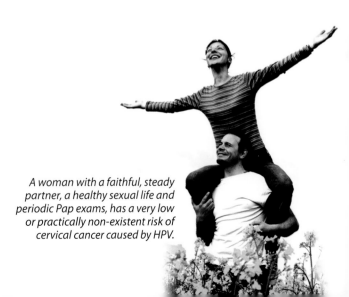

A woman with a faithful, steady partner, a healthy sexual life and periodic Pap exams, has a very low or practically non-existent risk of cervical cancer caused by HPV.

MENSTRUAL PAIN RELIEF

*In addition to the natural treatments in the previous unit,
these recommendations provide relieve for dysmenorrhea.*

RULE OUT ORGANIC CAUSES

Every woman who has dysmenorrhea should undergo a gynecological exam to rule out organic causes for her menstrual pain, including endometriosis, pelvic inflammatory disease (inflammation of the Fallopian tubes or adnexitis) or retroverted uterus (tipped uterus).

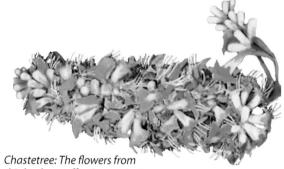

Chastetree: The flowers from this bush are effective against menstrual pain.

DIET

- Avoid refined sugars.
- Increase intake of seeds (squash, sunflower, sesame and flaxseed) and nuts –mainly walnuts, for their high essential fatty acid and vitamin E content.
- Take 400 IU per day of vitamin E supplements.
- Completely eliminate tobacco and caffeine, as they stimulate uterine contractions.

HEAT OVER THE PELVIC AREA

Any form of heat over the pelvic area, such as a hot water bottle or clay poultice, has a relaxing effect for uterine muscle spasms that cause menstrual pain.

Clay Poultice
Dissolve clay in extremely hot water until it forms a thick paste, and apply it onto the skin in a 1-2 cm layer. Cover with a wool blanket.
After half an hour, remove the poultice and cleanse completely with water, then apply a moisturizer.

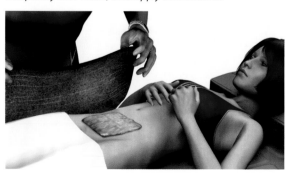

PLANTS

- **Chastetree** (*Vitex agnus-castus*): A Mediterranean bush that is found all over the world. It regulates female hormones, balancing the production of estrogen and progesterone in the ovaries. It is recommended by the German Commission E for treatment of dysmenorrhea. Due to its antispasmodic action, it is also good for fighting the migraine headaches associated with menstruation. It also prevents fluid retention and breast swelling the few days before the period and has a positive effect on mood.
  – How to Use: Take one 30-40 mg capsule of berry extract with water after breakfast each morning for 2-6 months.

- **Sage** (*Salvia officinalis*): Due to its mild estrogenic action, it balances the hormonal system and regulates menstruation. Take 3 or 4 cups of leaf infusion per day.

- **Common Yarrow or Milfoil** (*Achilea millefolium*): Has an antispasmodic action similar to chamomile, and relaxes the uterine muscles.

- **Lemon Balm** (*Melissa officinalis*): Sedating and antispasmodic. Take 3 or 4 cups of leaf infusion per day.

- **Evening Primrose Oil** (*Oenothera biennis*): Rich in essential fatty acids that promote the production of uterus-relaxing prostaglandins. Take 2-3 g per day.

PREVENTION OF YEAST INFECTIONS

A complete healing of vaginal candidiasis (yeast infections), the most common genital infection, requires much more than an antifungal medication.

Yeast infections caused by the *Candida* fungus family often improve with treatment, but soon return. In order to prevent them, these recommendations should be followed.

PREVENT OR CONTROL RISK FACTORS

- Diabetes.
- Obesity.
- Factors that cause local irritation of the vagina, such as tampons.
- Taking broad-spectrum antibiotics, oral contraceptives or corticoids. All promote yeast infections.
- HIV Infection: A woman with recurrent yeast infections of the vulva or vagina that are not responding well to antifungal treatment should be tested for AIDS.

GENERAL HYGIENE

- Wear cotton undergarments and avoid tight-fitting clothing.
- Keep external genitalia as dry and ventilated as possible.
- Wash undergarments with boiling water, as fungus survives normal washing. High-temperature ironing is recommended.
- Sitz baths with antiseptic products (see "Natural Treatments for the Female Genitalia").

SEXUAL HYGIENE

Yeast infections are not considered a venereal disease because the fungus usually comes from a person's own anus. However, a sexual partner can carry the *Candida* fungus on the glans without any symptoms, which contributes to the spread of the infection. For this reason, in cases of recurrent yeast infections, the following recommendations should be kept in mind when having sexual intercourse:

- Use a condom.
- Wash hands and genitals before and after intercourse.
- Have sexual partner examined and treated.

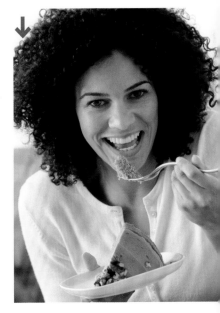

DIET

- Avoid sugar and sweets, as they promote growth of Candida fungus.
- Avoid aged cheese, beer, wine, cured meats and other fermented products.
- Increase intake of vegetable fiber, yogurt, garlic, broccoli, cabbage and radishes, as they fight fungus.

IDENTIFY THE FUNGUS

Many cases of recurring yeast infections are not caused by the most common fungus, *Candida albicans*, but rather by *Candida glabrata*, another emerging species that is resistant to the usual azole-type antifungal medications.

La *Candida glabrata* does respond to nystatin, boric acid (used as vaginal suppositories), tea tree oil and other natural antifungal treatments.

Lower Limbs

The body's support columns.

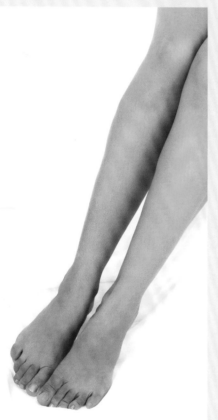

Stability, strength, and flexibility are the primary characteristics of the lower limbs. All of their joints, from the hip to the small joints of the feet, are under tremendous pressure and tension, especially with walking or running. However, along with bones, ligaments and tendons, these joints are designed for movement. In fact, idleness is more harmful than moderate exercise.

Indeed, the legs require movement to stay in good shape, whether it is through walking, running, jumping or swimming. When muscles contract, blood from the veins is pushed back up to the heart, which is very necessary for good circulation in the entire body. Due to this propelling function that the leg muscles perform while walking or running, it is said that they act as a true peripheral heart.

The most delicate part of each lower limb is, without a doubt, the foot. Blood must reach this area that is distant from the heart and return against gravity. Foot injuries and wounds, including the simplest abrasion, require special attention, especially in diabetics and the elderly who already have a certain amount of arterial blockage.

Caring for the lower limbs requires wise movement and attention to possible wounds; but it is well worth the effort, since they offer such a great service in permitting ambulation.

Facts and Figures About the Lower Limbs

2 mm (0.08 in)	Average thickness of the cartilage that comprises joints.
15 mm (0.59 in)	Diameter of the sciatic nerve at the gluteal level.
26	Number of bones that comprise the foot. One quarter of the body's bones are found in the feet.
100 000 km (62 137 mi)	Average distance that a person walks over a lifetime.

Restless Leg Syndrome

Restless leg syndrome is a hereditary chronic neurological disorder that causes an overwhelming need to move the legs. It is accompanied by discomfort such as pinprick sensations and tingling. Restless episodes of the legs tend to appear at night, causing insomnia and daytime fatigue.

Although it often goes undiagnosed, it is estimated that this syndrome affects 15% of the adult population.

WHEN AN EPISODE BEGINS

- Take a walk, even if it is short.
- Do leg muscle stretching exercises.
- Massage the legs.

PREVENTION

- Exercise more: Episodes of restless legs tend to appear after long periods of inactivity or sitting.
- Avoid alcoholic or caffeinated beverages, as they promote restless legs.
- Undergo a medical exam to detect any causation factor, such as iron-deficient anemia, neuropathies (nerve diseases), kidney disorders or diabetes.

(1) Pelvic Bones
(2) Hip Joint
(3) Femoral Neck
(4) Sciatic Nerve
The largest nerve in the body.
(5) Femur
(6) Knee Joint
(7) Tibia
(8) Fibula
(9) Calcaneus

Chapter Contents

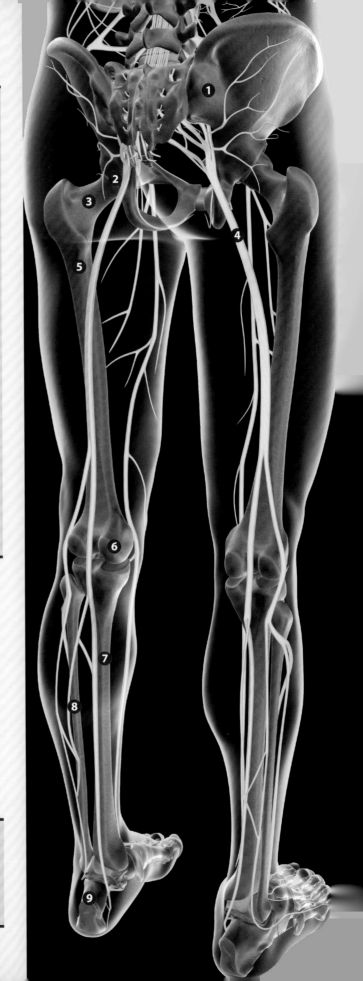

CARING FOR THE LOWER LIMBS

Avoiding injuries and stopping the normal joint deterioration process are the two major objectives.

LEG EXERCISES

Strenuous exercises are not required for shapely legs with firm muscles. It is enough to do the following exercises with each leg 10 about times per day.

Leg muscle strengthening promotes circulation, especially venous blood return.

CAREFUL WITH CERTAIN STRAINING MOVEMENTS

Each joint has a limited range of motion. When these limits are pushed, whether with daily activities or sports, different injuries appear –from pulled ligaments (sprain) to torn ligaments and tendons or broken bones.

Skiing and soccer are the sports that most often tend to exceed the limits of the knees and ankles.

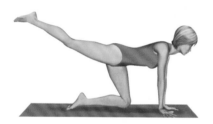

Buttock Strengthening Exercises
On hands and knees, lift each leg to align horizontally with the body.

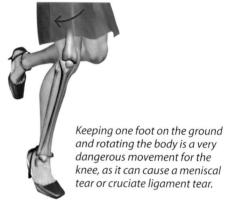

Keeping one foot on the ground and rotating the body is a very dangerous movement for the knee, as it can cause a meniscal tear or cruciate ligament tear.

Hip Strengthening Exercises
Lie on one side and lift each leg to a vertical position.

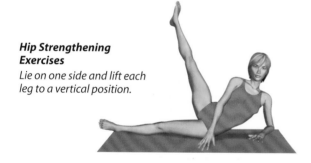

Thigh and Calf Strengthening Exercises
Keeping the back very straight, step up and down from the first rung on a ladder, one leg after the other.

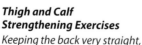

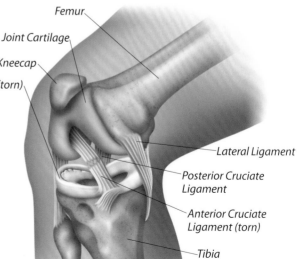

Femur
Joint Cartilage
Kneecap
Meniscus (torn)
Lateral Ligament
Posterior Cruciate Ligament
Anterior Cruciate Ligament (torn)
Tibia

STOPPING OSTEOARTHRITIS OF THE HIP AND KNEE

Osteoarthritis is a process of joint surface deterioration that causes pain and limited range of motion. Although the joint deterioration process is associated with age, it can be stopped by keeping the following recommendations in mind:

- **Reduce High-Impact Activities**
  - Going down stairs.
  - Weightlifting.
  - Walking or jogging on asphalt.
- **Increase Non-Impact Activities** for the hips and knees:
  - Swimming.
  - Bicycling or stationary biking.
  - Running on a treadmill.
- **Lose Weight**: The hip joints support greater pressure with walking. Losing weight is the best way to relieve these joints and stop the cartilage deterioration associated with osteoarthritis.
- **Diet**: The best diet for osteoarthritis is one that results in weight loss. In addition, the diet should be:
  - High in alkalinizing fruits and vegetables that reduce bone calcium loss.
  - Low in meat and meat products, as these promote calcium loss and joint inflammation.

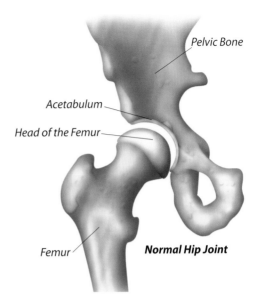

Pelvic Bone

Acetabulum

Head of the Femur

Femur

Normal Hip Joint

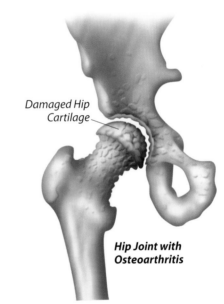

Damaged Hip Cartilage

Hip Joint with Osteoarthritis

CUSHIONED FOOTWEAR

Athletic or dress shoes with gel or air cushions absorb the impact of the feet hitting the ground with walking or running. This impact can be very intense when a person is overweight, promoting erosion of the knee and hip associated with osteoarthritis.

Cushioned footwear protects the deterioration of the lower limb joints.

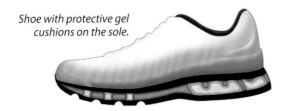

Shoe with protective gel cushions on the sole.

Reasons You Must See a Doctor

- Foot wound or abrasion in diabetics or patients with circulation disorders of the legs (can cause infection or gangrene).
- Skin ulcer on ankle or leg (not healing with usual treatment).
- Swelling, redness, and pain of the leg (could be thrombophlebitis).
- Loss of hip or knee strength (giving out).

NATURAL TREATMENTS FOR THE LOWER LIMBS

Applying water through baths and sprays, massage and medicinal herbs is beneficial for the legs.

ALTERNATING-TEMPERATURE LEG BATHS

Alternating-temperature leg baths provide a strong stimulus for arterial and venous circulation in the lower limbs, which is a type of gymnastics for arteries and veins. This treatment is recommended in cases of:

- Ischemia (lack of circulation) of the lower limbs, usually due to arteriosclerosis.
- Venous insufficiency (difficult venous return), usually accompanied by varicose veins.

Water Temperature: For the hot bath, 36-42 °C (97-108 °F); for the cold bath, 12-15 °C (54-59 °F).

Duration: Start by placing both feet in the hot water for 5 minutes, then 10-15 seconds in the cold water. Repeat the alternation 3-5 times, ending with the cold water.

Afterward: Rub feet with a cloth soaked in cold water and put on wool socks.

Frequency: Up to three times (sessions) per day.

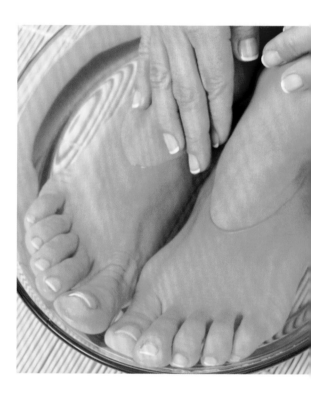

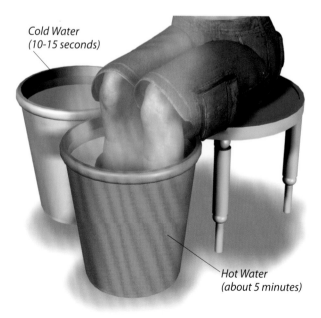

Cold Water
(10-15 seconds)

Hot Water
(about 5 minutes)

Start with the hot water, and end with the cold water. Repeat the alternation 3-5 times per session.

LYMPHATIC DRAINAGE

Lymphatic drainage is very effective in stimulating poor venous circulation and fluid retention that can cause leg heaviness.

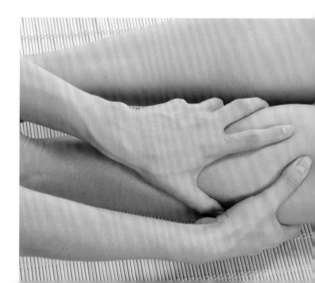

CIRCULATION TONICS

There are medicinal herbs that can improve blood circulation in the lower limbs. They can be taken as an infusion or applied directly onto the legs with herbal poultices and preparations. There are extracts, gels, creams, and other pharmaceutical preparations made from these herbs.

Arterial Circulation: *Ginkgo biloba* leaves are known for their vasodilator effect and for promoting blood flow to the tissues.

Venous Circulation: The bark and nuts of the horse chestnut tree (*Aesculus hippocastanum*) are known for their venous tonic effect, which can decongest veins and reduce leg swelling.

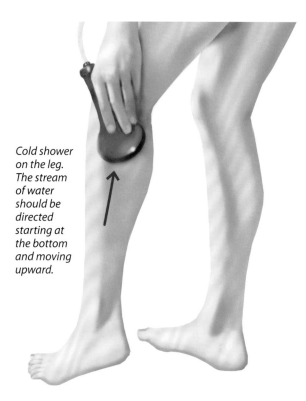

Cold shower on the leg. The stream of water should be directed starting at the bottom and moving upward.

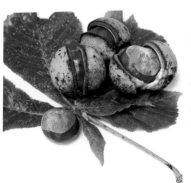

The leaves and nuts of the horse chestnut tree ("Aesculus hippocastanum"), a powerful venous tonic used to relieve fatigued legs and varicose veins.

COLD SHOWERS OR STREAMS OF WATER ON THE LEGS

The combination of mechanical stimulus produced by the water pressure along with that of the cold speeds up venous blood return from the legs to the heart. This decongests legs, relieves heaviness and stops progression of varicose veins.

SELF-LEG MASSAGE

Self-leg massage promotes venous blood return, which fights swelling and heaviness of the legs.

HOT WATER BOTTLE ON THE HIP

A hot water bottle applied to the hip relaxes contracted muscles and relieves hip pain caused by osteoarthritis (joint deterioration).

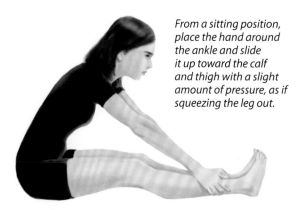

From a sitting position, place the hand around the ankle and slide it up toward the calf and thigh with a slight amount of pressure, as if squeezing the leg out.

Hip or Knee Prosthesis: When to Implant

- When pain occurs daily.
- When pain limits activities of daily living, such as putting on clothing and shoes, going up and down stairs.
- When joint instability causes stumbling while walking.

IMPROVING VENOUS CIRCULATION

*The blood in leg veins needs help to return up
to the heart against gravity.*

COMPRESSION STOCKINGS

Compression stockings worn on the legs keep blood from pooling due to venous insufficiency. There are now stocking models that are attractive and comfortable, both in knee- and thigh-high styles, in three compression strengths (light, normal or strong).

Benefits of Compression Stockings

- They relieve leg heaviness, especially during pregnancy.
- They stop the progression of varicose veins and development of phlebitis.
- They prevent clot formation in dilated veins, which cause embolisms.
- They contribute to healing of varicose ulcers.

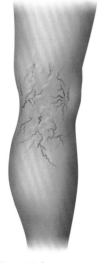

**Varicose Veins
(Dilated Veins)**
They promote nighttime cramping, thrombophlebitis and venous embolisms.

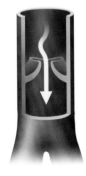

**Venous Valve
Insufficiency**
The valve remains open permanently, allowing blood to return downward instead of going up to the heart. Venous valves that have insufficiency are the primary cause of varicose veins.

SWIMMING AND WATER THERAPY

The pressure that water exerts on the legs contributes to venous blood return and improves circulation.

Swimming and water therapy are also good in cases of osteoarthritis of the hip or knee, as they relax muscles and relieve cramping and pain.

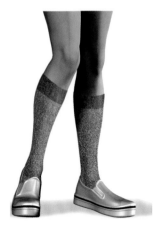

*Knee-High
Compression Stockings.*

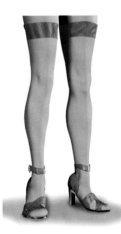

*Thigh-High
Compression Stockings.*

SEASIDE WALKS

Walking along the edge of the sea, with feet in the water, promotes venous return circulation in the legs, and is a very recommendable exercise for fatigued legs.

The massage that is produced naturally by bare feet walking on the sand combines with the toning effect of water on the feet and ankles, promoting leg circulation.

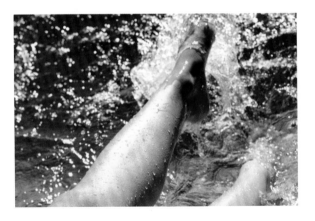

Cramp Prevention

Cramps are painful muscle contractions, generally associated with poor venous circulation in the lower limbs. They tend to occur at night, primarily affecting calf muscles, and are quite painful.

PREVENTION OF NIGHTTIME CRAMPS

- Prevent or control cramp-promoting factors such as:
  - Poor or inadequate venous circulation.
  - Excessive heat.
  - Muscle fatigue.
- Do stretching exercises during the day.
- Stay well-hydrated, drinking at least two liters of water per day.
- Avoid excessive sweating and fatigue.
- Minerals: Muscle cramps can be due to a mineral imbalance, usually due to a lack of calcium, magnesium, or potassium. Taking supplements of these minerals, or a vitamin and mineral complex, helps reduce frequency and severity of cramps.
- Watch for certain medications: Many diuretics increase loss of potassium and other minerals with urine, thereby promoting cramps.

MAINTAIN PROPER HYGIENE

Daily habits, posture and footwear can do a great deal to stop the progression of varicose veins.

No

Clothing, belts, bands or footwear that are too tight.

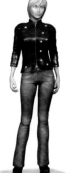

Yes

- Comfortable Clothing.
- Comfortable, flexible footwear.

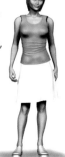

No

Prolonged leg-crossing or keeping a foot in a single position.

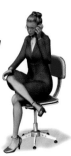

Yes

- Walk at least an hour per day and play an outdoor sport. Stand on toes and heels.
- Raise legs whenever possible.

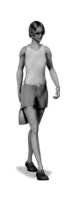

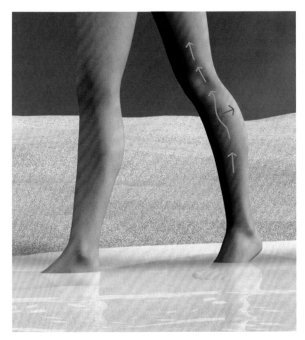

While walking, the leg muscles push blood through the veins up towards the heart, which contributes to good circulation. Water stimulus also helps circulation.

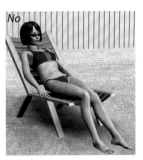

Prolonged exposure to the sun and avoiding excessive heat to the legs from stoves, electric blankets, or the hot ground.

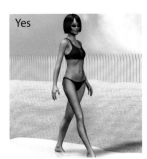

- Walk along the edge barefoot with feet in water.
- Apply cold showers to the legs.

CARING FOR THE FEET

*The feet are subjected to a great deal of pressure and require, in addition
to hygiene, constant observation for early detection of lesions.*

FOOT HYGIENE

- Foot Baths: Recommended daily, especially after walking
  or physical exercise. Once finished, dry feet well,
  especially between toes. Daily foot cleansing can be done
  with water alone. In some cases, certain substances can
  be added to the water:
  – An acidic soap or gel, with a maximum pH of 5.5.
  – Tea tree oil or essential thyme or oregano oil (10-15
    drops per liter of water), as antiseptics and antifungals.
- Massage with moisturizing cream daily to avoid skin
  dryness. A massage with sesame or olive oil is effective
  in healing cracked heels, which are more common in the
  summertime.
- Examine feet for early detection of abrasions, cracks,
  hard areas, calluses, moles or other lesions.
- Trim nails on a regular basis.

Caution: Any small foot lesion for a diabetic or patient
with arterial ischemia (lack of blood flow) in lower limbs
should be seen by a physician or podiatrist, as it can easily
become complicated and cause a serious infection.

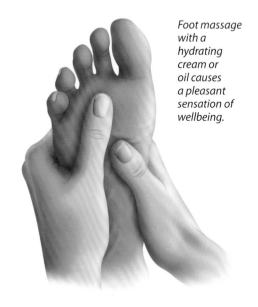

*Foot massage
with a
hydrating
cream or
oil causes
a pleasant
sensation of
wellbeing.*

PREVENTING INGROWN TOENAILS

- Trim nails in a straight line. Nails should never be trimmed on the sides or
  corners, as they then grow more and dig into skin.
- Use wide footwear that does not cause compression of the feet.
- Consult a podiatrist to determine if there is any anatomical condition or
  plantar support defect –such as flat feet or inturned feet– that can cause
  predisposition to ingrown toenails. Support insoles can be helpful.

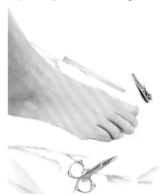

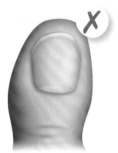

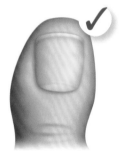

To prevent ingrown toenails, do not trim corners.

PROPER FOOTWEAR

- Footwear should
  be flexible and
  comfortable to avoid
  abrasions.
- A shoe should not
  compress the foot.
- The heel should
  not be over 2 or 3
  centimeters high, as
  it has been shown
  that anything higher
  causes pulling on
  ligaments, tendons
  and muscles of the
  legs and feet.

PREVENTING ATHLETE'S FOOT

Athlete's foot is an infection caused by dermatophyte filamentous fungi, usually located between the toes.

Athlete's foot is easily spread from person to person and usually takes several weeks to heal.

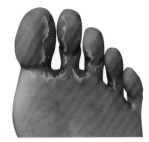

Athlete's Foot

The typical treatment consists of applying antifungal creams, lotions or powders.

Systemic antifungals (taken orally) are needed on a consistent basis and in cases of diabetes, circulatory disorders or weakened immune system.

Hygiene Guidelines for Preventing Athlete's Foot

- Do not walk barefoot on the ground around public pools, saunas, dressing rooms and athletic areas.
- After bathing or showering, dry carefully between toes and folds of the body, such as the groin and armpits. Fungus proliferates in moist areas of the skin.
- Avoid moisture on the feet, especially when using closed footwear. For this, change socks whenever they become moist, use antiperspirant powders, and do not wear plastic sandals that retain moisture.
- Disinfect floors in the shower, bathtub, and bath areas on a daily basis using 10% bleach (one part bleach to 10 parts water).
- Avoid taking certain medications whenever possible because fungal infections are promoted by:
  – Antibiotics, because they destroy beneficial bacteria of the skin and bowels that stop the development of fungi.
  – Oral or local corticosteroids.
  – Oral contraceptives and hormones.

VISIT THE PODIATRIST REGULARLY

A podiatrist should be visited regularly for early detection of foot conditions and prompt corrective measures.

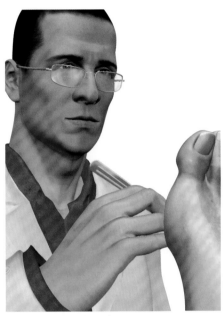

Foot pain is not the only reason to remember the podiatrist.

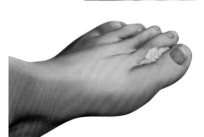

Antifungal Lotions

1. To protect feet against fungus, soak cotton with a few drops of tea tree oil ("Melaleuca alternifolia") diluted in even parts with olive or almond oil.

2. Rub the skin between toes with the cotton. Leave it between toes for a more lasting effect.

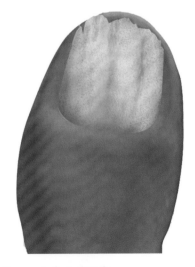

Fungus-Infected Nails

Many nail conditions are due to fungal infections that are similar to those that cause athletes' foot.

Dabbing tea tree oil and crushed garlic compresses on the nail are alternative remedies against fungus.

Epilogue

No matter how well the body is cared for, it eventually becomes weak and ceases to live. What will be its destination?

The proven, documented, eye witnessed fact of the resurrection Jesus is, for believers, the promise and the basis of resurrection of their body for eternal life.

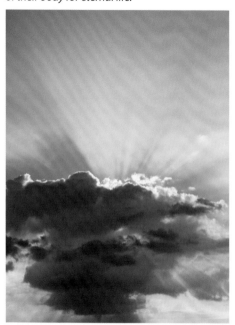

POSSIBLE DESTINATIONS FOR THE BODY

At some time or another in life, all human beings must face death. Although one does not want to think about it, the body must have a destination, whether foreseen or unforeseen. Here are some of them:

- **Burial or Interment**: A lifeless body goes through a process of decay due to the action of bacteria, fungus and worms, and eventually turns to dust. The body returns to the earth –the origin of its prime matter.

- **Cremation**: The body is subjected to high temperatures, up to 1 000 °C (1 832 °F) or more, for about two hours. Water vaporizes, proteins, fats and carbohydrates become oxidized, and eventually only minerals remain in the form of ashes, which do not evaporate or disappear. The calcium in bones is the primary component of ashes.

- **Mummification**: Body tissues are kept intact due to the action of a variety of chemical substances added after death (embalming). Mummification can occur spontaneously due to extreme dryness or cold that prevent the development of decay-causing bacteria.

- **Organ Donation**: In the majority of developed countries, all people who die are considered donors in the absence of express opposition by the deceased person. In any case, in order to proceed to remove organs from a cadaver, it must be authorized by a judge. Organ donation is an utterly altruistic gesture, considered by many as the ultimate act of kindness among human beings. Thanks to organ donation, others can continue living, or have an improved quality of life. The main organs that can be donated are the kidneys, liver, heart, pancreas and lungs. Bone marrow, corneas, bones and other body parts can also be transplanted.

- **Object of Anatomic Study**: Donating the body to science so that medical students can study anatomy.

- **Freezing**: There are companies that offer freezing of the body at extremely low temperatures, with the hope of bringing it back to life after a certain number of years. There is no confirmation that this is possible, and even if it were, one must question whether it would be worth it to come back to life under uncertain and possibly regrettable conditions.

Resurrection: Certain Hope

As much as it is repeated and expected, death is never accepted by loved ones or by oneself. Nobody feels comfortable with it. This is because all humans have "eternity in their hearts", as it is well expressed by the Preacher.[a]

Throughout history, many answers have been developed to satisfy the human longing to remain. Among them, the resurrection of the physical body, such as is presented in the Bible, offers a solution that is consistent to this universal aspiration to immortality.

A human being's immortality is not native or inherent, but rather conditional. This is the reason that once waking up from the unconscious sleep of death on the day of resurrection, a person receives the gift of immortality from the Creator.

RESURRECTION AND DNA

Resurrection of the righteous is the most glorious and transcendent destiny that the body could have and, for this reason, that a human being could have. The body is remade from the "deposit" mentioned by the Apostle Paul in his letter to Timothy, no matter where the material that made him ended up, no matter where the atoms and molecules that made up his flesh and bones are now. Everyone can be resuscitated, no matter what destiny his body had. *"...for I know whom I have believed and am persuaded that He is able to guard My deposit unto that Day".*[b]

For many, in light of modern science, that "deposit" could well be a copy of the genetic code contained in the DNA in the nucleus of every somatic cell. Today, we know that from this macromolecule of DNA, that weighs no more than a few millionths of a gram, it is possible to reconstruct every part of a living being. Science has made the belief in resurrection more possible.

A BODY REDONE

Paul was convinced that from that "deposit" the Creator will remake his mortal body, but no longer subject to current imperfections and weaknesses, but rather perfect and immortal, like it was in the beginning, and that this supernatural event will occur on "that promised day" of the second coming of Jesus to the Earth –this time in glory and majesty.

Many believers throughout history have been laid to rest and many others live today with the hope of the arrival of that day when those dead in Christ shall resurrect first and the living righteous shall be transformed. Both groups shall receive a new body from the Creator, no longer subject to disease and death. At that time, there will be no need to worry about how to achieve a "HEALTHY BODY".

a. Ecclesiastics 3:11 (NKJV)
b. 2 Timothy 1:12 (NKJV)

The desire to continue living and defy death is deeply rooted in the human being, irrespective of culture or condition. Nobody is satisfied with simply being the healthiest person in the cemetery.

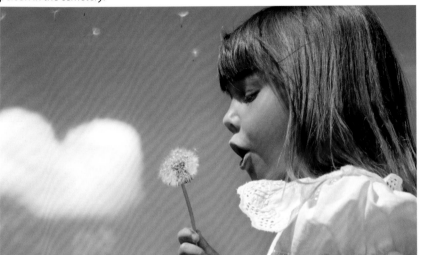

REASONS TO CARE FOR THE BODY NOW

If this body is temporal and eventually disappears, why worry about developing a healthy body? Why stay healthy? Here are just some of the answers to these challenging questions:

- To enjoy a fuller life and be closer to true happiness. The health care guidelines included in this book can bring a great deal of satisfaction to those who follow them.
- To achieve closeness with others and better assist them.
- To leave a model to younger people that motivates them to care for their health.
- To achieve the personal satisfaction of collaborating with life.

Believers have an additional reason: To honor the Creator of this body that, despite being subjected to the defects and weaknesses of its current condition, continues to be a reflection of the eternal wisdom of its Maker.

Alphabetical Index

POSITIVE MIND

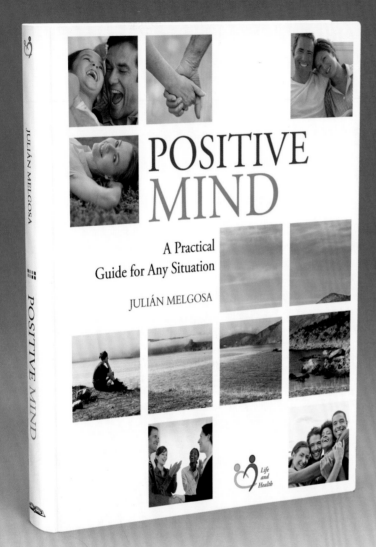

POSITIVE MIND provides tools for challenges that we sometimes seem unable to solve. In a single volume, this handbook offers an extensive inventory of problem situations that affect everyone. Adversities and behavioural options are analysed in an interesting yet scientific way by a recognised communicator with decades of success as professor and writer.

To address these situations, the book includes valuable self-help techniques, professional psychotherapeutic strategies, and a large number of natural treatments. This guide of holistic mental health provides counsel and practical remedies—many times for immediate application—about principles for better living, self-centred and interpersonal problems, resilience (or ability to face and overcome adversity), as well as major therapeutic techniques grouped by theoretical school.

"Whether or not the reader has a background in the behavioural sciences, I am sure that no-one will regret reading this excellent book. It will not protect them from all pain, but it will prevent evil from taking over their spirit" (From the Foreword by José Luis Pinillos, Spanish Royal Academy).

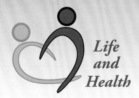

Life and Health